This handbook p~~rovides~~ ~~p~~hysician–
neurologist edito~~rs~~ ~~te~~xt *Emer-*
~~ergency~~
department~~~~ ~~osis, the text, table~~ ~~a~~nd illus-
trations guide the emergency physicia~~n~~ in the recognition, di~~ag~~nosis, and
management of neurological disorder~~s~~ both common and com~~pl~~ex. Inte-
~~damental neurological concepts with the ju~~ ~~ities and
demands of e~~~~ergency care, this handbook features managem~~nt algo-
~~ritms for dozens of conditions and~~ list of ~~pearls and~~ ~~at the
~~clusion of each~~ of the thirty-eight chapters. This ~~sur~~~~est prac-
~~tices in emergency neurology provide~~ ~~ecise~~ and crucial c~~ical infor-
~~mation~~ all emergency physicians w~~~~agnose and manage n~~urologic
~~nditions~~ such as headache, seizure, and spinal cord ~~injury, em~~hasizing
~~ficient neurological examination t~~echniques, this handb~~~~essential
~~for emergency physicians, neurologists, internists, and reside~~nts.

M M. Shah, M.D., is Assistant Clinical ~~Professor at Michigan State~~ Univer-
~~sity and a faculty member of Spartan Wide Emergency Medicine~~ ~~R~~esidency
Program in B~~ay City, Michigan, with a special interest in neu~~rological
emergencies. He is an attending emergency medicine physician at~~~~ Ingham
~~Regional Medical Center and~~ co-ed~~or~~ of the comprehensive ref~~~~ference,
Emergency Neurology: Principles and Practice (1999).

Kevin M. Kelly, M.D., Ph.D., is Associate Professor of Neurology at Drexel
~~University College of Medicine. He is an adult neurologist and~~ epileptol-
ogist at Allegheny General Hospital in Pittsburgh, Pennsylvania. He is the
director of coursework in Emergency Neurology and Basic Neuroscience for
residents in the clinical neurosciences and Emergency Medicine, and his
research at the Allegheny-Singer Research Institute focuses on brain aging
and the mechanisms of poststroke epilepsy. He is the co-editor of the comprehensive reference, *Emergency Neurology: Principles and Practice* (1999).

Principles and Practice of
EMERGENCY NEUROLOGY

Handbook for Emergency Physicians

Edited by

Sid M. Shah
Ingham Regional Medical Center
Michigan State University

Kevin M. Kelly
Allegheny General Hospital
Drexel University College of Medicine

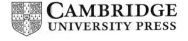

CAMBRIDGE
UNIVERSITY PRESS

PUBLISHED BY THE PRESS SYNDICATE OF THE UNIVERSITY OF CAMBRIDGE
The Pitt Building, Trumpington Street, Cambridge, United Kingdom

CAMBRIDGE UNIVERSITY PRESS
The Edinburgh Building, Cambridge CB2 2RU, UK
40 West 20th Street, New York, NY 10011-4211, USA
477 Williamstown Road, Port Melbourne, VIC 3207, Australia
Ruiz de Alarcón 13, 28014 Madrid, Spain
Dock House, The Waterfront, Cape Town 8001, South Africa

http://www.cambridge.org

First published 2003

Printed in the United States of America

Typefaces Stone Serif 9/12 pt. *and* Symbol   *System* LaTeX 2_ε [TB]

A catalog record for this book is available from the British Library.

Library of Congress Cataloging in Publication Data

Principles and practice of emergency neurology : handbook for emergency physicians /
edited by Sid M. Shah, Kevin M. Kelly.
    p. ; cm.
Includes bibliographical references and index.
ISBN 0-521-00980-4 (pbk.)
1. Nervous system – Diseases – Handbooks, manuals, etc.   2. Medical emergencies –
Handbooks, manuals, etc.   3. Neurological intensive care – Handbooks, manuals, etc.
I. Shah, Sid M.   II. Kelly, Kevin M.
[DNLM: 1. Nervous System Diseases – diagnosis – Handbooks.   2. Emergency Medicine –
Handbooks.   3. Neurologic Examination – methods – Handbooks. WL 39 P957 2003]
RC355 .P75   2003
616.8′0425–dc21   2002034812

ISBN 0 521 00980 4 paperback

To my parents Liza and Madhukar Shah
SMS

To my mother Rose and in memory of my father Thomas Kelly
KMK

Contents

Contents

Preface

After the publication of *Emergency Neurology: Principles and Practice*, many emergency medicine residents inquired whether a handbook based on the main text would be available. As a result, we developed a handbook to be carried by emergency physicians, extending our initial goal of disseminaing the principles of emergency neurology to emergency physicians and providing a ready resource in caring for patients with neurological emergencies. As we embarked upon the handbook project, we realized that this is a daunting challenge. Providing the relevant and necessary information in a form that is easily understood and to the point turned out to be much more difficult than we had anticipated. Brevity is a challenge when one is expressing complex ideas. As editors we honor the need of emergency physicians all over the country who work under increasing time constraints by trying to provide only the most essential information about a given topic in a focused manner. Each chapter is extensively updated with timely information. As in *Emergency Neurology: Principles and Practice*, most of the chapters are authored by a team of an emergency physician and a neurologist. Each chapter is organized with an introduction of the topic, emergency assessment and clinical findings, pertinent laboratory and radiographic studies, management, and disposition. Each chapter ends with a list of pearls and pitfalls pertaining to the topic reviewed.

The handbook is divided into eight sections. Section I contains the essentials of a focused neurologic examination and neuro diagnostic testing. As editors, we felt that even though EEG does not directly impact the daily emergency medicine practice, it is important for the ED physicians to know the importance of an emergent EEG when a condition such as nonconvulsive status epilepticus is suspected. Common neurological presentations are reviewed in Section II, whereas the specific neurological conditions are reviewed in Section III. Owing to the importance of the diagnosis and management issues of Guillain-Barré syndrome and myasthenia gravis, these are now reviewed in two separate chapters. Section IV deals with the three main components of neurological trauma: traumatic brain injury and spinal and peripheral nerve injuries. In Section V, those pediatric neurological emergencies likely to be encountered in an emergency setting are reviewed. The chapter on pediatric seizures has been extensively revised. Sections VI and VII review pregnancy-related neurological emergencies and selected topics in neuro-toxicology, respectively. The concluding section is a brief review of brain death.

The editors thank all the authors for their diligence and patience, without which this handbook would not have been possible. We also thank all our colleagues, friends, and emergency medicine and neurology residents for their comments, both critical and encouraging.

Contributors

James W. Albers, M.D., Ph.D.
Department of Neurology
University of Michigan
Ann Arbor, Michigan

Roger L. Albin, M.D.
Department of Neurology
University of Michigan
Ann Arbor, Michigan

Mara S. Aloi, M.D.
Department of Emergency
    Medicine
Allegheny General Hospital
Pittsburgh, Pennsylvania

Daniel M. Ammons, M.D.
Department of Emergency
    Medicine
Allegheny General Hospital
Pittsburgh, Pennsylvania

Moises A. Arriaga, M.D.
Department of Neuro-otology
Allegheny General Hospital
Pittsburgh, Pennsylvania

A. Sinan Baran, M.D.
Department of Psychiatry
University of Mississippi
Jackson, Mississippi

Mark E. Baratz, M.D.
Department of Orthopedic
    Surgery
Allegheny General Hospital
Pittsburgh, Pennsylvania

Susan M. Baser, M.D.
Department of Neurology
Allegheny General Hospital
Pittsburgh, Pennsylvania

Charles H. Bill II, M.D., Ph.D.
Sparrow Healthcare System
Lansing, Michigan

Paul Blackburn, D.O., FACEP
Maricopa Medical Center
Phoenix, Arizona

Amy Blasen, D.O.
Sparrow Healthcare System
Sparrow Hospital/MSU
Emergency Medicine Residency Program
Lansing, Michigan

Jon Brillman, M.D.
Department of Neurology
Allegheny General Hospital
Pittsburgh, Pennsylvania

Anthony Briningstool, M.D.
Sparrow/MSU
Emergency Medicine Residency Program
Lansing, Michigan

Christopher R. Carpenter, M.D.
Departments of Emergency and Internal
    Medicine
Washington University
St. Louis, Missouri

Marc Chimowitz, M.D.
Department of Neurology
Grady Memorial Hospital
Atlanta, Georgia

David M. Chuirazzi, M.D.
Department of Emergency Medicine
Allegheny General Hospital
Pittsburgh, Pennsylvania

Nick E. Colovos, M.D.
Department of Emergency Medicine

Allegheny General Hospital
Pittsburgh, Pennsylvania

Merle L. Diamond, M.D.
Diamond Headache Clinic
Chicago, Illinois

Ivo Drury, MB, Bch
Department of Neurology
Henry Ford Hospital
Detroit, Michigan

Eric R. Eggenberger, D.O.
Michigan State University
East Lansing, Michigan

Janet Eng, D.O.
Ingham Regional Medical Center
Sparrow Hospital/MSU
Emergency Medicine Residency
   Program
Lansing, Michigan

Norman L. Foster, M.D.
Department of Neurology
University of Michigan
Ann Arbor, Michigan

Michael R. Frankel, M.D.
Department of Neurology
Grady Memorial Hospital
Atlanta, Georgia

Kevin J. Gingrich, M.D.
Department of Anesthesiology
Thomas Jefferson University
Philadelphia, Pennsylvania

Andrew L. Goldberg, M.D.
Medical Director
Westside Imaging Center
Brook Park, Ohio

Stephen Guertin, M.D.
Sparrow Healthcare System
Lansing, Michigan

Dennis P. Hanlon, M.D.
Department of Emergency Medicine
Allegheny General Hospital
Pittsburgh, Pennsylvania

Rae R. Hanson, M.D.
Midelfort Clinic
Eau Claire, Wisconsin

Fred Harchelroad, M.D.
Department of Emergency Medicine
Allegheny General Hospital
Pittsburgh, Pennsylvania

Vanessa L. Harkins, D.O.
Sparrow Healthcare System
Sparrow Hospital/MSU
Emergency Medicine Residency Program
Lansing, Michigan

Oliver W. Hayes, D.O.
Ingham Regional Medical Center
Sparrow Hospital/MSU
Emergency Medicine Residency Program
Lansing, Michigan

Judith L. Heidebrink, M.D.
Department of Neurology
University of Michigan
Ann Arbor, Michigan

Mary Beth Hines, D.O.
Keweenaw Memorial Medical Center
Laurium, Michigan

J. Stephen Huff, M.D.
University of Virginia Health Systems
Charlottesville, Virginia

Mary Hughes, D.O.
Sparrow Healthcare System
Ingham Regional Medical Center
Sparrow Hospital/MSU
Emergency Medicine Residency
   Program
Lansing, Michigan

Imad T. Jarjour, M.D.
Department of Pediatrics and
   Neurology
Allegheny General Hospital
Pittsburgh, Pennsylvania

Sam Josvai, M.D.
Kalamazoo Center for Medical Studies/
MSU Emergency Medicine Residency
   Program
Kalamazoo, Michigan

Patricia B. Jozefczyk, M.D.
Department of Neurology
Allegheny General Hospital
Pittsburgh, Pennsylvania

Robert G. Kaniecki, M.D.
Department of Neurology
University of Pittsburgh
Pittsburgh, Pennsylvania

Kevin M. Kelly, M.D., Ph.D.
Department of Neurology
Allegheny General Hospital
Pittsburgh, Pennsylvania

Rashmi U. Kothari, M.D.
Kalamazoo Center for Medical Studies/
MSU Emergency Medicine Residency
  Program
Kalamazoo, Michigan

Lara J. Kunschner, M.D.
Department of Neurology
Allegheny General Hospital
Pittsburgh, Pennsylvania

Michael G. Millin, M.D.
Oregon Health Sciences University
Portland, Oregon

Herbert B. Newton, M.D.
Department of Neurology
Ohio State University
Columbus, Ohio

David Overton, M.D.
Kalamazoo Center for Medical Studies/
MSU Emergency Medicine Residency
  Program
Kalamazoo, Michigan

Page B. Pennell, M.D.
Department of Neurology
Emory University
Atlanta, Georgia

Sandeep S. Rana, M.D.
Department of Neurology
Allegheny General Hospital
Pittsburgh, Pennsylvania

Marsha D. Rappley, M.D.
Michigan State University
East Lansing, Michigan

Earl J. Reisdorff, M.D.
Ingham Regional Medical Center
Sparrow Hospital/MSU
Emergency Medicine Residency Program
Lansing, Michigan

Mont R. Roberts, M.D.
Sparrow Healthcare System
Sparow Hospital/MSU
Emergency Medicine Residency Program
Lansing, Michigan

David Rossi, M.D.
Kalamazoo Center for Medical Studies/
MSU Emergency Medicine Residency
  Program
Kalamazoo, Michigan

Thomas F. Scott, M.D.
Department of Neurology

Allegheny General Hospital
Pittsburgh, Pennsylvania

L. R. Searls, D.O.
Ingham Regional Medical Center
Sparrow Hospital/MSU
Emergency Medicine Residency Program
Lansing, Michigan

Sid M. Shah, M.D.
Ingham Regional Medical Center
Sparrow Hospital/MSU
Emergency Medicine Residency Program
Lansing, Michigan

George A. Small, M.D.
Department of Neurology
Allegheny General Hospital
Pittsburgh, Pennsylvania

Liza A. Squires, M.D.
Devos Childrens Hospital
Grand Rapids, Michigan

Thomas M. Stein, M.D.
Department of Emergency Medicine
Allegheny General Hospital
Pittsburgh, Pennsylvania

Craig A. Taylor, M.D.
Southwood Psychiatric Hospital
Pittsburgh, Pennsylvania

Steven A. Tellan, M.D.
Department of Otolaryngology
University of Michigan
Ann Arbor, Michigan

Jane Turner, M.D.
Michigan State University
East Lansing, Michigan

James P. Valeriano, M.D.
Department of Neurology
Allegheny General Hospital
Pittsburgh, Pennsylvania

John J. Wald, M.D.
Department of Neurology
University of Michigan
Ann Arbor, Michigan

W. Lee Warren, M.D.
Department of Neurology
Wildford Hall Air Force Medical Center
San Antonio, Texas

James E. Wilberger, Jr., M.D.
Department of Neurology

Allegheny General Hospital
Pittsburgh, Pennsylvania

David G. Wright, M.D.
Department of Neurology
Pittsburgh, Pennsylvania

David K. Zich, M.D.
Department of Emergency and Internal
    Medicine
Northwestern University
Chicago, Illinois

1 Neurological Examination

Thomas F. Scott and Sid M. Shah

INTRODUCTION

The neurological history and examination provide information to help localize lesions of the nervous system. The neurological examination is incorporated in the context of the patient's overall health history and general physical examination. Evidence of systemic disease is considered in the interpretation of the neurological findings.

Goals of an emergency neurological examination:
1. Is there a neurological condition?
2. Where is (are) the lesion(s) located?
3. What are the possible causes?
4. Can the patient be discharged safely from the emergency department or is hospitalization required?

Neurological History

A detailed neurological history allows one to focus on important components of the neurological examination, thus saving time and resources. The more specific and detailed a history, the greater is the likelihood of making a definite diagnosis in the emergency department. About 75% of neurological diagnoses are made from the history alone. An account from family members and bystanders can be an important source of information. A detailed description of the event is more important than the patient or a bystander volunteering a diagnosis such as "I had a seizure." The history obtained from the patient can be considered a part of the mental status examination.

Important Historical Elements of a Focused Neurological Examination

1. Onset of symptoms: time and mode (Look beyond the symptoms, to the context in which they occur.)
2. Temporal relationships of symptoms

Table 1.1. The Brief Mental Status Examination

Item	Number of errors × Weight		= Total
	Score		
What year is it now?	0 or 1	× 4	=
What month is it?	0 or 1	× 3	=
Present memory phrase: "Repeat this phrase after me and remember it: *John Brown, 42 Market Street, New York.*"			
About what time is it? (Answer correct if within one hour)	0 or 1	× 3	=
Count backwards from 20 to 1.	0, 1, or 2	× 2	=
Say the months in reverse.	0, 1, or 2	× 2	=
Repeat memory phrase (Each underlined portion is worth 1 point.)	0, 1, 2, 3, 4, or 5	× 2	=
Final score is the sum of the total			=

Possible score range, from 0 to 28. 0–8 normal; 9–19 mildly impaired; 20–28 severely impaired.
Source: Kaufman DM, Zun L. A quantifiable, brief mental status examination for emergency patients. *J Emerg Med.* 1995;13:449–56.

3. Progression of symptoms
4. Associated symptoms (neurological and nonneurological)
5. Exacerbating and alleviating factors
6. Symptoms that indicate involvement of a particular region of central nervous system
7. History of similar event
8. History of medication use: illicit drug use, exposure to toxins, head trauma

Neurological Examination

Mental status
Cranial nerve function
Motor function
Deep tendon reflexes, cutaneous reflexes, and miscellaneous signs
Sensory modalities
Pathological reflexes

Mental Status

See Table 1.1.

Six elements of mental status evaluation, modified from Zun and Howes (1988), are:

1. Appearance, behavior, and attitude
    Is dress appropriate?
    Is motor behavior at rest appropriate?
    Is the speech pattern normal?
2. Disorders of thought
    Are the thoughts logical and realistic?
    Are false beliefs or delusions present?
    Are suicidal or homicidal thoughts present?

Table 1.2. Glasgow Coma Scale

Eye opening
Opens eyes spontaneously	4
Opens eyes to verbal command	3
Opens eyes to pain	2
Does not open eyes	1

Verbal response
Alert and oriented	5
Converses but disoriented	4
Speaking but nonsensical	3
Moans or makes unintelligible sounds	2
No response	1

Motor response
Follows commands	6
Localizes pain	5
Movement or withdrawal from pain	4
Abnormal flexion (decorticate)	3
Abnormal extension (decerebrate)	2
No response	1
Total	3–15

---

3. Disorders of perception
   Are hallucinations present?
4. Mood and affect
   What is the prevailing mood?
   Is the emotional content appropriate for the setting?
5. Insight and judgment
   Does the patient understand the circumstances surrounding the visit?
6. Sensorium and intelligence
   Is the level of consciousness normal?
   Is cognition or intellectual functioning impaired?

The Glasgow Coma Scale is often used as a method of briefly quantitating neurological dysfunction (see Table 1.2).

More specific testing of higher cortical functions is often added to the mental status examination in patients with evidence of focal lesions. Delineation of aphasias can involve detailed testing but is usually limited to gross observation of speech output, conduction (ability to repeat), and comprehension. Other tests include naming objects, distinguishing between right and left, and testing for visual and sensory neglect (especially important in parietal and thalamic lesions).

Cranial Nerve Function

Evaluating the Cranial Nerves

➤I. Olfactory

Evaluate: Smell

Anatomic Location: Olfactory bulb and tract

Tests: Odor recognition

Significant Findings: Lack of odor perception in one or both sides

Lesions of the olfactory groove (typically meningioma) can have associated psychiatric symptoms related to frontal lobe injury.

➤ II. Optic

Evaluate: Vision

Anatomic Location: Optic nerve, chiasma, and tracts

Tests: Visual acuity

Significant Findings: Reduced vision

Tests: Pupillary light reflex

Significant Findings: Afferent pupillary defect (Marcus-Gunn pupil +/−)

Tests: Visual field testing

Testing visual acuity is important when primarily ocular lesion(s) are suspected. Papilledema: increased intracranial pressure due to tumor, hydrocephalus, or other causes. Hollenhorst plaque: a bright-appearing cholesterol or atheromatous embolus visualized by funduscopic examination of the retinal vessels, implies an embolic process. Optic nerve lesions: monocular visual disturbance.
See comment 1.

➤ III. Oculomotor

Evaluate: Eye movement, pupil contraction and accommodation, eyelid elevation

Anatomic Location: Midbrain

Tests: Extraocular eye movements (EOM)

Significant Findings: Impairment of one or more eye movements or disconjugate gaze

Tests: Pupillary light reflex

Significant Findings: Pupillary dilatation, ptosis

Cranial nerves III, IV, VI – Check for EOM.
Dysfunction of these nerves can be localized by noting the direction of gaze, which causes or worsens a diplopia, and any loss of upgaze, downgaze, or horizontal movements in either eye. Diplopia that worsens on lateral gaze suggests an ipsilateral palsy of cranial nerve VI or lateral rectus weakness.
See comment 2.

➤ IV. Trochlear

Evaluate: Eye movement

Anatomic Location: Midbrain

Tests: Extraocular eye movements

Significant Findings: Impairment of one or more eye movements or disconjugate gaze

➤ V. Trigeminal

Evaluate: Facial sensation, mastication

Anatomic Location: Pons

Tests: Sensation above eye, between eye and mouth, below the mouth to angle of jaw

Significant Findings: Reduced sensation in one or divisions of cranial nerve V

Tests: Corneal reflex

Significant Findings: Impaired

Tests: Palpation of masseter muscles

Significant Findings: Reduced strength in masseter or pterygoid muscles

If an abnormality is found in only one or two divisions of cranial nerve V (V_1–V_3), the findings imply a lesion distal to the gasserian ganglion.
See comment 3.

➤VI. Abducens

Evaluate: Ocular movement

Anatomic Location: Pons

Tests: Extraocular eye movements

Significant Findings: Reduced eye abduction

➤VII. Facial

Evaluate: Facial expression secretions, taste, visceral and cutaneous sensibility

Anatomic Location: Pons

Tests: Facial expression

Significant Findings: Weakness of upper or lower face or eye closure

Tests: Corneal reflex

Significant Findings: Impaired

Tests: Taste on anterior $\frac{2}{3}$ tongue

Significant Findings: Impaired

Seventh cranial nerve lesions can be either central or peripheral. In central lesions, located proximal to the seventh nerve nucleus and contralateral to the resulting facial droop, the upper face (periorbital area and forehead) will be relatively spared. The palpebral fissure may be slightly larger ipsilateral to the facial droop. In peripheral lesions, weakness is ipsilateral to the lesion of the seventh cranial nerve nucleus or the nerve itself. Other brainstem signs are seen typically when a lesion involves the nerve nucleus; the term Bell's palsy commonly refers to lesions of the nerve distal to the nucleus. Eye closure may be lost in severe cases of peripheral seventh nerve lesions. Hyperacusis is due to loss of the seventh nerve's dampening influence on the stapes.

➤VIII. Acoustic

Evaluate: Hearing, equilibrium

Anatomic Location: Pons

Tests: Auditory and vestibular

Significant Findings: Reduced hearing

The eighth cranial nerve consists of an auditory component and a vestibular component. Deafness rarely results from cortical lesions, which more often cause difficulty with

sound localization. Common bedside testing involves comparison for gross symmetry with a high-pitched tuning fork (512 or 256 Hz) or by finger rubbing near the ear, and the Weber and Rinne tests (for air conduction compared to bone conduction of sound). Lesions of the vestibular nuclei and the vestibular portion of the eighth cranial nerve can produce vertigo, nausea, vomiting, and nystagmus.

➤IX. Glossopharyngeal

Evaluate: Taste, glandular secretions, swallowing, visceral sensibility (pharynx, tongue, tonsils)

Anatomic Location: Medulla

Tests: Gag reflex

Significant Findings: Reduced gag

Tests: Speech (phonation)

Significant Findings: Dysarthria

Tests: Swallowing

Significant Findings: Dysarthria

Lesions of cranial nerve IX may be undetected clinically.

➤X. Vagus

Evaluate: Involuntary muscle and gland control (pharynx, larynx, trachea, bronchi, lungs, digestive system, heart), swallowing, phonation, visceral and cutaneous sensibility, taste

Anatomic Location: Medulla

Tests: Phonation

Significant Findings: Hoarseness

Tests: Coughing

Significant Findings: Impaired

Hoarseness and dysphagia can be seen with unilateral or bilateral injury to cranial nerve X.

➤XI. Accessory

Evaluate: Movement of head and shoulders

Anatomic Location: Cervical

Tests: Resisted head turning

Significant Findings: Weakness of trapezius and sternocleidomastoid muscle

The loss of strength is often greater with nuclear or peripheral lesions as opposed to a supranuclear injury of cranial nerve XI.

➤XII. Hypoglossal

Evaluate: Tongue movement

Anatomic Location: Medulla

Tests: Tongue protrusion

Significant Findings: Deviation, atrophy of tongue, fasciculations of tongue

On protrusion, a unilateral weak tongue deviates toward the side of weakness in lesions of the nucleus and peripheral nerve injury, but away from supranuclear lesions. Nuclear and peripheral lesions are associated with atrophy when chronic.

Comment 1. Visual field defects include (a) homonymous hemianopsia, a large hemispheric lesion or lesion of the lateral geniculate ganglion, (b) bitemporal hemianopsia, a lesion of the pituitary area compressing the optic chiasm, (c) central scotoma, a lesion of the optic nerve that typically occurs with optic neuritis, (d) superior quadrantanopsia, a contralateral temporal lobe lesion.

The pupillary light reflex includes the swinging flashlight test that may reveal a consensual response (contralateral pupillary constriction with stimulation) despite a relatively poor direct response ipsilaterally (afferent pupillary defect, also known as a Marcus-Gunn pupil) due to an optic nerve lesion.

Bilateral pinpoint pupils in a comatose patient with apneustic or agonal respirations imply a pontine lesion or a narcotics overdose. Loss of the oculocephalic reflex, or "doll's eyes," is rarely seen in drug overdose and implies brainstem injury (normally, eye movements are opposite to rotary movements of the head performed by the examiner). A unilateral dilated pupil in a comatose patient implies brainstem herniation, usually related to contralateral hemispheric mass effect. Bilateral dilated and fixed pupils and loss of all brainstem reflexes and respiratory drive occur in brain death. Paralytic agents can produce a similar clinical presentation, but typically pupils are not affected.

Comment 2. Cranial nerve III and sympathetic fibers are responsible for eye opening; consequently, ptosis, without or with a Horner's syndrome (ptosis, miosis, anhidrosis), is recorded as part of the extraocular muscle examination (although the pupil abnormalities associated with these syndromes can be recorded as part of the visual examination). A classic finding of abnormal ocular motility is referred to as an internuclear ophthalmoplegia (INO). See Chapter 18, "Neuro-Ophthalmological Emergencies," for definition of INO. Abnormal ipsilateral adduction with visual tracking of the eye is seen with lacunar infarcts of the medial longitudinal fasciculus (MLF) or with multiple sclerosis plaques in the MLF.

Comment 3. Distinct splitting of sensory function at the midline face can imply a functional disorder. Vibration is not tested for cranial nerve V function, but splitting of vibratory sensation across the forehead or skull is further evidence of a functional component in a clinical presentation.

Motor Function

Tone and Power

Muscle tone is evaluated by passively moving joints through a range of motion at varying velocities. Rigidity occurs in extrapyramidal disorders such as Parkinson's disease. Tremor plus rigidity yields "cogwheel" rigidity. Muscle tone can be increased in both pyramidal and extrapyramidal disturbances. Acute central nervous system (CNS) lesions involving the pyramidal tracts often produce hypotonia. This finding evolves over days, producing hyperreflexia and hypertonicity, referred to as spasticity. Hypertonicity can occur acutely in brainstem lesions (decorticate or decerebrate posturing). Hypotonicity may be present chronically in neuromuscular disease.

Muscle group power is graded on a scale of 0 to 5:

Grade 0	No muscle contraction
Grade 1	Muscle contraction without joint movement
Grade 2	Partial movement with gravity eliminated
Grade 3	Movement against gravity
Grade 4	Movement against some resistance
Grade 5	Normal strength

The two most commonly performed tests for detection of mild weakness:

Pronator drift	Patient with arms extended and supinated tends to pronate and lower the whole arm with flexion at the elbow
Gait observation	Includes heel and toe walking

Coordination

Equilibrium refers to the coordination and balance of the whole body. The presence of ataxia and the result of tests for Romberg sign and tandem gait are sensitive markers of dysequilibrium.

Truncal ataxia is tested by observing sitting, balance when standing, and gait (classically "wide-based" in cases of mild to moderate ataxia).

Limb ataxia (appendicular ataxia) can be present in a single extremity (usually an arm) but is more often seen in an ipsilateral arm and leg pattern, with the patient exhibiting a tendency to fall to that side. Limb ataxia is demonstrated by testing finger-to-nose and heel-to-shin movements. Limb ataxia causes intention tremor (see below) and dysdiadochokinesia (impairment of rapid alternating movements), classic indicators of lesions of the cerebellar system.

When limb ataxia is combined with weakness, the term *ataxic hemiparesis* is used. Ataxic hemiparesis is a classic finding for an internal capsule or pontine lacunar stroke when presenting as a pure motor stroke syndrome. Limb ataxia in the absence of weakness suggests a lesion of the cerebellar hemispheres and their projections, whereas truncal ataxia in isolation suggests a lesion of midline cerebellar structures and their projections.

Abnormal Movements

See Chapter 13, Movement Disorders.

Deep Tendon Reflexes, Cutaneous Reflexes, and Miscellaneous Signs

When deep tendon reflexes (DTR) are increased or hyperactive, reflex "spread" occurs in other local muscles, resulting in an increased intensity of muscle contraction.

Deep Tendon Reflexes

Deep tendon reflexes are generally graded on a 0 to 4 basis.

Grade 0	Reflex is not elicited
Grade 1	Hypoactive reflex or one that is present only with reinforcing maneuvers
Grade 2	Normal reflex
Grade 3	Reflexes that appear to be hyperactive but may not necessarily be pathological
Grade 4	Clonic reflexes that may or may not be pathological

Cutaneous Reflexes

Abdominal reflex	Abdominal wall muscle contraction
Cremasteric reflex (stimulation of the skin over the scrotal area)	Testicular elevation
Anal wink reflex	Anal contraction with stimulation

Sensory Modalities

Objective findings of a sensory examination are difficult to interpret, particularly in a concise emergency department (ED) examination, since the response of both the patient and the examiner can be subjective. A quick and effective ED examination consists of checking for recognition of numbers written on the palms of hand with eyes closed. A major sensory deficit is unlikely if the patient is able to recognize the numbers and letters. A cooperative patient can outline the area of sensory deficit by marking or with pinpricks. A "sensory level" can be outlined by the patient by having the patient run his or her own finger up the body until there is a sensory change.

The sensory examination is documented as a response to five modalities: light touch, pinprick, vibration, joint position, and temperature.

Light touch and pinprick sensation assesses the integrity of the peripheral nervous system and spinal cord sensory tracts. It can also be used to assess the presence of a cortical lesion (e.g., "extinction" in parietal lobe lesions occurs when bilateral stimuli are presented and the sensory stimulus is neglected contralateral to the lesion).

Perception of temperature or pain requires integrity of unmyelinated peripheral nerves (which originate as bipolar neurons in the dorsal root ganglia), the spinothalamic tracts of the spinal cord and brainstem, the ventral posterolateral and ventral posteromedial thalami, and thalamic projections to the parietal lobes.

Sensation of light touch is transmitted similarly, but it is also likely transmitted through the posterior columns. Sensory loss to light touch and pinprick can occur in the distribution of a single nerve, nerve root, plexus pattern, hemi cord pattern, transverse cord pattern, or crossed brainstem pattern (see later), or it can occur somatotopically, corresponding to lesions above the brainstem (e.g., contralateral face-arm-leg). A lesion is localized to the brainstem when sensory loss occurs on one side of the face and contralateral body. A "stocking-glove" pattern is usually seen with polyneuropathy, often due to diabetes. Perception of vibratory and position sense requires integrity of myelinated nerve fibers (originating as bipolar neurons in the dorsal root ganglion), the posterior columns, the medial lemniscus, ventral posterolateral nucleus of the thalamus, and cortex. Lesions of the posterior columns are demonstrated by loss of vibratory and position sense disproportionate to the loss of other modalities (e.g., B_{12} deficiency). Vibratory sensation is best tested with a 128-Hz tuning fork, and position sense is tested by small excursions of the distal digits.

Pathological Reflexes

Pathological reflexes can be associated with the following signs:

- ➤ Frontal release signs consist of glabellar, snout, suck, root, grasp, and palmomental reflexes. These signs usually indicate bilateral frontal lobe disease.
- ➤ Hoffmann's sign indicates hyperreflexia in the upper extremities, elicited by brisk tapping of the distal digits in the hand and observing for flexion of the thumb.
- ➤ Babinski sign occurs when plantar stimulation of the foot with a blunt object produces extension of the great toe and fanning of the other toes. This reflex is synonymous with an extensor plantar response and is a sign of upper motor neuron dysfunction. Other methods of eliciting an "upgoing toe" involve stimulation of the lateral foot (Chaddock's sign) or pinprick over the dorsum of the foot (Bing's sign).

Anatomical Basis of Neurological Examination

A simple method to remember the anatomic basis of neurological examination is to focus on five "levels" of the CNS, which are the brain, the brainstem, the spinal cord, the peripheral nerves, and the muscles.

Brain (hemispheres)	(a) Alteration of thought processes or consciousness, language problems (dysphasia/aphasia), neglect. (b) Seizures and involuntary movements. (c) When motor and sensory deficits are present, they occur on the same side.
Brainstem	(a) Cranial nerve(s) deficits in association with motor and sensory deficits (b) Diplopia, vertigo, dysarthria, dysphagia, disequilibrium
Spinal cord	(a) Well-demarcated "level" – sensory or motor. Normal function above and below the level. (b) Sensory dissociation – decreased pain on one side and decreased vibration and position on the other side;

	sensory deficits on one side and motor deficits on the opposite side. (c) Mixed upper and lower motor neuron signs.
Nerves	(a) Motor (weakness) or sensory (pain, sensory loss) deficits. (b) Reflexes are generally decreased or absent. (c) Findings can be limited to a nerve root or a specific nerve. (d) Distal symptoms are more often prominent than proximal.
Muscles	(a) Weakness – the most prominent symptom – is usually bilateral and symmetrical. (b) Sensation is usually normal. (c) Reflexes are generally preserved.

PEARLS AND PITFALLS

- Examination findings for patients with neurological disease can be mistaken for hysteria.

- Abnormal findings on neurological examination can result from one or more disease processes. Findings are considered in isolation and in combination.

- An age-associated loss of upgaze and vibratory sensation is normal in elderly patients.

- A detailed neurological examination evaluating the entire neuraxis is not practical in the emergency department setting; therefore, the examination is tailored to the patient's specific complaints in order to localize lesions.

- An abnormal gait can be the only sign of serious neurological disease.

SELECTED BIBLIOGRAPHY

Adams RD, Victor M. *Principles of Neurology*, 3rd ed. New York, NY: McGraw-Hill; 1985.

American College of Emergency Physicians. Clinical policy for the initial approach to patients presenting with altered mental status. *Ann Emerg Med.* 1999;33:251–81.

Haerer AF. *DeJong's The Neurologic Examination*, 5th ed. Philadelphia, Pa: JB Lippincott; 1992.

Kaufman DM, Zun L. A quantifiable, brief mental status examination for emergency patients. *J Emerg Med.* 1995;13:449–56.

O'Keefe KP, Sanson TG. Elderly patients with altered mental status. *Emerg Med Cl N Am.* 1998;16:701–15.

Mancall E. *Alpers and Mancall's Essentials of the Neurologic Examination*, 2nd ed. Philadelphia, Pa: FA Davis; 1981.

Plum F, Posner JB. *The Diagnosis of Stupor and Coma*, 3rd ed. Philadelphia, Pa: FA Davis; 1982.

Zun L, Howes DS. The mental status examination: application in the emergency department. *Am J Emerg Med.* 1988;6:165–72.

2 Neuroradiology

Andrew L. Goldberg and Sid M. Shah

INTRODUCTION

Contemporary trends emphasize the importance of a definitive diagnosis and treatment plan of many neurological conditions prior to hospitalization, which poses a unique challenge to the emergency physician. Computerized tomography (CT) and magnetic resonance imaging (MRI) are paramount among the tools that are available today.

The clinical presentation directs the choice of diagnostic procedure, usually CT or MRI. The CT of the brain remains the most frequently performed emergent neuroimaging study. Commonly suspected conditions that prompt emergent brain CT scans include acute intracranial injury, intracranial hemorrhage, and occlusive vascular disease (e.g., stroke).

Myelography is utilized primarily for patients with symptoms of myelopathy or radiculopathy, in whom MRI is contraindicated. Contraindications for MRI include pacemakers and virtually all cerebral aneurysm clips. Cerebral angiography is an important, but no longer primary, neuroradiological procedure. It is performed frequently on an emergency basis, after CT or MRI, to evaluate the possibility of ruptured aneurysm or arteriovenous malformation or to exclude acute intracranial arterial occlusion.

Computerized Tomography Versus Magnetic Resonance Imaging

CT is sensitive to acute hemorrhage and is the procedure of choice for acute trauma. CT can clearly depict skull base, facial, and calvarial fractures. CT is readily adaptable to patients requiring life support equipment. MRI can identify acute hemorrhage, particularly within the brain parenchyma, but it is typically unreliable in the diagnosis of subarachnoid hemorrhage.

The superb soft tissue contrast sensitivity of MRI provides an excellent means to diagnose both intra- and extraaxial mass lesions, especially when supplemented by intravenous contrast. Hemorrhagic brain lesions have a characteristic appearance with MRI, and chronic subdural collections are more easily

12

distinguished from adjacent bone with MRI than with CT. Magnetic resonance angiography (MRA) can image flowing blood without intravenous contrast, thus evaluating arterial or venous pathology.

Indications for Emergent Brain CT Scan

Emergent imaging is recommended for new focal deficits, persistent altered mental status, fever, recent trauma, intractable headache, history of cancer, history of anticoagulation, or suspicion of AIDS. An increased likelihood of a structural lesion is also present in patients over the age of 40 years and in those presenting with partial-onset seizure. Emergent neuroimaging in patients presenting with vertigo or dizziness is not generally indicated unless accompanied by focal neurological findings. MRI with or without contrast is the study of choice when cerebellar, brainstem, or internal auditory meatus pathology is suspected. Similarly, the yield of CT brain scans is minimal in patients with syncope or near syncope. However, persistent altered mental status requires an emergent study.

Indications of Emergent MRI

Suspected spinal cord compression is best defined by MRI. Similarly traumatic or atraumatic myelopathy should be investigated with emergent MRI. In case of nontraumatic myelopathy, the entire spine must be evaluated by MRI. Other conditions that require emergent MRI include suspected dural sinus thrombosis and arterial dissection.

Selected Neurological Conditions

Vascular Disease

Ready access to CT and its accurate interpretation is essential in evaluating the patient presenting with a new ischemic neurological deficit. Acute hemorrhage or hemorrhagic infarction must be excluded prior to initiating anticoagulant therapy. Thrombolytic intervention can proceed only if the symptoms are less than 3 hours in duration and the emergent CT scan does not reveal any hemorrhage. This requires that CT study be done very expeditiously.

Early CT signs of cerebral infarctions (Figure 2.1) include:

1. Insular ribbon sign (loss of gray–white interfaces)
2. Sulcal effacement
3. The "hyperdense middle cerebral artery sign" (This is insensitive but has strongly positive predictive value for the onset of major hemispheric infarction.)

Most CT scans are normal in the early stage of cerebral infarction. Cytotoxic edema develops within 6 hours of onset of stroke that is visible on MRI. Vasogenic edema, which is detectable by CT at 12–24 hours, develops later. See also Chapter 23, "Increased Intracranial Pressure and Herniation Syndromes."

MRA is useful in the evaluation of the posterior circulation in patients with vertebrobasilar transient ischemic attacks (TIAs). Typically, these are elderly

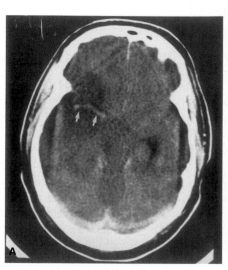 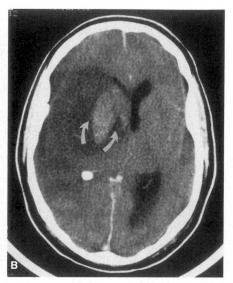

Figure 2.1. A. CT scan showing a linear hyperdensity (arrows) corresponding to thrombus in the M1 segment of the right middle cerebral artery. Surrounding edema indicates the incipient infarction in this vascular territory. **B.** CT scan showing extensive infarction in the right middle cerebral artery territory. There is a hemorrhagic component in the basal ganglia (curved arrows). There is mass effect on the ventricular system, and midline structures are shifted from right to left.

patients for whom selective catheterization of the vertebral arteries presents a relatively high risk. MRA can support the clinical impression of posterior circulation TIA by revealing vertebrobasilar stenoses and/or occlusions (Figure 2.2). The carotid bifurcations can be evaluated at the same time.

Arterial Dissection

Arterial dissection is the other major but infrequent vascular emergency. Selected nontraumatic causes of arterial dissection include fibromuscular dysplasia (Marfan's syndrome), hypertension, and collagen vascular diseases.

Transcatheter angiography may be needed for definitive diagnosis of internal carotid artery dissection, although the diagnosis can be made with MRI and MRA. This entity can be an unexpected cause of stroke, particularly after apparent minor trauma (Figure 2.3).

Cerebral Venoocclusive Disease

Cerebral venoocclusive disease (dural sinus thrombosis) is an important entity that can present with misleading or nonspecific symptoms and signs. Oral contraceptives, pregancy or puerpuerium, dehydration (particularly in children), any hypercoaguable state, connective tissue diseases, systemic neoplasia, parameningeal inflammation (e.g., otomastoiditis), and trauma are predisposing factors. A CT scan can be normal or show subtle postcontrast abnormalities such as the "delta" sign. This consists of a triangular hypodensity representing thrombus, surrounded by the enhancing wall of the superior sagittal (or other dural) sinus.

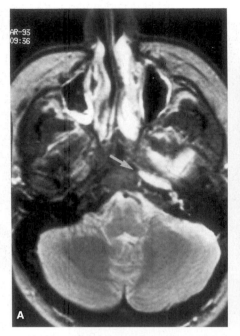

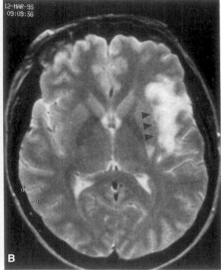

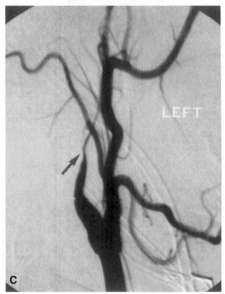

Figure 2.2. A. T2-weighted axial MRI of the skull base showing asymmetrical hyperintensity in the petrous portion of the left internal carotid artery (arrow) suggestive of thrombosis. By contrast, flow-void is seen in the basilar artery. **B.** T2-weighted axial MRI showing hyperintensity in the left insular cortex (arrowheads) indicating ischemic infarction in the left middle cerebral artery territory. **C.** Selective angiography showing tapered occlusion of the left internal carotid artery (arrow) characteristics of intimal dissection.

Intracerebral hemorrhage occurs in many cases. Emergent MRI with magnetic resonance venography is the procedure of choice (Figure 2.4).

Subarachnoid and Intracerebral Hemorrhage

Emergency CT scanning is used in the evaluation of a sudden headache. Acute subarachnoid hemorrhage (SAH) is readily diagnosed when blood is

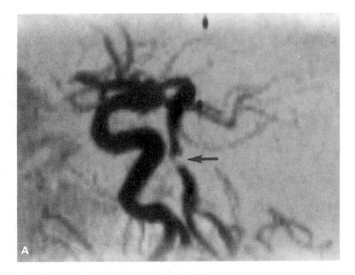

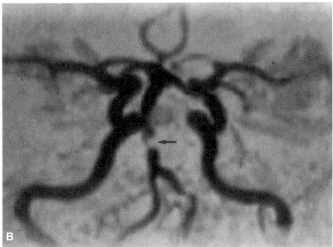

Figure 2.3. Three-dimensional time-of-flight MRA, in both (A) frontal and (B) lateral projections. There is focal stenosis (arrow) in the proximal basilar artery.

abundant; however, a CT scan is also crucial to detect smaller traces of hemorrhage, as many of these patients have no neurological deficits (Figure 2.5). CT detects over 90% of all SAH within the first 24 hours. Most CT scans return to normal within approximately 3 days after the hemorrhage. Dilatation of the temporal horns of the lateral ventricles often indicates impending hydrocephalus.

Transarterial angiography or MRA is the next step in the evaluation of SAH. MRA is used more frequently to detect unruptured aneurysms after CT scanning has demonstrated an abnormality, or in patients being screened for higher than average risk of subarachnoid hemorrhage (e.g., polycystic kidney disease).

Cavernous angioma is a specific vascular malformation that is imaged particularly well by MRI (Figure 2.6).

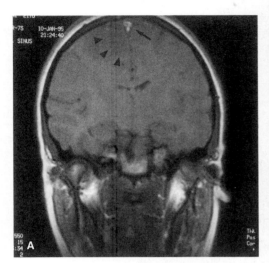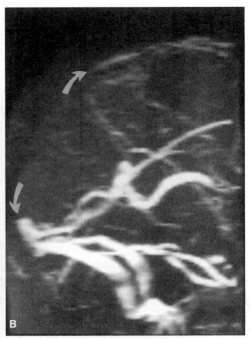

Figure 2.4. A. Coronal T1-weighted MRI. There is focal hyperintensity in the superior sagittal sinus (arrow). It is difficult to distinguish thrombus from artifact (flow-related enhancement); however, surrounding edema (arrowheads) strongly favors thrombus. **B.** Magnetic resonance venography using two-dimensional time-of-flight technique and arterial presaturation. Absence of flow (arrows) in the mid and distal superior sagittal sinus is demonstrated.

Spontaneous intracerebral hemorrhage can occur as a result of coagulopathy, toxins, hypertensive vasculopathy or amyloid angiopathy or with primary or metastatic tumors (Figure 2.7). It is difficult to exclude the possibility of an underlying tumor with CT findings of acute intracerebral hemorrhage, particularly if the density and margins of the hematoma are irregular. MRI without and with contrast can help when there is an enhancing component distinct from the intensity changes due to hemorrhagic breakdown products. In metastatic disease, additional lesions that are remote from the hematoma can exist.

Craniospinal Trauma

Expeditious diagnosis of acute traumatic epidural and subdural hematomas is critical. Epidural hematomas are often associated with skull fractures, which should be evaluated with CT bone settings and the plain radiography. Most of epidural hematomas result from laceration of the meningeal arteries and/or dural venous sinuses. The shape is typically biconvex, and the margins typically stop at the sutures (Figure 2.8).

A subacute subdural hematoma can appear isodense on CT. MRI is particularly sensitive in demonstrating subacute subdural hematomas because of

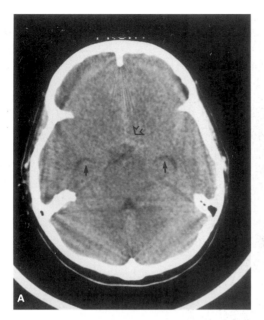

Figure 2.5. A. CT scan showing minimal hyperdensity in the anterior aspect of the suprasellar cistern extending into the interhemispheric fissure (open arrow). There is associated moderate enlargement of the temporal horns of the lateral ventricles for a young patient (closed arrows). These findings are consistent with a "sentinel" subarachnoid hemorrhage with early hydrocephalus. **B.** Three-dimensional time-of-flight MRA centered on the circle of Willis. There is a saccular aneurysm (arrows) arising from the anterior communicating artery.

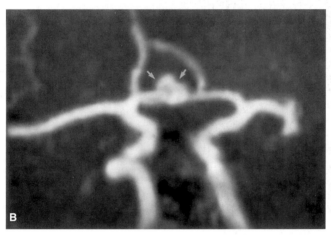

its inherent soft tissue contrast characteristics and its multiplanar capability. Free dilute methemoglobin creates panhyperintensity in these collections on all MRI sequences (Figure 2.9).

Traumatic brain injury resulting from shearing forces causes diffuse axonal injury. This can be better visualized on MRI than on CT. T2-weighted spin echo, T2*-weighted gradient echo, or fluid-attenuated inversion recovery (FLAIR) images show multiple small tissue tear hemorrhages (Figure 2.10).

Intracranial trauma can also precipitate cerebral infarction. For example, uncontrolled intracranial hypertension can lead to caudal herniation with compression of the posterior cerebral arteries. Transfalcine herniation can compromise the anterior cerebral arteries. These herniation syndromes result in infarction in the involved vascular territories. Radiographic signs of increased

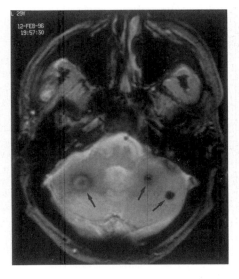

Figure 2.6. MRI susceptibility-weighted gradient echo image shows well-demarcated hypointense lesions (arrows) without surrounding edema in the cerebellum. There are multiple additional lesions (not shown) in the supratentorial region. These findings are characteristic of cavernous angiomata.

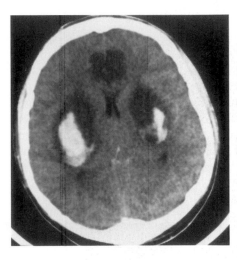

Figure 2.7. CT scan showing hemorrhagic infarction in the putamina of a young patient who ingested methanol. There is nonhemorrhagic infarction in the medial frontal lobes.

ICP are listed in Chapter 23, "Increased Intracranial Pressure and Herniation Syndromes."

Spinal Trauma

Evaluation of acute spinal trauma begins with plain radiographs. Unilateral facet lock can be difficult to discern on plain radiographs. CT and MRI allow diagnostic accuracy. MRI is able to detect a wide spectrum of spinal cord injuries, including cord contusions, hemorrhage, and transection in severe cases. The sagittal and parasagittal images generated by MRI are useful in evaluating alignment abnormalities.

Cervical sprains due to hyperextension injuries can result in serious neurological deficits, which may not be evident on plain radiographs. MRI

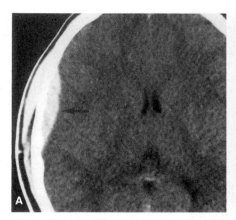
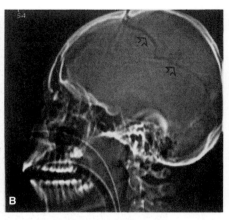

Figure 2.8. A. CT scan showing the typical lentiform hyperdensity of a right convexity epidural hematoma (arrow). **B.** Lateral digital radiograph shows the associated fracture extending from the coronal to the lambdoidal suture (open arrows). The fracture's parallel orientation to the plane of section made its identification difficult with CT scanning that included bone windows (not shown).

shows anterior ligamentous disruption, discovertebral separation, extrinsic cord compression, and intrinsic cord contusion (Figure 2.11). In contrast, flexion injuries cause anterolisthesis and posterior longitudinal ligament disruption.

At the craniocervical junction, a combination of CT and MRI is useful to assess fractures (Figure 2.12). MRI is superior in defining nonosseous compressive lesions such as epidural hematoma and herniated nucleus pulposus. CT more clearly depicts bony disruption of the neural arch. Thus CT and MRI complement each other in the evaluation of burst fractures and flexion-distraction injuries (chance or seat belt–type fractures) at the thoracolumbar junction (Figure 2.13).

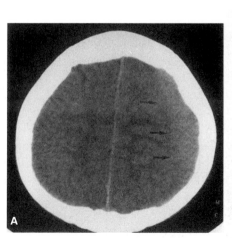
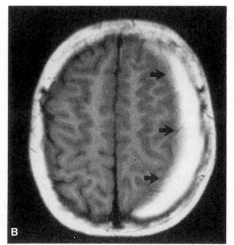

Figure 2.9. A. CT scan showing a left convexity subdural hematoma (arrows) that is virtually isodense to the underlying brain. **B.** T1-weighted MRI shows a hyperintense hematoma (arrows) due to the paramagnetic effect of free-dilute methemoglobin.

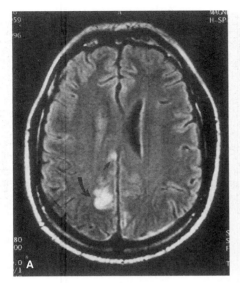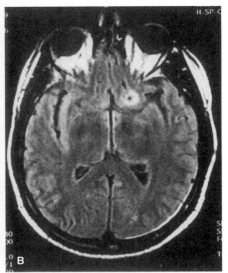

Figure 2.10. A, B. Fluid-attenuated inversion recovery axial MRIs following head trauma showing hyperintense foci of shearing injury that were not visible on preceding CT scan (not shown). The most prominent high signal abnormality is in the right medial occipital lobe (curved arrow). Additional sites of diffuse axonal injury are noted in the splenium of the corpus callosum and the left inferior frontal lobe (small arrows).

Degenerative Disease of the Spine

Radiologic evaluation of lumbar and/or cervical radiculopathy frequently begins with plain radiographs that provide little diagnostic information. In many cases, no imaging is necessary for radicular symptoms, which are often self-limited or respond to conservative measures. See Chapter 17, "Musculoskeletal and Neurogenic Pain," for indications of plain radiography in a patient with back pain.

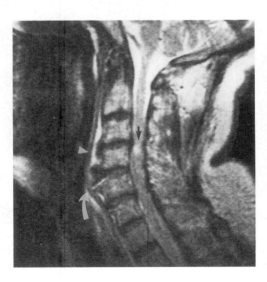

Figure 2.11. Midsagittal T2-weighted MRI showing hyperextension sprain. There is a hyperintensity consistent with a prevertebral hematoma in the high cervical region (arrowhead). There is disruption of the anterior longitudinal ligament at the C4–5 level (curved arrow). The anterior aspect of the disc space is widened abnormally. A linear hyperintensity that reflects blood and/or edema defines the superior endplate of C5. A focal intramedullary hyperintensity represents spinal cord contusion (small arrow).

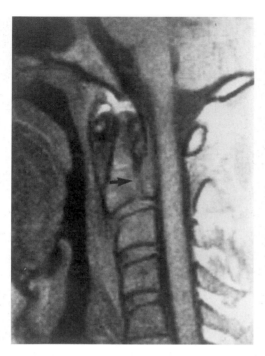

Figure 2.12. A fracture extending vertically from the dens through the body of C2 is noted on this midsagittal T1-weighted MRI (arrow). There is prevertebral hematoma. There is no cord compression.

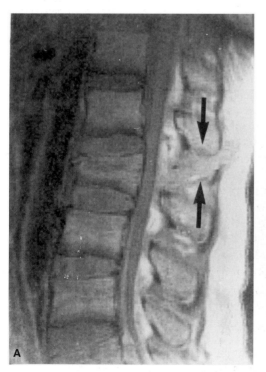

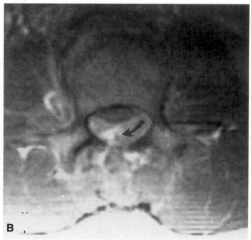

Figure 2.13. A. Midsagittal T1-weighted MRI showing a compression deformity of the L2 vertebral body and disruption of the interspinous ligament (black arrows) consistent with a flexion distraction (seat belt–type) injury. **B.** Axial T1-weighted MRI showing the thecal sac displaced anteriorly by an epidural hematoma. Conversion to methemoglobin resulted in a focal hyperintensity (curved arrow).

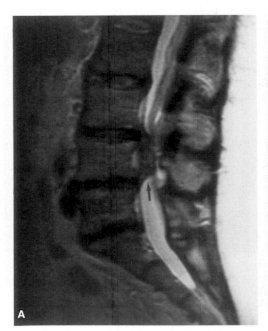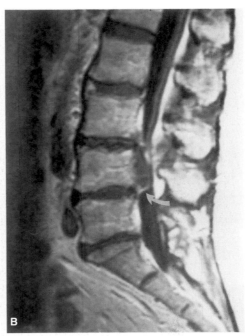

Figure 2.14. A. T-2 weighted midsagittal MRI showing a mass (arrow) that fills much of the epidural space between the L3–4 and L4–5 interspaces. **B.** T1-weighted midsagittal MRI following intravenous contrast administered to exclude a neoplastic lesion. The image shows rim enhancement of the herniated disc (curved arrow). A cleavage plane is seen between the disc material and the L4–5 interspace, further suggesting an L3–4 disc herniation with caudal migration.

When indicated, cross-sectional imaging can demonstrate abnormalities such as disc herniation and spinal stenosis. (See Figure 2.14.) CT scanning may be adequate for the lumbar region, particularly when there is sufficient epidural fat, which acts as a natural contrast agent between the extruded disc and the thecal sac. However, MRI has superior contrast resolution and remains the study of choice.

Spondylolisthesis usually results from a stress phenomenon that causes spondylolysis of the pars interarticularis, typically at the L5 level. Spondylolisthesis can be seen on plain radiographs, but CT or MRI are useful in assessing possible associated disc herniation at the involved or adjacent level. When anterolisthesis is seen at a level other than L5–S1, it is usually due to degenerative facet arthropathy rather than spondylolysis and is frequently associated with canal stenosis.

Inflammatory Disease of the Central Nervous System

Imaging performed for suspected bacterial meningitis is typically normal and excludes hydrocephalus or a focal mass lesion prior to lumbar puncture. CT scanning, and especially MRI, can reveal infarction, cerebritis, subdural empyema, or a mass in complicated cases (Figures 2.15 and 2.16).

Herpes simplex encephalitis is an acute viral inflammatory process that has specific imaging abnormalities affecting the temporal lobes, insular cortex, and

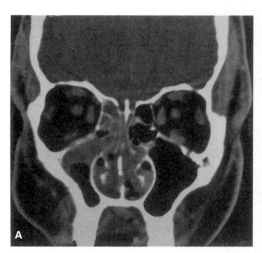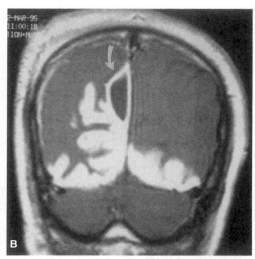

Figure 2.15. A. Coronal CT scan showing asymmetrical soft tissue density consistent with right maxilloethmoid sinusitis. **B.** Coronal postcontrast T1-weighted MRI showing gyriform enhancement associated with cerebritis. The rim-enhancing extraaxial collection in the interhemispheric fissure (curved arrow) is a subdural empyema.

orbitofrontal region. The putamen is spared. MRI shows greater evidence of bilateral involvement (areas of T2 hyperintensity) than has CT. Contrast enhancement is variable, but a gyriform pattern is typical (Figure 2.17).

HIV infection can result in an encephalitis that affects deep gray matter and periventricular white matter and is seen as hyperintensity on T2-weighted images and as low density on CT images. HIV is associated with cytomegalovirus, toxoplasmosis, progressive multifocal leukoencephalopathy, and primary central nervous system lymphoma. A mass lesion suggests toxoplasmosis or lymphoma. Differentiating these two entities can be difficult clinically, but certain imaging features are helpful. Lymphoma has higher density on noncontrast CT and lower signal intensity on T2-weighted MRI than does toxoplasmosis, which is usually hyperintense (Figure 2.18).

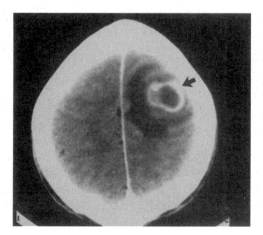

Figure 2.16. Axial CT scan showing a ring-enhancing left frontal lesion with surrounding edema (arrow). Although abscess and neoplasm (particularly metastatic) are diagnostic possibilities, a candida albicans abscess was determined following surgery.

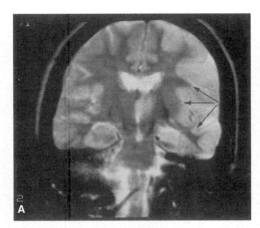

Figure 2.17. A. Coronal T2-weighted MRI showing gyral swelling of the left frontotemporal region with constriction of the normal ramifying subcortical white matter tracts (arrows) compared to the right side. **B.** Contiguous coronal T1-weighted postcontrast MRIs extending from the parieto-occipital region through the frontotemporal area showing a pattern of gyriform enhancement that extends to the tentorial surface. The findings are consistent with blood–brain barrier breakdown due to the inflammatory process.

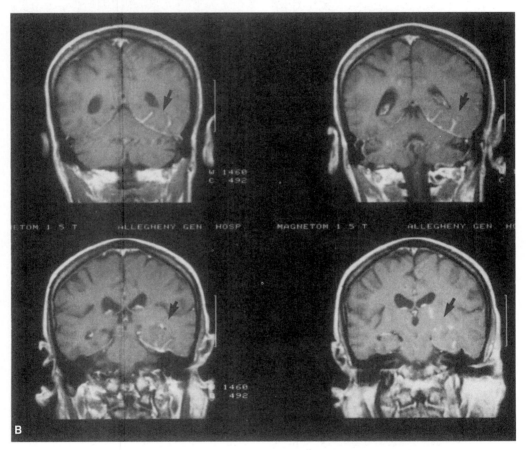

MRI provides important clues in the diagnosis of multiple sclerosis. Proton density, T2-weighted, and FLAIR images show deep white matter hyperintensities that tend to have a periventricular orientation in the periventricular region (ovoid lesions) (Figure 2.19). Contrast enhancement provides a measure of lesion activity by demonstrating blood–brain barrier disruption.

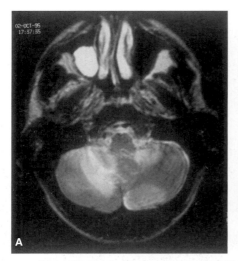
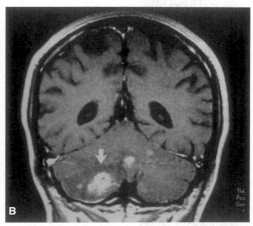

Figure 2.18. A. T2-weighted axial MRI showing abnormal hyperintensity in the cerebellar hemispheres in a nonvascular distribution. Right maxillary sinusitis is present in this HIV-positive patient. **B.** Postcontrast T1-weighted coronal MRI showing enhancement of the lesions, with edema noted surrounding a large right cerebellar mass (arrow), and a smaller vermian mass – in this case, of cerebellar toxoplasmosis.

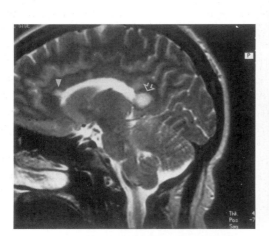
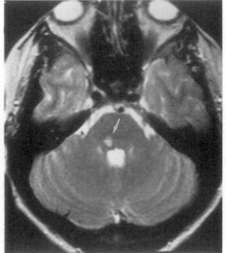

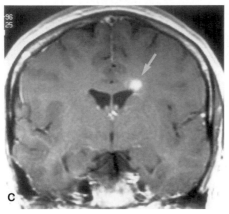

Figure 2.19. A. Midsagittal T2-weighted MRI showing abnormal hyperintensity involving the corpus callosum at multiple foci along the callosal septal interface including the rostrum (arrowhead) and the splenium (open arrow). **B.** Midsagittal T2-weighted MRI showing a focal lesion in the pontine tegmentum (arrow) probably involving the medial longitudinal fasciculus. **C.** Coronal postcontrast MRI showing asymmetrical enhancement involving the left forceps minor (arrow) indicating active blood–brain barrier breakdown in a plaque of multiple sclerosis.

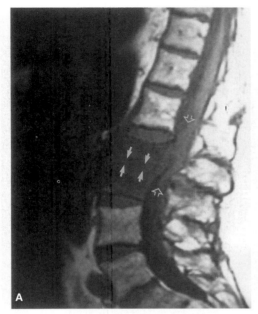
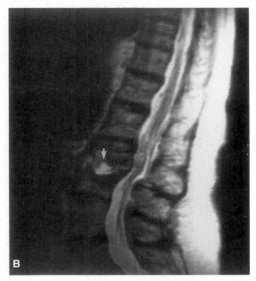

Figure 2.20. A. Midsagittal T1-weighted MRI showing marked hypointensity in the L2 and L3 vertebral bodies and obliteration of the intervertebral disc (solid arrows). **B.** T2-weighted midsagittal MRI showing marked hyperintensity in the L2–3 interspace. Findings on T1- and T2-weighted MRIs are characteristic of discitis-osteomyelitis. The proximal cauda equina is obscured by amorphous soft tissue intensity consistent with abscess or phlegmon. Extension of abnormal signal (intermediate between spinal cord substance CSF) into the spinal canal is seen (open arrows).

Acute disseminated encephalomyelitis is an infrequent monophasic illness that occurs after a viral illness or vaccination and results in neurological deficits. Multiple ring-enhancing or solidly enhancing lesions are seen on brain MRI.

Vertebral discitis/osteomyelitis can occur following surgery for lumbar disc disease and in septicemia. On MRI, findings of T1 hypointensity in adjacent vertebral bodies, T2 hyperintensity in the intervening disc space, and irregularity of the end plates are diagnostic (Figure 2.20). Following administration of intravenous contrast, patchy enhancement is seen in the disc space and spreads into the vertebral bodies.

Brain Tumors

The brain and meninges are sites of benign and malignant neoplasia. Primary gliomas are common and generally easy to diagnose by CT or MRI. Glioblastoma multiforme is observed as a mass of heterogeneous density or intensity associated with contrast enhancement and surrounding edema. Acoustic Schwannoma is a benign extraaxial lesion that can cause sensorineural hearing loss in an adult. Newer three-dimensional sequences of MRI with thin sections through the internal auditory canals provide excellent anatomical detail. Patients with intraaxial posterior fossa masses can present with nausea, vomitting, and headache. MRI is the study of choice when posterior fossa pathology is suspected. The spinal cord and vertebral column are sites for a variety of tumors. Vertebral metastases, which

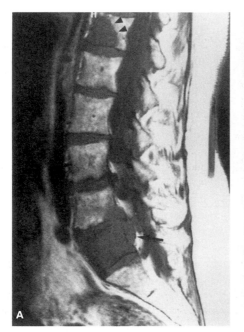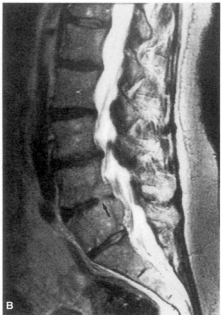

Figure 2.21. A. Midsagittal T1-weighted MRI showing abnormal hypointensity consistent with marrow infiltration by metastatic carcinoma in the L5 and T12 (arrowheads) vertebral bodies. Canal encroachment by an epidural mass is seen at the L5 level (arrow). **B.** T2-weighted midsagittal MRI showing a lesion at L5 that has the unusual feature of disc space invasion (arrow).

compress the spinal canal and/or spinal cord, occur more frequently than intrinsic cord lesions. The noncontrast T1-weighted MRI best demonstrates these lesions (Figure 2.21). Phased array surface coil technology has facilitated metastatic survey of the entire spinal axis; sensitivity is similar to radionuclide bone scanning, and specificity is superior.

PEARLS AND PITFALLS

- CT, not MRI, is essential in the diagnosis of sudden headache because CT is sensitive to subarachnoid hemorrhage.
- The "dense middle cerebral artery sign" can indicate an impending hemispheric infarction.
- Isodense subdural hematomas on CT are hypointense of all MRI sequences.
- Hyperextension sprain without associated fracture can result in spinal cord contusion, which is demonstrated on MRI.
- Lateral disc herniations are diagnosed by CT or MRI; these herniations are inapparent on myelography.
- MRI demonstrates that herpes simplex encephalitis frequently involves both cerebral hemispheres.

SELECTED BIBLIOGRAPHY

Daffner RH. *Imaging of Vertebral Trauma*, 2nd ed. Philadelphia, Pa: Lippincott-Raven; 1966.

Doezema D, King JN, Tandberg D, et al. Magnetic resonance imaging in minor head trauma. *Ann Emerg Med*. 1991;20:1281–5.

Gomori JM, Grossman RI, Goldberg HI, et al. Intracranial hematomas. Imaging by high field MR. *Radiology*. 1985;157:87–93.

Greenberg MK, Barsan WG, Starkman S. Neuroimaging in the emergency patient presenting with seizure. *Neurology*. 1996;47:26–32.

Kelly AB, Zimmerman RD, Snow RB, et al. Head trauma: Comparison of MR and CT – experience in 100 patients. *AJNR*. 1988;9:699–708.

Modic MT, Masaryk TJ, Ross JS, et al. Imaging of degenerative disk disease. *Radiology*. 1988;168:177–86.

Ross JS, Masaryk TJ, Modic MT, et al. Intracranial aneurysms: Evaluation by MR angiography. *AJNR*. 1990;11:449–56.

Shellock FG, Kanal E. Policies, guidelines, and recommendations for MR imaging safety and patient management. *J Magn Reson Imaging*. 1991;1:97–101.

Tomsick T, Brott T, Barsan W, et al. Prognostic value of the hyperdense middle cerebral artery sign and stroke scale score before ultraearly thrombolytic therapy. *AJNR*. 1996;17:79–85.

Von Kummer R, Meyding-lamade' U, Forstung M, et al. Sensitivity and prognostic value of early CT in occlusion of the middle cerebral artery trunk. *AJNR*. 1994; 15:9–15.

3 Electroencephalography

Ivo Drury

INTRODUCTION

The electroencephalogram (EEG) measures temporal changes in summated post-synaptic potentials from the superficial layers of the cerebral cortex. Today, use of the EEG has evolved to two major areas: the investigation of (1) patients with seizure disorders and (2) patients with altered states of consciousness. There are few indications for obtaining an EEG emergently; however, an EEG is considered in cases of unexplained altered mental status especially when nonconvulsive status epilepticus is suspected.

The Normal Electroencephalogram

The appearance of the normal EEG changes significantly from birth through the teenage years and then remains relatively unchanged until at least age 80. Unlike most imaging studies of the brain, the EEG also changes markedly depending on the behavioral state of the patient. In the normal awake adult whose eyes are closed, the background rhythms consist of sinusoidal activity of 9–10 Hz over the parieto-occipital region, which attenuates when the eyes are open. A mixture of faster and slower frequencies over the more anterior head regions is relatively unaffected by eye opening or closure. Drowsiness and sleep result in characteristic changes in the EEG background including increasing amounts of slower frequencies.

The Abnormal Electroencephalogram

EEG abnormalities can be reduced to two fundamental types: (1) changes seen in patients with seizure disorders and (2) various types of slow-wave abnormality. EEG findings in certain clinical conditions are summarized in Table 3.1.

Electroencephalogram Changes in the Epilepsies

Nearly every epileptic syndrome can be defined according to the following four categories: generalized or partial (i.e., due to a diffuse or more focal brain

Table 3.1. EEG Findings in Major Neurological Conditions

Diagnosis	EEG Findings
Metabolic encephalopathies (e.g., renal or hepatic) with depression of mental status	Generalized background slowing; intermittent rhythmic delta, triphasic waves; severity of slowing correlates
Focal brain lesions (e.g., stroke, tumor, inflammatory)	Focal slowing; PLEDs if acute
Encephalitis	PLEDs or Bi-PLEDs; generalized or multifocal slowing
Anoxic brain injury:	
Mild to moderate	Slowing with or without reactivity
Severe	Alpha coma; burst suppression; periodic generalized sharp waves
Brain death	Isoelectric EEG
History of seizures:	
Focal epilepsy	Focal slowing; focal epileptiform discharges
Idiopathic generalized epilepsy	Normal background; generalized epileptiform discharges
Symptomatic generalized epilepsy	Slowing of background; generalized epileptiform discharges
Status epilepticus:	
Nonconvulsive	Recurrent focal seizures (complex partial SE) Generalized spike-wave activity (nonconvulsive generalized SE)
Convulsive	Generalized spike-wave activity with periods of voltage attenuation
Syncope	Normal EEG; EKG abnormalities
Psychogenic unresponsiveness	Normal background
Pseudostatus epilepticus	Normal background; muscle and movement artifacts

abnormality, respectively) and idiopathic or symptomatic (i.e., usually benign and commonly occurring on a heredofamilial basis, or due to some underlying insult, respectively). EEG findings parallel the clinical features. Patients with idiopathic epilepsies have normal background; patients with symptomatic epilepsies have an abnormal background. Epileptiform discharges seen in patients with generalized epilepsies are generalized; those in patients with focal (partial) epilepsies are focal.

Epileptiform abnormalities on the EEG may be either interictal (i.e., occurring between seizures) or ictal (i.e., seen during the course of a clinical seizure). Interictal epileptiform discharges are spikes, sharp waves, or spike-wave complexes. Their morphology, topography, frequency, appearance in different states of behavior and in response to different activation procedures will vary depending on the patient's underlying epileptic syndrome. Acute cortical insults may lead to periodic lateralized epileptiform discharges (PLEDs), which are high-amplitude, regularly recurring sharp waves on a markedly attenuated background. PLEDs are most commonly seen in patients with stroke or encephalitis. Ictal EEG discharges are more prolonged than interictal activity and, especially in the partial epilepsies, show an evolution in frequency, morphology, and topography during a clinical seizure.

Status Epilepticus

Status epilepticus (SE) is defined as a continuous seizure lasting 30 minutes or more, or the occurrence of two or more seizures without full recovery of the baseline level of consciousness. Although a variety of classifications exists, a simple and practical one describes SE as either convulsive or nonconvulsive. The nonconvulsive types may be either complex partial SE or nonconvulsive (absence) generalized SE. EEG recordings are of value in the pharmacological management of patients with convulsive SE. An EEG should be obtained as quickly as possible, but treatment is never delayed while awaiting an EEG recording.

Nonconvulsive SE can occur in patients with a known history of epilepsy, or it may be the de novo manifestation of a seizure disorder. This diagnosis is always considered in patients who demonstrate a relatively acute onset of mental status changes without medical, psychiatric, or toxic/metabolic explanation. Nonconvulsive SE should be considered in patients with an unexpectedly prolonged postictal state. A conclusive diagnosis of either complex partial SE or absence SE can be made only by concurrent EEG recording (Figure 3.1).

Slow-Wave Abnormalities

EEG abnormalities that are slower than expected for the age and behavioral state of the patient are referred to as slow-wave abnormalities. These may be generalized or focal, and intermittent or persistent, the latter defined as present for greater than 80% of an EEG. Focal slow-wave abnormalities imply a local disturbance of cortical and sometimes adjacent subcortical structures. Generalized intermittent slowing occurs most commonly in diverse encephalopathies. The frequency of the slowing and the percent to which it is present in the EEG correlate with the severity of the encephalopathy. EEG slowing in a comatose patient is marked and persistent and typically does not change with stimulation. In the heavily sedated patient or the patient paralyzed with neuromuscular blocking agents, the EEG can be an extremely useful bedside measure of the integrity of brain function. EEG is useful in establishing a diagnosis of brain death; it should be used as such only when the patient has met all clinical criteria for the absence of any brain or brainstem function due to a known and irreversible cause.

PEARLS AND PITFALLS

- EEG is used in the evaluation of patients with seizure disorders and patients with altered states of consciousness.
- Interictal epileptiform discharges occur between seizures and consist of spikes, sharp waves, or spike-wave complexes.
- PLEDs are most commonly observed in patients with acute stroke or encephalitis.
- EEG is very useful in the diagnosis and management of status epilepticus.
- EEG slowing in a comatose patient is marked, persistent, and typically does not change with stimulation of the patient.

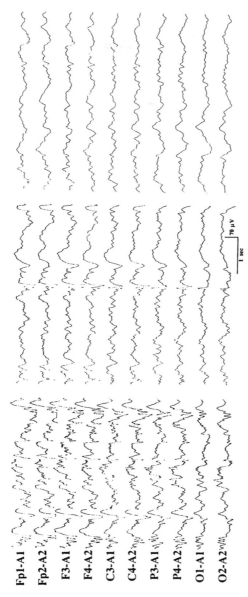

Figure 3.1. Three discontinuous samples of EEG from a 65-year-old woman in nonconvulsive generalized SE. The patient experienced repeated episodes of intermittent stupor, some associated with generalized tonic–clonic seizures, since age 50. The first EEG sample occurred after several hours of a confusional state and showed generalized irregular polyspike-and-wave activity. The next two samples were obtained 90s and 115s, respectively, after intravenous administration of 7.5 mg diazepam and showed prompt resolution of the epileptiform activity. (Reprinted with permission from Drury I, Henry TR. Ictal patterns in generalized epilepsy. *J Clin Neurophysiol.* 1993; 10:268–80, New York, NY: Raven Press.

SELECTED BIBLIOGRAPHY

Drury I, Henry TR. Ictal patterns in generalized epilepsy. *J Clin Neurophysiol.* 1993;10:268–80.

Lee SI. Nonconvulsive status epilepticus. Ictal confusion in later life. *Arch Neurol.* 1985;42:778–81.

Privitera MD, Strawsburg RH. Electroencephalographic monitoring in the emergency department. *Emerg Med Clin North Am.* 1994;12:1089–100.

4 Lumbar Puncture

James Valeriano and Daniel Ammons

INTRODUCTION

Two clinical entities (meningitis and subarachnoid hemorrhage) account for most of the lumbar punctures performed in the emergency department. Both subarachnoid hemorrhage and an infectious process are variable enough in presentation and serious enough in consequence (especially if the diagnosis is missed) that a fairly low threshold for lumbar puncture (LP) is prudent. When performed by an experienced operator an LP is a safe and simple procedure, but it is still not without its risks.

Indications

The two main indications for lumbar puncture in the emergency department are meningitis and spontaneous subarachnoid hemorrhage (SAH). Symptoms of meningitis, discussed more thoroughly in Chapter 11, "Central Nervous System Infections in Adults," include fever, headache, neck stiffness, photophobia, and mental status changes. Symptoms of SAH, also covered in Chapter 11, include sudden, "thunderclap"-type headache, mental status changes, photophobia, neck stiffness, and photophobia.

In assessing the possibility of one of these two processes, a thorough neurological examination is essential. In the absence of any focal neurological deficits, papilledema, or altered mental status, LP can be done prior to brain computerized tomography (CT) scan. The presence of any focal neurological deficits (unequal pupil size, focal weakness, aphasia, etc.) should prompt a more thorough exam with radiological imaging. The concern in this clinical setting is for a space-occupying lesion within the cranial cavity. Space-occupying lesions, such as a brain abscess (often with a high fever mimicking meningitis) or intraparenchymal hemorrhage (often associated with a "thunderclap" headache mimicking a SAH) can greatly increase the intracranial pressure (ICP). When ICP is increased in a balanced fashion (i.e., the ICP increase in the cranial cavity is approximately equal to the pressure increase in the spinal canal, such as in meningitis), the anatomical positioning of the central nervous system (CNS) is maintained. Space-occupying lesions, however, increase pressure in an unbalanced fashion, preferentially raising ICP over spinal cord pressure. Lumbar puncture performed in such a setting can induce or exacerbate a transtentorial herniation.

Contraindications

The only absolute contraindication to performance of a lumbar puncture is the presence of infection over the puncture site. Performance of the procedure in such a circumstance carries a high risk of *creating* meningitis where there may not have been one before. The procedure can be performed at a spinal level distant from the infection site if available; otherwise, it must be foregone until the superficial infection is resolved.

A relative contraindication to the performance of a lumbar puncture is the presence of a space-occupying lesion within the cranium. As already stated, such lesions tend to create an unbalanced increase in pressure in the different compartments of the central nervous system. These lesions can at times induce herniation on their own. When lumbar puncture is performed in the presence of such a lesion, the pressure in the spinal canal has a sudden "escape valve," which can lead to rapid decompression if the canal is under high pressure. This decompression increases the pressure gradient across the tentorium and across the foramen magnum, allowing herniation of the cranial contents past these structures. The compression of vital structures in the brain thus produced can lead to rapid clinical deterioration and death. The value of the information to be gleaned from the procedure must be carefully considered against the risks in such a situation.

Coagulopathy is another relative contraindication to performance of a lumbar puncture. The potential risk of creating a spinal subdural or epidural hematoma must again be weighed against the value of information to be gleaned from performance of the procedure. In cases of severe coagulopathy and when the patient's clinical status permits, replacement of deficient clotting factors and/or platelets through transfusion of blood products prior to performance of the procedure is recommended.

Risks and Complications

Potential side effects of lumbar puncture range from minor to life threatening. The most serious potential complications such as transtentorial herniation have been discussed.

Even in the absence of infection in the region of the puncture site, there is a risk of introducing an infection into the spinal canal. Strict sterile precautions must therefore be maintained to minimize this risk.

Meningitis can develop following LP in a bacteremic patient. Teele et al. reported that 7 of 46 bacteremic patients developed meningitis following an (initially negative) diagnostic LP. Generally, the benefits of cerebrospinal fluid (CSF) analysis in a bacteremic patient outweigh the risk of iatrogenic meningitis.

Bleeding following this procedure is normally mild and not of clinical consequence. The exception to this rule occurs in the setting of coagulopathy as previously discussed.

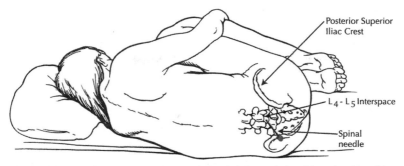

Figure 4.1. Lumbar puncture in an adult – left lateral decubitus fetal position.

Post-LP headaches are fairly common but, in most cases, minor. The risk, severity, and longevity of such headaches appear to be more closely related to the size of the dural rent created than to any persistent leak of CSF, as has often been proposed. The headache can therefore be minimized by using as small gauge a needle as is feasible; 22-gauge is often recommended for its strength and ability to avoid deflection off the midline despite its small size.

Procedure

See Figures 4.1, 4.2, and 4.3.

The lateral decubitus position is recommended for positioning of the patient – with the patient laying on his or her left for right-handed operators and vice versa.

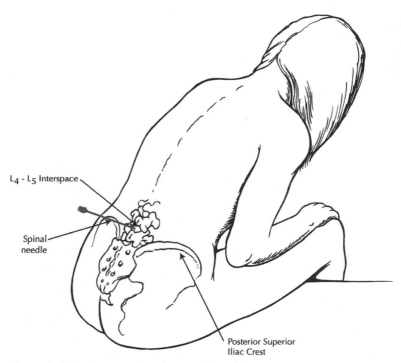

Figure 4.2. Lumbar puncture in an adult – sitting.

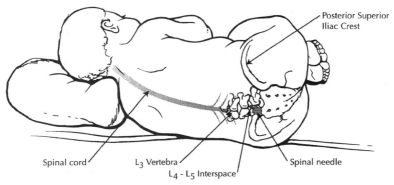

Figure 4.3. Lumbar puncture in an infant – left lateral decubitus fetal position.

The patient is asked to curl up in as near a fetal position as possible and to arch the back outward. It is helpful to have an assistant standing on the opposite side of the bed to help guide the patient into the proper position or to help restrain an uncooperative patient (such as an infant). It is not necessary nor is it helpful to force the patient's head and neck inward toward the chest; this does not help to expose the lumbar vertebra further and only succeeds in increasing the discomfort of the patient.

The patient is asked to flex at the hips and shoulders in order to push the lumbar spine outward and open up the intervertebral spaces. Such movements often result in the patient rotating the superior shoulder and hip forward relative to the positioning of the other side; the operator or the assistant should then gently redirect the patient back into the proper position.

Some operators prefer to have the patient sitting upright, which aids in identification of the midline. It is more difficult, however, for the patient to flex sufficiently for the procedure while in this position.

Following proper positioning, the area is prepped with povidone-iodine solution starting at the proposed site of skin puncture and spiraling outward, making sure to paint all the skin in the area. This is then repeated two more times. Allow the povidone–iodine solution to dry before proceeding as the drying of the povidone–iodine solution provides the bactericidal effect.

The best site for puncture is the L3–L4 or L4–L5 interspaces. The spinal cord in adults extends to the level of the L1–L2 interspace so either of these sites allows for sufficient space below the termination of the cord to avoid injuring it. The L4–L5 interspace is easily identifiable as being at the same height as the iliac crests. Following identification of the puncture site and the prep, the back is covered with a commercial towel with a center cutout, included with commercial LP kits. In infants and young children, the cord extends to the level of the L3 vertebral body, so the preferred sites for the tap are the L4–L5 or L5–S1 interspaces.

After donning sterile gloves, infiltrate 1% Lidocaine just under the skin to raise a small weal: 1–2 cc is sufficient. Use a long ($1\frac{1}{2}$ inch) needle to further infiltrate another 3–4 cc into the deeper tissues. While waiting for the local anesthetic to take effect, assemble the rest of your equipment: four collection tubes (three in infant kits), which should be uncapped and laid out in order for easy retrieval, and pressure manometer, which often requires assembly. When assembling the manometer attach a three-way stopcock (included in most kits) to the manometer base to control the flow. Most kits also come with a length of flexible tubing that can be used to connect the stopcock to the needle hub without worrying about dislodging the needle.

A 20- to 22-gauge spinal needle is best, though very muscular patients may need an 18-gauge for added strength. The standard length is $3\frac{1}{2}$ inches for adults and $1\frac{1}{2}$ inches for infants; larger sizes are available for obese patients. Insert the needle with the bevel facing toward the patients' left or right flank as appropriate. The fibers of the ligamentum flavum are oriented longitudinally such that inserting the needle in this way separates rather than cuts the ligament fibers. It is best to insert the needle at the midpoint of the spine between the appropriate spinous processes. The needle is advanced perpendicularly to the skin, withdrawing the stylet frequently to test for fluid flow. If bone is encountered, withdraw the needle almost to the surface, redirect slightly cephalad.

Once CSF flow is obtained, reinsert the stylet. Have the patient relax from the fetal position and stretch his or her legs out straight; this is the proper position for measuring opening pressure. Attach the manometer to the hub of the needle and adjust the stopcock so that CSF flows into the manometer tubing. Maximum CSF pressure (i.e., opening pressure or ICP) is obtained when the CSF no longer continues to rise but rather rises and falls with expiration and inspiration, respectively.

Once opening pressure is measured, adjust the stopcock to close off the manometer. Remove the tubing from the needle hub, and replace the stylet to prevent unnecessary runoff of CSF. Use the stopcock to empty approximately 3 cc CSF into each of the four collection tubes. If necessary, remove the stylet and collect CSF in the tube directly from the needle to get approximately 3 cc in each tube. This ensures adequate CSF volume to run all necessary tests.

Results

The initial appearance of the CSF is described as clear, turbid, bloody, etc. CSF samples are sent for evaluation of cell counts, glucose, protein, gram stain, and bacterial culture. Certain clinical scenarios require testing for fungal stain (India Ink stain) and culture, cytology, bacterial and/or viral antigens, and so on. Some CSF (such as tube 4) should be saved for further studies.

Cell Counts

CSF is generally acellular, but a few white blood cells (WBCs), predominately lymphocytes, can be normal. The presence of red blood cells (RBCs) in the CSF indicate either a traumatic tap or SAH (see later).

Glucose

Normal CSF glucose is approximately 60 mg/dl. This can vary according to serum glucose levels but tends to remain at approximately 60% of serum glucose until serum glucose rises above 250 mg/dl, at which point the ratio of CSF glucose to serum glucose tends to decline. Infectious pathological processes tend to cause a decrease in CSF glucose levels secondary to disruption of the carrier-mediated

Table 4.1. Timing of CSF Changes After Subarachnoid Hemorrhage

	RBCs	Xanthochromia
First appearance (range)	≤ 30 minutes	2–24 hours
Present in all patients	0–12 hours	12 hours–2 weeks
Disappearance by (range)	1–24 days	2–7 weeks
	(Avg.: 3–9 days)	(Avg.: 3–4 weeks)

system for transporting glucose across the blood–brain barrier and due to increased use of glucose by CSF polymorphonuclear neutrophils.

Protein

Normal CSF protein is approximately 45 mg/dl. This tends to elevate in conditions of CSF inflammation (such as meningitis) due to "leaking" of the blood–brain barrier.

Opening Pressure

As noted earlier, opening pressure is measured with the patient relaxed and fully extended in the lateral decubitus position. Normal pressure is less than 200 mm water. Elevated CSF opening pressure can be seen in multiple processes including meningitis, SAH, pseudotumor cerebri, tumor, and brain abscess.

Traumatic Tap Versus SAH

It is often difficult to discern whether blood in the CSF is due to a traumatic tap or SAH. The best way to distinguish between these is to centrifuge the CSF immediately following the procedure and look for xanthochromia. Xanthochromia is a yellowish or orangish discoloration of the supernatant following centrifugation caused by the presence of hemoglobin and hemoglobin breakdown products in the CSF. Xanthochromia appears in the CSF approximately 12 hours after an SAH, lasts approximately 2 weeks, and would not be expected in a traumatic tap alone (unless there is also an underlying SAH). See Table 4.1. Xanthochromia is best distinguished by comparing the CSF supernatant to a sample of water against a white background or by spectometry.

Another widely used method for distinguishing these two events is to perform cell counts on the first and last tubes and to look for "clearing" of the RBCs, which would be expected in a traumatic tap but not in SAH. No guidelines exist for determining what is sufficient clearing, however, unless the RBCs decline to near zero in the final tube. An existing SAH can be missed if this method is relied on.

Elevation in CSF glucose and/or WBCs above that expected by simple infiltration of blood into the CSF provides additional evidence in favor of SAH as the source of blood in the CSF. In SAH, inflammation causes an increase in WBC count and protein above that predicted by the WBC : RBC ratio (or protein : RBC ratio) from a peripheral blood sample.

Table 4.2. Cerebrospinal Fluid Findings in Different Pathological Conditions

	Protein (mg/dl)	Glucose (mg/dl)	Cell Count/mm^3 WBCs
Viral meningitis	Mild ↑	↔	10–200 Mainly lymphocytes
Bacterial meningitis	↑-↑↑	↓-↓↓	1,000–10,000 Mainly PMNs
Fungal meningitis	↑-↑↑	↓	100–1,000 Mainly lymphocytes
Tuberculosis meningitis	↑-↑↑	↓-↓↓	100–5,000 Mainly lymphocytes
Acute subarachnoid hemorrhage	↑	↔-↓	Markedly ↑ RBCs; often >100,000; ↑ WBCs with PMN predominance

Bacterial Versus Viral Meningitis

WBC counts greater than 5 are considered to be abnormal. A count of less than 100, however, makes bacterial meningitis unlikely. Within the range of WBC from 100 to 1,000, it can be difficult to reliably distinguish viral from bacterial meningitis. The WBC differential is unreliable in this cell-count range. Bacterial meningitis can often have a lymphocytic predominance whereas viral meningitis may demonstrate a neutrophilic predominance, especially early in the course of the infection. See Table 4.2.

Glucose tends to be markedly lowered in bacterial meningitis, with protein markedly elevated. Viral meningitis, by contrast, usually shows a low-normal to slightly lower-than-normal glucose with a mildly elevated protein. There is sufficient overlap in these measurements to make a definitive diagnosis based on them alone impossible.

In a patient with equivocal test results and a negative Gram stain, empiric antibiotics therapy is begun until culture results are available. In cases where the examiner has a high pretest probability of bacterial meningitis, the patient should receive appropriate antibiotics before or immediately after LP is performed, without waiting for results to become available. There is a 2–4 hour window of opportunity following administration of antibiotics before CSF results change appreciably. Bacterial meningitis carries such risk of rapid clinical deterioration and long-term sequelae, including death, that there is no excuse for delaying antibiotics when the clinician strongly suspects this disease.

PEARLS AND PITFALLS

■ The site of LP in infants and young children is lower (L4–L5 or L5–S1 vertebral level) than in adults (L3–L4 or L4–L5 vertebral level).

■ In patients suspected of having SAH, LP and examination of CSF are necessary when CT scanning of the brain fails to demonstrate SAH.

■ The traditional practice of obtaining a CT scan of the brain prior to performing LP is tempered with clinical reasoning and a comprehensive neurological examination.

- Papilledema observed on funduscopic examination is a readily accessible bedside finding of increased ICP. Papilledema is not an absolute contraindication for an LP.

- Papilledema depends on the absolute increase in ICP and the chronicity of ICP elevation.

- There is no ideal test to distinguish traumatic from nontraumatic LP. Although direct visual inspection can be unreliable, it is the usual method of determining xanthochromia.

- There is no single clinical or laboratory parameter that can reliably distinguish between viral and bacterial infections when the CSF WBC count is in the intermediate range of 100–1,000 cells/ml.

SELECTED BIBLIOGRAPHY

Fedor HM, Adelman AM, Pugno PA, Dallman J. Meningitis following normal lumbar puncture. *J Fam Pract*. 1985;20:437.

Krishra V, Liu V, Singleton AF. Should lumbar puncture be routinely performed in patients with suspected bacteremia? *J Nat Med Assoc*. 1983;75:1153.

Sengupta RP, McAllister VL, Gates P. Differential diagnosis. In: Sengupta RD, McAllister VL, eds. *Suberachnoid Haemorrhage*. Berlin: Springer-Verlag, 1986:79–92.

Swartz MN, Dodge PR. Bacterial meningitis – a review of selected aspects, I: general clinical features, special problems and unusual meningial reactions mimicking bacterial meningitis. *N Engl J Med*. 1965;272:725–31, 779–87, 842–8, 898–902.

Talan DA, Guterman JJ, Overturf GD, Singer C, Hoffman JR, Lambert B. Analysis of emergency department management of suspected bacterial meningitis. *Ann Emerg Med*. 1989;18:856–62.

Teele DW, Dashefsky B, Rakusan T, Klein JO. Meningitis after lumbar puncture in children with bacteremia. *N Engl J Med*. 1981;305:1079–81.

Vermeulen M, van Gijn J. The diagnosis of subarachnoid haemorrhage. *J Neurol Neurosurg Psychiatry*. 1990;53:365–72.

Vermeulen M, Hasan D, Blijenberg BG, Hijdra A, van Gijn J. Xanthochromia after subarachnoid haemorrhage needs no revisition. *J Neurol Neurosurg Psychiatry*. 1989;52:826–8.

Victor M, Ropper AH, Eds. *Adams and Victors Principle of Neurology*, 7th ed. New York: McGraw Hill; 2001.

Weir B. Headaches from aneurysms. *Cephalalgia*. 1994;14:79–87.

5 Altered Mental Status

Lara J. Kunschner and J. Stephen Huff

INTRODUCTION

Central nervous system dysfunction (either decreased function leading to obtundation and eventually coma or the converse, hyperactivity leading to delirium) can be due to a primary neurological condition or secondary to a medical condition. Determination of the patient's baseline mental status is crucial to identifying mild disturbances in mental status. More severe disturbances are more obvious in presentation, but for all cases from mild to severe, the clinical history of onset, course, and coexisting features are crucial to identify the underlying cause.

Coma can be described as an eyes-closed, unresponsive state. There is no verbal response, and a failure to localize noxious stimuli. Milder forms of depressed mental status have been termed obtundation (a blunting of consciousness) or stupor (a sleep-like state from which the patient can be aroused with vigorous stimulation). It is best however to simply describe the degree and type of stimulation needed to elicit a response, if any can be obtained, as these terms describe a continuum of symptomology that may fluctuate and change rapidly.

Comalike conditions that may be mistaken include the "locked-in state" in which the patient is alert but has lost all voluntary motor control to the body except for vertical extraocular eye movements; akinetic mutism in which bilateral deep, medial, frontal lobe disease results in an awake, attentive state devoid of verbal or motor output; and the "vegetative state" in which the patient has a chronic state of unresponsiveness, but may have intact sleep–wake cycles and at times appear to be awake. The opposite end of the spectrum includes delirium in which there is abnormally excessive motor and verbal activity, including agitation and hallucinations.

Coma and delirium can be due to global, diffuse central nervous system dysfunction, bilateral cerebral hemisphere dysfunction, unilateral hemisphere dysfunction with impaired brainstem function (usually due to compression), or primary brainstem dysfunction. Consciousness consists of two components: arousal generated in the brainstem and meaningful content of thought mediated through the cerebral hemispheres. Altered mental status is due to neuronal dysfunction on a cellular level due primarily to inadequate oxygenation or glucose delivery to the cell. Ischemia initiates a cascade of neurotransmitter and chemical changes within the neuron leading to cell loss.

Adequate neuronal function depends heavily on electrolyte balance, especially glucose, calcium, and sodium. Neuronal dysfunction can also result from deficiencies of thiamine (B_{12}) and from toxic substances that interfere with synaptic transmission such as ammonia, lead, exogenous benzodiazepines, and other drugs.

Evaluation

Abnormal *vital signs* are noted. Arrhythmias, especially atrial fibrillation and ventricular tachycardias, suggest an ischemic, toxic, or multifocal embolic etiology but also occur in dehydration or stress. Bradyarrhythmias occur from a primary cardiac dysfunction, and as part of Cushing's syndrome of bradycardia, or hypertension, as the result of brainstem autonomic dysfunction due to increased intracranial pressure. Hypertension when extreme (diastolic greater than 120 mm Hg) can cause coma in hypertensive encephalopathy. Hypertension is commonly seen at more moderate elevations after intracranial hemorrhage and ischemic stroke. Fever is noted in coma due to sepsis, meningitis, heat stroke,

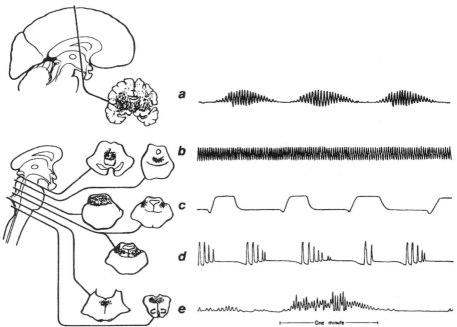

Figure 5.1. Abnormal respiratory patterns in coma and cerebral localization. Tracings are recorded by chest-abdomen pneumograph. (a) Cheyne-Stokes respiration typical of bilateral hemispheric lesions of deep structures of the cerebral hemispheres or diencephalon. (b) Central neurogenic hyperventilation due to hypothalamic-rostral midbrain damage. (c) Apneustic breathing seen with mid to lower pontine damage. (d) Cluster breathing seen with either low pontine or medullary damage. (e) Ataxic breathing seen with medullary dysfunction. (From Plum F, Posner JB. *The Diagnosis of Stupor and Coma*, 3rd ed. Philadelphia, Pa: FA Davis; 1980:41. © 1966, 1972, 1980 by Oxford University Press. Used by permission of Oxford University Press.

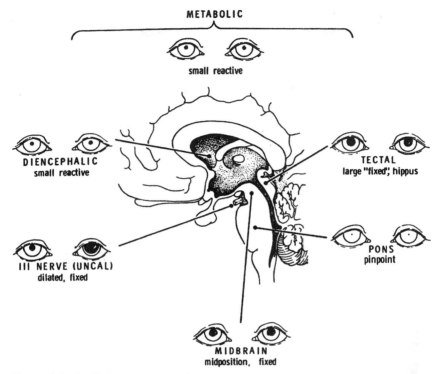

Figure 5.2. Pupils in comatose patients. From Plum F, Posner JB. *The Diagnosis of Stupor and Coma,* 3rd ed. Philadelphia, Pa: FA Davis, 1984. © 1966, 1972, 1980 by Oxford University Press. Used by permission of Oxford University Press.

neuroleptic malignant syndrome, and intoxications. Hypothermia is present in sepsis, intoxications, and hypoglycemia.

Respiratory abnormalities can be primary as in hypoxic coma due to asthmatic attack, or due to central nervous system impairment. Cheyne-Stokes respiration, alternating smooth crescendos of rapid, deep breathing for several seconds that transitions to shallow, slower breathing with brief apneic periods, usually suggests bi-hemispheric dysfunction due to ischemic or metabolic causes, or a primary congestive pulmonary pathology. Hyperventilation suggests either a metabolic disturbance, such as acidosis, pulmonary congestion, increased intracranial hypertension, or a hypothalamic-midbrain process with compensatory central hyperventilation. Apneustic breathing consists of end-inspiratory pauses lasting 2–3 seconds and occurs in midcaudal pontine injury. Ataxic breathing, irregular rhythm and depth of respiration with variable pauses, and gasping respiration is present with medullary dysfunction. Figure 5.1 demonstrates the various breathing patterns and cerebral localizations.

Focal neurologic findings must be sought. Brainstem reflexes can be helpful in localizing the cause of coma and may be of some prognostic value. The pupillary reflex is a critical reflex because it is relatively resistant to metabolic insult, and the presence of pupillary dysfunction or asymmetry is the single most important sign to distinguish structural from metabolic coma. Pupillary abnormalities corresponding to the area of brain insult are shown in Figure 5.2. Pupillary asymmetry is best understood by determining which pupil is abnormal and whether

> **Table 5.1.** Pharmacologic Agents That Can Affect
> Pupillary Responses
>
> Atropine/scopolomine: fully dilated and relatively fixed pupils
> Opiates: pinpoint, poorly reactive pupils
> Glutethimide: midposition or dilated, unequal, fixed pupils
> Barbiturates: relatively fixed pupils of varying sizes

the asymmetry is due to a parasympathetic dysfunction (third nerve palsy) or sympathetic dysfunction (Horner's syndrome). For patients who are able to open their eyes, the side with ptosis is usually the abnormal side. In the comatose patient, ptosis is not assessable. A limited number of drugs/toxins can affect the pupils (Table 5.1).

The *ocular reflexes*, oculocephalic and oculovestibular, lie in the brainstem adjacent to areas critical for maintenance of consciousness. Physical examination of these reflexes is demonstrated on Figure 5.4. The oculocephalic response in coma is normal if there is rotation of the eyes symmetrically contralateral to the direction of head turning. Medullary damage produces no rotation of the eyes, while pontine damage (medial longitudinal fasciculus) prevents medial movement of the eye unilateral to the side of damage. Symmetric eye deviation suggests either a frontal lesion unilateral to the side of deviation or a pontine lesion contralateral to the side of deviation. Roving eye movements, symmetric slow deviations to either side, are often present and indicate bilateral hemispheric dysfunction with intact oculomotor function in the brainstem. Disconjugate eye positions at rest suggest damage to the third, fourth, or sixth nerves or nuclei. Spontaneous blinking indicates an intact pontine reticular formation. The corneal response tests the integrity of the facial nerve and the third nerve. A normal response is eye closure and upward deviation of the eye (Bell's phenomenon). Metabolic processes do not generally affect reflex eye movements.

Motor response to stimulation can have a range of responses in coma and delirium. Asymmetric responses suggest a focal neurologic lesion; they can be seen with metabolic encephalopathy or in the postictal phase. Localization, reaching to grab a hand that pinches, suggests higher cortical functioning opposite to the side of stimulation. Simple flexion away from the stimulus can be purposeful but is more often a reflex movement. Decorticate posturing is flexion and pronation of the arm and hand with simultaneous extension of the leg in response to a stimulus and indicates hemispheric cortical dysfunction. Decerebrate posturing is simultaneous in upper and lower extremity extensor movement in response to noxious stimulation and indicates brainstem dysfunction. Both types of posturing have been seen with injury at multiple sites in the brain. Deep tendon reflex asymmetries also point to a lateralizing intracranial process, although the side of abnormality may not be clear if examined in isolation. Extensor plantar responses indicate dysfunction along the corticospinal tracts but are relatively nonlocalizing.

Differential Diagnosis

The differential diagnosis of delirium and coma is quite extensive. The most common causes of coma presenting to the emergency department (ED) include

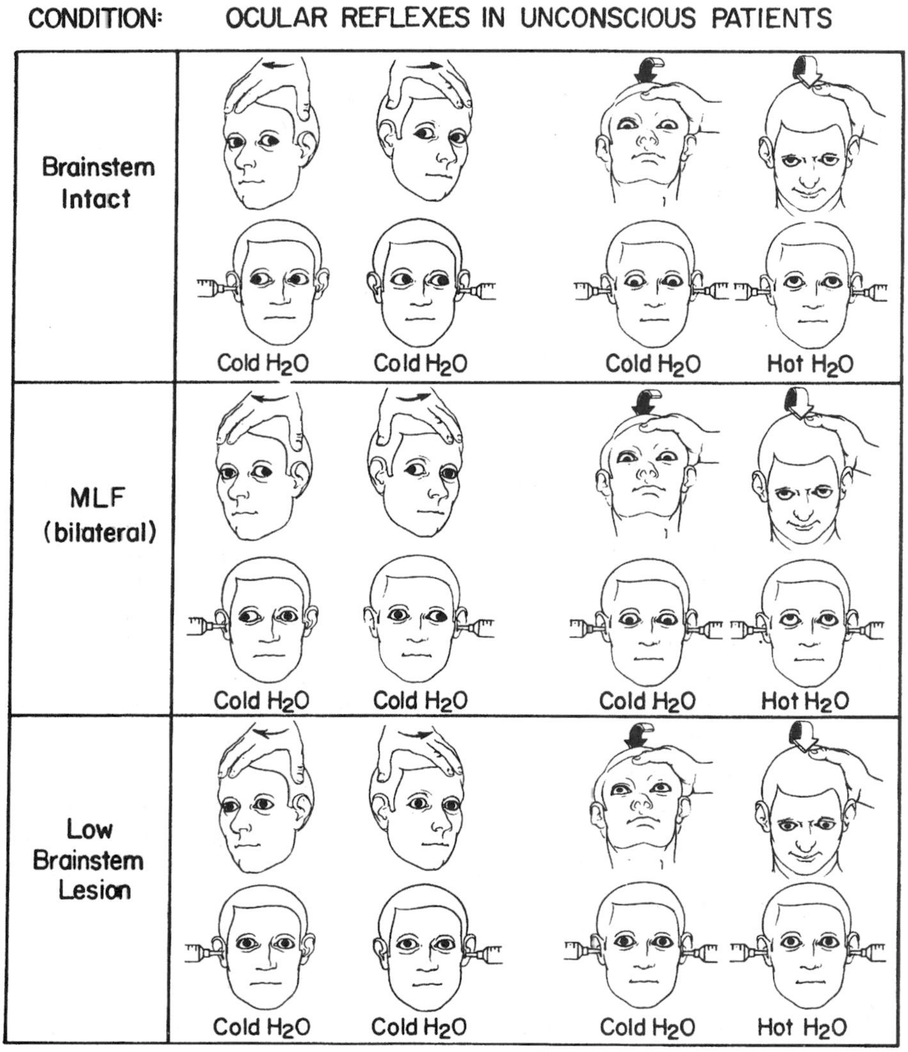

CONDITION: OCULAR REFLEXES IN UNCONSCIOUS PATIENTS

Figure 5.3. Ocular reflexes in unconscious patients. From Plum F, Posner JB. *The Diagnosis of Stupor and Coma*, 3rd ed. Philadelphia, Pa: FA Davis, 1984. © 1966, 1972, 1980 by Oxford University Press. Used by permission of Oxford University Press.

trauma, hemorrhagic and ischemic stroke, seizure, resuscitated cardiopulmonary arrest patients, sepsis, and intoxication.

A nonfocal neurological exam directs the work-up toward an etiology affecting the cortex diffusely, causing encephalopathy. The causes of global central nervous system (CNS) dysfunction are myriad medical conditions; some of the more common are listed on Table 5.2. Primary neurological causes of global dysfunction include generalized seizures, including nonconvulsive status epilepticus, the postictal state, subarachnoid hemorrhage, head trauma resulting in diffuse axonal injury, and increased intracranial pressure due to obstructive or (much less commonly) communicating hydrocephalus. Focal neurological signs direct the evaluation toward intracranial pathology. Coma due to either bilateral hemisphere dysfunction and/or brainstem dysfunction is usually to a primary neurological cause, such as those in Table 5.3.

Table 5.2. Differential Diagnosis of Coma, Stupor, and Delirium

Global cerebral dysfunction without focal neurological signs:

Trauma
  Multifocal/multiorgan trauma
  Isolated cranial trauma
Metabolic encephalopathies
  Electrolyte abnormalities
    Hypoglycemia
    Hyperglycemia/ diabetic ketoacidosis/ nonketotic hyperosmalor coma
    Hyponatremia
    Hypernatremia
    Hypercalcemia
  Organ system dysfunction
    Hepatic/ hyperammonemia
    Renal/ uremia
    Endocrine/ myxedema coma/ Addison's disease (hyperthyroidism can
    cause delirium)
Hypertensive encephalopathy
Toxic encephalopathy
  Sedative medication/ alcohol/ tricyclics/ opioids
  Carbon monoxide/ inhalants
  Neuroleptic malignant syndrome
Environmental causes
  Hyperthermia
  Hypothermia
Nutritional
  Wernicke's syndrome
Anoxic/hypoxic encephalopathy
  Multiple etiologies with decreased oxygen delivery to the brain as common
  pathway, i.e. cardiac failure, respiratory arrest, drowning, severe anemia, shock
Seizures/postictal state
Psychiatric causes

Table 5.3. Differential Diagnosis of Coma
or Delirium with Focal Neurological Signs

Stroke
  Ischemic/ hemorrhagic
  Subarachnoid hemorrhage
  Subdural/epidural hematomas
  Venous sinus occlusion
Seizure
  Postictal state
  Subclinical status epilepticus
Intracranial trauma
Meningitis/encephalitis
Intoxications

Ancillary Tests

Initial laboratory testing includes basic chemistries, glucose, creatinine, blood urea nitrogen, urinalysis and urine culture, and arterial blood gases. Toxicology screening is considered and tailored, if possible, to potential offending agents. Liver, thyroid, and adrenal function testing are also considered. Brain imaging is indicated clinically whenever focal neurologic signs are noted on initial exam. Computerized tomography (CT, without contrast enhancement) is obtained to exclude the possibility of hemorrhagic events. Cerebral edema and mass effect, hydrocephalus, and ischemia can be readily detected. Very early ischemia may not be evident on CT. The role of magnetic resonance imaging (MRI) in the ED is limited but has seen an expanding role in the evaluation of ischemic stroke, since ischemia can be detected after very few minutes on MRI compared to several hours after onset on CT. Magnetic resonance angiogram and venogram can occasionally add diagnostic information as well.

Lumbar puncture is indicated in any suspected case of meningitis and in any patient with a suspected subarachnoid hemorrhage in whom a screening CT is negative.

Electroencephalogram (EEG) testing is not routinely obtained in the ED; however, it can prove diagnostic in certain conditions. See Chapter 3, "Electroencephalography." Coma and sleep share many EEG characteristics, typically with slow background rhythms of 1–5 Hz. Nonconvulsive status epilepticus can only be accurately diagnosed via an EEG. Pontine stroke or hemorrhage will often show a normal background on EEG, whereas medullary damage will produce an EEG that resembles deep sleep. The EEG in persistent vegetative state shows normal sleep–wake cycles with several stages of sleep as in normal patients. Metabolic coma, classically hepatic encephalopathy, may show triphasic waves, which are bilateral, synchronous 2–4 Hz waves emanating from the frontal regions. Typically with metabolic coma there is a generalized slowing of the EEG from the normal 9–13 Hz. Delirium due to intoxication or alcohol withdrawal may show excess fast rhythms, low-voltage 13- to 20-Hz beta activity. Atropine used during a cardiac resuscitation temporarily slows the EEG.

Electrocardiogram (ECG) abnormalities are sought to detect cardiac ischemia and arrhythmias. Severe subarachnoid hemorrhage produces ECG abnormalities, often ventricular arrhythmias, presumably due to massive catecholamine release. Acute stroke patients also frequently show arrhythmic changes, typically conduction defects, atrial fibrillation, premature ventricular beats, or ischemia.

Management

Depressed level of consciousness requires airway protection and adequate ventilation. Administration of dextrose and thiamine is warranted in those patients in whom the etiology of the mental status change is unclear and the neurological examination is nonfocal. Naloxone is given for depressed respiratory effort; however, this can result in acute narcotic withdrawal in chronic narcotic users. Flumazenil is not routinely administered because arrhythmias and generalized seizures can be induced in cases of benzodiazepine or tricyclic overdose.

Anticonvulsant administration is quickly delivered when status epilepticus is suspected. When appropriate, antibiotic therapy for meningitis, sepsis, or fever is initiated.

Table 5.4. Glosgow Coma Scale, see Table 1.2

Eye opening

Opens eyes spontaneously	4
Opens eyes to verbal command	3
Opens eyes to pain	2
Does not open eyes	1

Verbal response

Alert and oriented	5
Converses but disoriented	4
Speaking but nonsensical	3
Moans or makes unintelligible sounds	2
No response	1

Motor response

Follows commands	6
Localizes pain	5
Movement or withdrawal from pain	4
Abnormal flexion (decorticate)	3
Abnormal extension (decerebrate)	2
No response	1
Total	3–15

Increased intracranial pressure is aggressively treated. (see Chapter 23, "Increased Intracranial Pressure and Herniation Syndromes.")

Ischemic and hemorrhagic intracranial events require initiation of therapy in the ED tailored to the specifics of the situation.

Prognosis

The overall prognosis depends on the etiology of coma. Coma scoring systems can be used to estimate the severity and depth of coma. The Glasgow Coma Scale, (Table 5.4), has been shown to help prognosticate recovery in coma resulting both from trauma and out-of-hospital cardiac arrest. The score at day 2 is most predictive with those patients scoring 10 or higher having a greater chance of satisfactory recovery, and those scoring 4 or less, with an extremely poor chance of recovery. Additionally, duration of coma (not due to trauma) without recovery

Table 5.5. Brain Death Diagnostic Features

1. No localization, flexion, or extension to noxious stimuli
2. Body temperature greater than 34°C
3. The following movements are absent: spontaneous movement, shivering, decorticate posturing, decerebrate posturing
4. The following reflexes are absent bilaterally: papillary light reflex, corneal reflex, oculovestibular reflex, oculocephalic reflex
5. Serum ethanol and CNS depressant medication levels are negligible
6. Apnea test confirmatory; no evidence of spontaneous ventilatory effort for at least 3 minutes and the Pa_{CO_2} is greater than 60 mm Hg at end of test
7. Many institutions suggest that repeat examinations at least two hours apart be performed in adults, and in children at least 12 hours apart, prior to determining brain death.

of focal or localizing signs postresuscitation is prognostic. Longer duration coma is associated with diminishing likelihood of meaningful survival. Coma in the immediate postresuscitation period; however, it has no predictive value. Recovery, or lack thereof, of brainstem reflexes after cardiopulmonary arrest can add prognostic information as well. Absence of recovery of pupillary or corneal reflexes after 24 hours after cardiopulmonary resuscitation was correlated with 0% recovery of patients to an independent lifestyle in one large study.

Brain death determination may be required. See Table 5.5.

PEARLS AND PITFALLS

- Evaluation and management proceed simultaneously in a comatose patient.
- An abnormal pupillary reflex is the most important physical sign distinguishing structural neurologic coma from metabolic coma.
- "Focal" localizing signs have been described in drug overdoses and other metabolic causes of coma.
- Prognosis for neurological recovery cannot be made in the emergency department in patients in coma after cardiopulmonary arrest.
- Brain death is the absence of detectable function of the cerebrum and the brainstem.

SELECTED BIBLIOGRAPHY

Cerebral Resuscitation Study Group of the Belgian Society for Intensive Care. Predictive value of Glasgow Coma Score for awakening after out-of-hospital cardiac arrest. *Lancet.* 1988;1:137–40.

Huff JS, *Ann Neurol.* 1997;42 (3):471.

Koehler RC, Mitchell JR. Cardiopulmonary resuscitation, brain blood flow, and neurologic recovery. *Crit Care Clin.* 1985;1:205–22.

Levy DE, Bates D, Caronna JJ, et al. Prognosis in non-traumatic coma. *Ann Int Med.* 1981;94:293–301.

Levy DE, Caronna JJ, Singer BH, Lapinski RH, Grydman H, Plum F. Predicting outcome from Hypoxic-ischemic coma. *JAMA.* 1985;253:1420–6.

Plum F, Posner JB. *The Diagnosis of Stupor and Coma*, 3rd ed. Philadelphia, Pa: FA Davis; 1980:41.

6 Headache

Robert G. Kaniecki and Merle L. Diamond

INTRODUCTION

Headache is a nearly universal experience and a serious health concern. The life-time prevalence of headache is 93%, with severe headache impacting 20% of the population each year and 40% of the population over a lifetime. It is among the top complaints of patients seen in primary care and neurology, and it is responsible for approximately 2% of all visits to the emergency department (ED).

Due to the myriad of potential causes, ranging from the benign to the cata-strophic, headache seems to pose diagnostic and therapeutic challenges to the clinician (Table 6.1). Migraine, with an annual prevalence of 12.6% of adults and approximately 5% of children, is the most common severe headache in the popu-lation. It accounts for over two thirds of headache presentations to the ED.

Evaluation

History

The patient with headache often presents to the ED because the headache is new, different from former headaches in intensity or quality, or refractory to standard treatment. Separating the benign disorders from the serious secondary headache conditions requires a complete and detailed history. A thorough analysis of the presenting headache, a careful review of prior headaches, and a subsequent out-line of the past medical history are all critical. While evaluation needs to be timely, it also needs to be thorough. One cannot overemphasize the critical na-ture of the history in the distinction of primary and secondary headache disorders. Important historical elements include:

1. Length of headache history, and subsequent course
2. Provocative or palliative factors
3. Warning symptoms such as prodromes or auras
4. Headache duration, both treated and untreated

Table 6.1. Differential Diagnosis of Headache

I. Primary Headaches
  A. Migraine
  B. Tension-type
  C. Cluster
  D. Other benign headaches
II. Secondary Headaches
  A. Head/neck trauma
  B. Cerebrovascular disease
    1. Ischemic stroke
    2. Intracranial hematoma
    3. Cerebral aneurysm/AVM (arterio-venous malformation)
    4. Arterial dissection
    5. Arteritis
  C. Intracranial tumor
    1. Parenchymal
    2. Meningeal
  D. Intracranial infection
    1. Meningitis
    2. Encephalitis
    3. Abscess
  E. CSF abnormalities
    1. Hydrocephalus
    2. Pseudotumor cerebri
    3. Low-pressure syndromes
  F. Substance abuse or withdrawal
  G. Systemic disease
    1. Hypoxia or hypercapnia
    2. Dialysis (chronic renal failure)
    3. Hypoglycemia
    4. Hypothyroidism
  H. Disease of extracranial structures
    1. Glaucoma
    2. TMJ or dental disease
    3. Sinus disease
    4. Cervical spondylosis/disc disease
  I. Cranial neuralgias
    1. Trigeminal neuralgia
    2. Occipital neuralgia

---

5. Headache location, quality, intensity, onset, development
6. Associated symptoms such as nausea, sensitivity to sensory exposures, visual changes, neck stiffness, tearing, or rhinorrhea
7. Medication or toxin exposure
8. Postdrome or "hangover" symptoms
9. Prior response to medication
10. Prior testing and results

Physical Examination

In addition to neurological examination, vital signs, palpation of the sinuses, temporomandibular joint and cervical musculature, and auscultation of the carotids are included in the typical evaluations. The neurological examination includes

---

Table 6.2. Indications for the Diagnostic Evaluation of Headache Nasty Nine

1. First/worst severe headache
2. Abrupt-onset headache
3. Progressive or changing headache pattern
4. Headache with neurologic symptoms > 1 hour
5. Abnormal examination findings
6. Headache with syncope or seizures
7. New headaches in children < 5 years of age, adults > 50 years of age
8. New headaches in patients with cancer, immunosuppression, or pregnancy
9. Headache worsening with exertion, sex, Valsalva maneuver.

---

assessments of visual acuity and fields, optic discs, extraocular movements, gait, and segmental sensory, motor, reflex, and coordination exams. Signs of meningismus or temporal artery tenderness are investigated in certain circumstances as warranted.

Findings of the history and physical examination dictate appropriate diagnostic testing. The presence of certain clinical clues, here grouped as the "Nasty Nine," help alert to the presence of a secondary or "organic" headache disorder (Table 6.2).

Diagnostic Testing

Imaging Studies. Although plain films of the sinuses, temporomandibular joint, or cervical spine are occasionally helpful, brain computerized tomography (CT) or magnetic resonance imaging (MRI) are the imaging studies of choice. A noncontrasted CT scan of the brain is useful in presentations involving abrupt-onset headache or trauma, since acute fracture and blood are best visualized by CT. MRI scanning due to its greater sensitivity and capability of visualization of the sinuses, posterior fossa, and skull base is preferable for all subacute or chronic presentations of headache. Magnetic resonance angiography may be added in cases where vascular dissection, malformation, occlusion, or aneurysm is suspected.

Lumbar Puncture. Lumbar puncture (LP) is mandatory in cases of possible subarachnoid hemorrhage (when neuroimaging alone is only 90% sensitive), infectious or neoplastic meningoencephalitis, or pseudotumor cerebri. Cerebrospinal fluid (CSF) is analyzed for cell counts, protein, glucose, cultures, cytology, or special studies when warranted. In cases of possible hemorrhage, the CSF should be centrifuged to detect the presence of xanthochromia. An opening pressure is recorded in any headache patient undergoing lumbar puncture.

Serum Studies. Serum studies are indicated in specific clinical circumstances. A complete blood count (CBC) is indicated on patients with fever, meningismus, or suspected anemia. An erythrocyte sedimentation rate (ESR) is checked in all individuals over age 50 with new or different headaches. A carboxyhemoglobin level is checked in cases of carbon monoxide exposure, while arterial blood gases (ABGs) are performed in cases where symptoms or signs indicate hypoxia, hypercapnia, or acidosis. If systemic illness is suspected, liver, renal, and thyroid studies are helpful. Toxicology profiles also are of occasional benefit.

EKG and EEG. Electro cardiography (EKG) and electroencephalography (EEG) are indicated in cases of headache with any loss of consciousness. The former is routine if performed, while the latter is often done outside the confines of many departments. Appropriate referral will then be necessary.

Intraocular Pressure. In cases of suspected ocular etiology, intraocular pressure should be measured by tonometry or slit lamp.

Differential Diagnosis and Management

Secondary Headache Syndromes

Once a patient has been determined to suffer from a secondary headache disorder, it is imperative that appropriate therapeutic interventions be instituted immediately. The treatment is generally based on the specific etiology for the headache condition and the status of the patient at the time of evaluation.

Subarachnoid Hemorrhage

Subarachnoid hemorrhage (SAH) afflicts nearly 30,000 Americans each year, the majority suffering a ruptured intracranial aneurysm. Such hemorrhages are uncommon in children and adolescents, peaking between the ages of 40 to 60. The mortality rate is 50%, with half of survivors severely disabled. Most aneurysms are found in the anterior circulation and the Circle of Willis at the base of the brain, with 20% to 25% of patients harboring multiple aneurysms. Although classically described as "the worst headache of my life," the abrupt nature of the headache is actually more characteristic than its severity. Syncope or seizure, confusion, neck stiffness, focal deficits, or coma can be presenting features. Approximately half of patients have warning symptoms within a month of rupture, including generalized headache, cranial nerve palsies, and "sentinel bleeds." Emergency CT is the procedure of choice initially, but if unremarkable (10% of cases), a lumbar puncture is mandatory. A centrifuged sample of CSF will yield a yellow or "xanthochromic" supernatant that helps differentiate hemorrhage from a traumatic tap.

Treatment of patients with SAH begins with supportive measures and nimodipine 60 mg orally every 4 hours. Neurosurgical consultation is necessary to determine the optimal timing of angiography and surgery.

Meningitis

Meningitis may result from infectious, malignant, hemorrhagic, or toxic causes. Symptoms aside from headache may include fever, neck stiffness, photophobia, and nausea, while the presence of Kerning and Brudzinski's signs on examination may help establish meningeal irritation.

Intracranial Mass Lesions

The headache of an intracranial mass lesion is best characterized by its persistent and progressive nature. A history of trauma suggests the possibilities of epidural and subdural hematomas, although subdural hematoma is also seen in cases where trauma is minimal or nonexistent. Brain abscesses may present subacutely often with other symptoms suggestive of infection, while brain tumors may present with a more chronic picture. (See Chapter 11, "Central Nervous System Infections in Adults.") Impairment in the level of consciousness, particularly when accompanied by focal neurologic findings or papilledema, is an ominous sign. Emergent CT scanning generally confirms the diagnosis, and immediate neurosurgical consultation is warranted. Measures to lower intracranial pressure are reviewed in Chapter 23, "Increased Intracranial Pressure and Herniation Syndromes."

Disorders of CSF Volume or Flow

Both *hydrocephalus* and *pseudotumor cerebri* (see Chapters 24, "Idiopathic Intracranial Hypertension," and 25, "Normal Pressure Hydrocephalus") can present with symptoms and signs of increased intracranial pressure. Acute obstructive hydrocephalus may present as a sudden increase in intracranial pressure with headache, gait and visual disturbances, incontinence, and syncope. Chronic hydrocephalus and pseudotumor cerebri have a subacute presentation.

The headache of *intracranial hypotension* is characterized by its postural nature. It is aggravated in the upright position and often accompanied by complaints of nausea, dizziness, visual change, or neck stiffness. Such headaches may rarely occur spontaneously, but most follow trauma, surgery, spinal anesthesia, or lumbar puncture. Young age, female sex, and large diameter spinal needles are the essential risk factors for a "spinal" headache. Bed rest itself has no impact on the occurrence. Symptoms last for several days before spontaneous resolution. Treatment generally involves hydration with caffeinated beverages, bed rest, analgesics, and if necessary epidural blood patch placement or surgical repair of a persistent CSF leak.

Cerebrovascular Disease

Acute vascular occlusion, either arterial (stroke) or venous (*cerebral vein/sinus thrombosis*), may result in acute headache and neurologic symptoms. Symptoms that help distinguish vascular compromise from migrainous aura include rapid development, isolation to a single vascular territory, presence of negative phenomena without positive (numbness without paresthesias, visual loss without scintillation) component, and duration greater than 60 minutes.

Arterial dissection can be spontaneous or traumatic in nature and is more common among migraineurs. Headache from carotid dissection is severe, periorbital, and accompanied by anterior neck pain, transient or persistent neurologic complaints, and often a carotid bruit or ipsilateral Horner's syndrome. Vertebral dissection often involves posterior headache that may be unilateral, accompanied by neck pain and transient or persistent neurologic complaints. Neuroimaging studies and vascular investigation (angiography magnetic resonance angiography, or ultrasound) are warranted, and anticoagulation or thrombolytic therapy may be necessary in appropriate clinical settings.

Inflammatory Disorders

Giant cell arteritis, or temporal arteritis, is considered in all individuals over age 50 presenting with new or different headaches. Headache occurs in 70% of such patients, often unilateral and temporal, and two characteristic complaints are temporal soreness and jaw claudication. Approximately half present with symptoms of polymyalgia rheumatica: arthralgias, myalgias, fever, night sweats, and weight loss. The most important laboratory finding is an elevated ESR, often in the range of 50–100. Prednisone must be instituted immediately in a daily dose of 1 mg/kg, but admission for intravenous steroids is considered if visual complaints of amaurosis or obscuration are registered. A temporal artery biopsy may be arranged within a few days, but this must not delay therapy.

Temporomandibular and *cervical spine joint* disorders occasionally present with headache. Provocation with joint motion, local joint tenderness with restricted range, and abnormalities on imaging studies may help confirm the diagnosis. Joint rest and nonsteroidal analgesia are often helpful.

Acute bacterial sinusitis is characterized by headache with facial tenderness and pain, purulent or colored nasal discharge with congestion, and often fever. Maxillary pain is often in the cheek or upper jaw, ethmoid pain between the eyes, frontal pain in the forehead, and sphenoid pain at the vertex or any other cranial location. Sinus CT scan is more sensitive than plain films. Initial treatment is empiric with 10–14 days of broad-spectrum antibiotics, while frontal or sphenoid sinusitis is often a therapeutic urgency warranting intravenous antibiotics and surgical drainage.

Primary Headache Syndromes

Tension-Type Headache

Tension-type headache is the most common headache in the population, afflicting 63% of men and 86% of women each year. It is characterized by its steady nature, bilateral location, modest intensity, and paucity of associated symptoms. Episodic tension-type headache is rarely disabling enough to warrant evaluation in the ED. Chronic tension-type headache, affecting 2% of the population, is more likely to appear due to the frustration exhibited by the afflicted. Simple analgesics and prudent muscle relaxant use are frequently satisfactory for episodic tension-type headache, while patients with the chronic variant must be treated with daily prophylactic medication – most often an antidepressant.

Cluster Headache

Although much more uncommon than tension-type or migraine headaches, cluster headache present to the ED due to its marked severity. It afflicts less than 1% of the population, generally men (M:F ratio of 5:1) between the ages of 30 and 50 years. Cigarette smoking is commonly associated with the development of cluster, while alcohol and REM (rapid eye movement) sleep may act as triggers for attacks during cycles of activity. Roughly 10% of cluster patients experience chronic symptoms without remission. The headaches are characterized by sequential episodes of brief, strictly unilateral, excruciating pain with ipsilateral nasal or orbital autonomic changes. The brevity of each attack (20–120 minutes) is typical and often results in spontaneous improvement prior to full evaluation in the ED. During an acute attack, the examination often reveals a restless, agitated adult with ipsilateral Horner's syndrome, conjunctival injection, and discharge from the eye or nose.

The pain of an acute cluster headache is first managed with inhalation of 100% oxygen through high-flow face mask. Should this be ineffective, and in the absence of contraindications, the most reliable treatment option is 6 mg of subcutaneous sumatriptan. Ipsilateral sphenopalatine ganglion block can be

Table 6.3. Contraindication for Triptan/DHE Therapy

Coronary artery disease or Prinzmetal angina
Cerebrovascular disease
Peripheral vascular disease
Significant risk factors for vascular disease
Uncontrolled hypertension
Pregnancy
Prior serious adverse events reaction with the drug
Triptan or ergot/DHE within preceding 24 hours

achieved with the instillation of 4% topical lidocaine in the ipsilateral nostril of a supine patient. At the time of discharge, patients not only should receive such acute measures for future use but should also receive medication to prevent recurrence. A 7- to 14-day course of prednisone (1 mg/kg followed by taper) is often recommended. Standard prophylactic agents such as verapamil, methysergide (if sumatriptan is not used), or lithium can be instituted at the same time, with continuation a few weeks beyond cessation of the cluster headache cycle.

Migraine Headache

General Approach. Migraine headache presents to the ED for diagnostic purposes when it is new or different. Such patients require a thorough examination and often neuroimaging studies. However, the much more common presentation is of a patient who describes a migraine refractory to typical measures. If extension beyond 72 hours is identified, the label of status migrainosus is applied.

Once the diagnosis of migraine is confirmed, appropriate therapy is instituted. Since prophylactic agents for migraine require weeks to establish efficacy, their role in an ED treatment protocol is limited. However, their role in the management of patients with frequent (2 days per week or more) or disabling migraine must not be ignored. Acute intervention with specific or symptomatic migraine medications remains the focus of ED treatment of migraine, with the goals being complete relief of pain and associated symptoms and a return to normal function if possible.

Nonpharmacologic measure, which assists in treatment, should be employed immediately. Attempts to create a quiet, dark, cool environment are helpful. Local application of ice may ease the discomfort. Intravenous hydration itself is often therapeutic, restoring electrolyte balance and reversing dehydration.

Migraine-Specific Therapy. Migraine-specific therapeutic intervention is the next step in management. Two injectable preparations are presently available: subcutaneous sumatriptan and intravenous or subcutaneous dihydroergotamine. In the absence of contraindications (Table 6.3), these agents are the drugs of choice for refractory migraine.

Sumatriptan is a selective serotonin (5-hydroxytryptamine) receptor agonist that rapidly relieves the pain of migraine while also improving nausea, photophobia, phonophobia and restoring normal function. It works directly on key elements in the pathogenesis of migraine, reversing the dilation of intracranial arteries while also blocking release of vasoactive and inflammatory peptides from activated trigeminal nerve terminals. Approximately 80% of patients respond, often within 10–20 minutes. Its strengths include speed, ease of administration, overall efficacy, and reversal of the entire symptom complex of migraine. It requires no premedication, is neither sedating nor addictive, and may easily be administered at home. Weaknesses include transient flushing, dizziness or chest pressure, relative expense, and recurrence of headache in up to 40% of patients. Such recurrences often respond to a second dose of the drug or symptomatic therapies.

Dihydroergotamine, or DHE-45, is another extremely useful agent in the termination of refractory migraine. Although it is delivered intramuscularly or subcutaneously, it is most effective when given intravenously. In order to limit an exacerbation of nausea, pretreatment with 10 mg of intravenous metoclopramide or prochlorperazine is advised. A dose of 0.5 mg DHE-45 can be delivered intravenously 15–30 minutes later. If the headache persists, a second dose of 0.5 mg DHE-45 may then be administered in an additional 30 minutes. This regimen is superior to butorphanol and meperidine/hydroxyzine combinations in clinical trials. Strengths include efficacy of 80% and, like sumatriptan, a reversal of all symptoms of migraine. Its weaknesses include a requirement for premedication, a recurrence rate of up to 26%, and side effects including muscle/abdominal cramps, diarrhea, chest pressure, and nausea.

Nonspecific Pharmacologic Therapy. If migraine-specific therapies are contraindicated or unsuccessful, nonspecific agents are then employed. Table 6.4 outlines the various therapeutic options available. In addition to their role as antiemetics when administered with other migraine medications, *prochlorperazine, metoclopramide, chlorpromazine*, and *promethazine* are themselves effective in reducing or eliminating migraine pain. This effect appears to occur exclusively with parenteral administration. Controlled trials have established efficacy similar to that of DHE-45 and ketorolac given intramuscularly, and superior to that of meperidine or lidocaine given intravenously. Sedation, anxiety, motor restlessness, acute dystonia, and occasional hypotension with chlorpromazine are the most common adverse events.

A number of traditional approaches to acute migraine management have less convincing data. Intramuscular *ketorolac* provided relief of migraine headache in several clinical trials. It is avoided in patients with renal or gastrointestinal disease, and nausea may require codelivery of an antiemetic. Two small studies have investigated the use of intravenous *dexamethasone* for acute treatment of migraine, and there is extensive anecdotal support. Parenteral corticosteroid is followed by a rapid taper (dexamethasone 12 mg, 8, mg, 4 mg) over 3 days. Intravenous *diphenhydramine, diazepam, lidocaine*, and *magnesium* all have primarily anecdotal or open-label data.

A relatively new approach has garnered interest in emergency departments around the country. Intravenous *valproate* has been shown to abort migraine attacks with great speed and minimal side effects, but the data remain preliminary. *Occipital nerve blockade* may also help abort an intractable migraine attack.

Cardiotoxicity (prolongation of Q-T interval) has been recently reported with the use of droperidol.

Table 6.4. Acute Migraine Management

A. Nonpharmacologic steps
   1. Bedrest in quiet, dark, cool environment
   2. Local application of ice
   3. Intravenous hydration
B. Migraine-specific therapy (if no contraindication)
   1. Sumatriptan, 6 mg SQ (may be repeated in 1 hour)
   2. Dihydroergotamine, 0.5 mg IV (may be repeated in 30 minutes)
     • Premedication required: Metoclopramide 10 mg IV
                or
                Prochlorperazine 10 mg IV
C. Nonspecific pharmacologic therapy
   1. Neuroleptic agents
     • Prochlorperazine, 10 mg IV
     • Metoclopramide, 10 mg IV
     • Chlorpromazine, 12.5–25 mg IV (slowly) or 25–50 mg IM
     • Promethazine, 25–50 mg IV
     • Droperidol, 2.5 mg IV (slowly) (may repeat every 30, minutes up to 10 mg)
   2. Ketorolac, 30–60 mg IM
   3. Dexamethasone, 6–10 mg IV
   4. Valproate 300–1000 mg IV
   5. Occipital nerve blockade
     • Local anesthetic/saline delivery
   6. Narcotic analgesics
     • Butorphanol, 2 mg IM
     • Meperidine, 75–100 mg IM
   7. Other agents
     • Diphenhydramine, 50–100 mg IV
     • Magnesium sulfate, 1 g IV

Role of Narcotics. Given the wide array of newer treatment options for acute migraine, the role of narcotics has become more limited. However it is compassionate and necessary to treat occasional patients who have failed all reasonable options with potent narcotic analgesics. Studies have documented equivalent efficacy of intramuscular *butorphanol* and *meperidine/hydroxyzine*. The risks of narcotic management are analgesic rebound and chemical dependence, so such treatment must be minimized. Should injections be required monthly or more frequently, other steps to manage headache must be taken.

PEARLS AND **PITFALLS**

- Focus on "new" or "different" headaches, not merely the "worst" attacks.
- Hemorrhagic and traumatic spinal fluids are best distinguished by the presence of xanthochromia.
- All suspected cases of subarachnoid hemorrhage require CT and LP.
- New or different headaches in patients over age 50 should generate suspicion for temporal arteritis and an immediate ESR evaluation.
- Most migraine headaches may be aborted with parenteral sumatriptan, dihydroergotamine, or neuroleptic agents.

SELECTED BIBLIOGRAPHY

Barton CW. Evaluation and treatment of headache patients in the emergency department: a survey. *Headache*. 1994;34:91–4.

Couch JR. Headache to worry about. *Med Clin North Am*. 1993;77:141–65.

Edmeads JF. Emergency management of headache. *Headache*. 1998;28:675–9.

Ferrari MD, Haan J. Acute treatment of migraine attacks. *Curr Opin Neurol*. 1995;8:237–42.

Klapper JA, Stanton J. Current emergency treatment of severe migraine headaches. *Headache*. 1992;32:143–6.

Mitchell CS, Osborn RE, Grosskreutz SR. Computed tomography in the headache patient: is routine evaluation really necessary? *Headache*. 1993;33:82–6.

Silberstein SD. Evaluation and emergency treatment of headache. *Headache*. 1992;32:396–407.

Weakness

George A. Small and David M. Chuirazzi

INTRODUCTION

Weakness is a condition involving muscles that cannot exert a normal force. This is in contrast to fatigue, a vague complaint that is best defined as a diminution in strength with repetitive actions. Most patients respond affirmatively to questions about whether they are weak because they may interpret pain, cramping, fatigue, depression, and psychiatric issues as weakness. The inability to perform a specific normal activity suggests weakness, which can be readily distinguished from loss of stamina or endurance.

Evaluation

See Figure 7.1.

Onset

Weakness of acute onset can be the initial manifestation of new onset disease or an exacerbation of a known progressive disease such as myasthenia gravis. Slowly progressive disorders, causing profound weakness such as amyotrophic lateral sclerosis (ALS; Lou Gehrig's disease), can present with airway compromise in the terminal stages of the disease.

Location

One of the most common presentations of weakness is gait instability with frequent falls. Location of symptoms is divided into three categories: (1) proximal, (2) distal, and (3) cranial. Each of these locations is further subdivided into symmetrical and asymmetrical categories.

1. Proximal muscle weakness manifests as trouble combing hair, climbing stairs, or arising from a chair, toilet, or bathtub.

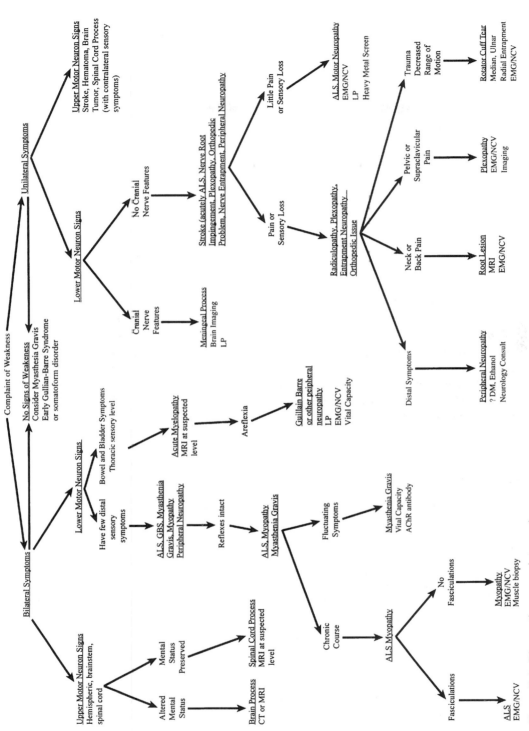

Figure 7.1. Diagnostic approach to weakness.

2. Distal weakness is found when patients complain of difficulty manipulating small objects, typing, buttoning clothes, or tripping over a curb or a high-pile rug.
3. Cranial weakness affecting the extraocular, facial, and oropharyngeal muscles, frequently manifesting as ptosis, ophthalmoparesis, diplopia, or dysphagia, can suggest two disorders of the neuromuscular junction: myasthenia gravis and botulism.

Associated Symptoms

Pain, cramping, and gastrointestinal complaints frequently accompany weakness. The collagen-vascular diseases and inflammatory myopathies are likely to produce myalgia and muscle tenderness; however, the absence of these symptoms does not exclude the diagnosis of an inflammatory myopathy. Muscle cramps, although usually benign, occur with hypothyroidism, overuse, hypocalcemia, hypomagnesemia, metabolic or respiratory alkalosis, and ALS. Nausea and vomiting can occur from an ingested toxin: botulism, heavy metal poisoning, or one of the various marine toxins.

Medical History

Medical history elicits risk factors for stroke that include, smoking, hypertension, hypercholesterolemia, diabetes, and coronary artery disease. Patients with human immunodeficiency virus (HIV) have a higher frequency of Guillain-Barré syndrome, myelopathy, and myopathy. Knowledge of current medications or recreational substance abuse assists in diagnosing toxic peripheral neuropathy, neuromuscular junction dysfunction, or muscle disorders. Certain medications that adversely affect the neuromuscular junction can lead to deterioration in a patient with myasthenia. Insect envenomation, such as tick paralysis, can result in an acute neuromuscular junction disorder with areflexia, mimicking Guillain-Barré syndrome. A history of travel to areas with known toxins from seafood may point to an accurate diagnosis of paralysis resulting from these poisons.

The degree of weakness is assessed for each muscle group; serial examinations can provide evidence of improvement or worsening in the condition. See Chapter 1, "Neurological Examination," for details of motor strength evaluation.

Differential Diagnosis and Specific Conditions

Cerebral Hemispheric Lesions

Patients with intracranial hemorrhage, ischemic stroke, or expanding neoplasms can present with unilateral weakness of the face, arm, and leg. These unilateral symptoms can be accompanied by sensory impairment. An abrupt onset signifies cerebral vascular disease of either ischemic or hemorrhagic cause. Other brain lesions such as central nervous system (CNS) lymphoma or toxoplasmosis occur in HIV-positive patients that present with progressive focal weakness.

Spinal Cord Disorders

The hallmark of myelopathy resulting in weakness includes bilateral symptoms with hyperreflexia, the Babinski sign, and symptoms of urinary dysfunction. If the condition evolves rapidly, areflexia can occur. Back pain is typical at the level of the spinal cord lesion. The most frequent cause of myelopathy is compression of the spinal cord by an extradural lesion due to vertebral trauma, disc herniation, epidural abscess, or metastatic carcinoma of the breast, lung, or prostate. Spine radiographs are often diagnostic in cases of trauma and can be helpful in suggesting other causes such as metastasis or osteomyelitis. Magnetic resonance imaging (MRI) is the neuroimaging modality of choice for diagnosing many of these diseases and establishes the lesion at the appropriate level of the spinal column. See Chapters 2, "Neuroradiology," and 29, "Spinal Cord Injury."

Transverse myelitis can be considered a primary intramedullary inflammatory process that can result in severe disability. The typical patient is a young woman who has experienced a viral syndrome in the preceding month, followed by back pain and typical signs of myelopathy. The term *transverse* is a misnomer, as the inflammatory process is clearly three-dimensional and can be patchy in nature. MRI reveals spinal cord hyperintensity and patchy enhancement in areas of blood–brain barrier breakdown. (See Chapter 23, "Increased Intracranial Pressure and Herniation Syndromes.")

Anterior Horn Cell Disorders

These devastating causes of weakness present without sensory disturbance. Poliomyelitis, which has been virtually eradicated, is an acquired degeneration of the anterior horn cells. The most frequently encountered anterior horn cell disorder in the emergency department is ALS. Patients with undiagnosed ALS can present with a diagnosis of "failure to thrive" or with severe respiratory insufficiency. Recent reports suggest West Nile Virus causes a poliomyelitis-like illness.

Nerve Root Disorders

Acute inflammatory demyelinating polyneuropathy, also known as Guillain-Barré syndrome, is the most common primary lesion of nerve roots seen in the emergency department. The criteria necessary for the clinical diagnosis of Guillain-Barré syndrome are weakness of a fairly symmetrical distribution and hyporeflexia or areflexia. (See Chapter 15, "Guillain-Barré.")

Isolated pathology of motor nerves distal to the nerve roots is rare and usually due to heavy metal intoxication. Acute poisonings of arsenic and other heavy metals can mimic Guillain-Barre syndrome.

Neuromuscular Junction Disorders

Myasthenia gravis and botulism are two of the most difficult to recognize and potentially life-threatening causes of weakness. Because both diseases can produce rapidly progressive pharyngeal and diaphragmatic dysfunction, a high index of suspicion is necessary for a quick and efficient assessment of a patient's risk of imminent respiratory failure. (See Chapter 16, "Myasthenia Gravis.")

Myopathies

Rarely acute, the most common myopathic disorders to present to the emergency department include polymyositis, dermatomyositis, steroid myopathy, and alcoholic myopathy. Prototypical distribution of proximal muscle weakness is common. No sensory loss occurs, but cramping can be a symptom. Swallowing can become a problem with polymyositis or dermatomyositis. Double vision, ptosis, or facial weakness is unlikely to occur. The patient often present with repeated falls, bruises, or broken bones. The presence of reflexes and the demonstration of proximal muscle weakness in a fairly symmetrical distribution around the shoulders and hip girdle, without sensory loss, generally allow for an accurate diagnosis. An elevated creatine phosphokinase (CPK) helps confirm the diagnosis; however, these levels can be normal in chronic myopathy. Ultimately, an electromyogram or muscle biopsy is necessary for definitive diagnosis of these disorders.

Severe electrolyte disturbances including hypophosphatemia and hypokalemia can cause an acute quadriparesis with areflexia. In addition to rare metabolic disturbances, electrolyte disturbances occur in patients with laxative abuse or diuretic use.

Acute Neuromuscular Respiratory Failure

In the emergency department, the most serious presentation of severe muscle weakness is acute respiratory failure. The three most common primary neurological causes of acute respiratory failure are previously unrecognized ALS, myasthenia gravis, and Guillain-Barré syndrome. Respiratory failure due to a neuromuscular cause is a form of restrictive pulmonary disease. This is in contrast to respiratory failure from chronic obstructive pulmonary disease in which the P_{CO_2} rises, heralding respiratory failure. Weakness of diaphragmatic and intercostal muscles causes ventilation–perfusion mismatch, usually occurring over a period of days or weeks. Respiratory failure is not reflected in arterial blood gases until extremely late in the course of respiratory muscle failure. The precipitous rise in P_{CO_2} occurs with much greater rapidity and is not a reliable indicator of when to provide ventilatory support. In general, a vital capacity of less than 1.0 liter in an adult (<15 cc/kg) indicates the likely need of endotracheal intubation and assisted ventilation. This can be assessed at the bedside by noting a rapidly rising respiratory rate, paradoxical breathing, or inability to generate a cough.

PEARLS AND PITFALLS

- Weakness implies an inability to perform usual activities due to loss of muscle, nerve, or upper motor neuron function, not a loss of stamina or endurance.
- Hip girdle weakness may be the only sign on examination in a weak patient who has myopathy or Guillain-Barré syndrome.
- Tick paralysis and heavy metal poisonings may mimic Guillain-Barré syndrome.
- ALS causes weakness due to dysfunction of upper and lower motor neurons.
- The varied presentation of myasthenia gravis can mimic other disorders and present a diagnostic challenge in the emergency department.
- The inability to generate a cough or handle oral secretions is a bedside marker of the need for assisted ventilation.

SELECTED BIBLIOGRAPHY

Dyck P, Thomas PK, eds. *Peripheral Neuropathy*, 3rd ed. Philadelphia, Pa: WB Saunders; 1993.

Engel AG, Franzini-Armstrong C, eds. *Myology*, 2nd ed. New York, NY: McGraw-Hill; 1994.

Lewis P, Rowland MD, eds. *Merritt's Textbook of Neurology*, 9th ed. Baltimore, Md: Williams & Wilkins; 1995.

Swanson PD, ed. *Signs and Symptoms in Neurology*. Philadelphia, Pa: JB Lippincott; 1984.

8 Dizziness

Kevin M. Kelly, Steven A. Tellan, Moises A. Arriaga, and Thomas M. Stein

INTRODUCTION

The evaluation of patients with the complaint of "dizziness" is a frequent occurrence in the emergency department (ED). The word *dizziness* is a nonspecific term used by patients and health care professionals to describe a disturbed sense of well-being, usually perceived as an altered orientation in space. Vertigo is defined as an illusion of movement of oneself or one's surroundings. It is usually experienced as a sensation of rotation or, less frequently, as undulation, linear displacement (pulsion), or tilt. Although vertigo usually suggests a vestibular disorder that can involve the inner ear or brain, this symptom itself cannot reliably localize the disorder. Dizziness or vertigo can result from numerous disorders of a complex human balance system. Despite the inherent complexities, the ED evaluation of dizziness or vertigo can be simplified by taking a systematic approach to history, physical examination, and laboratory tests. A useful diagnostic method is to determine whether the patient's symptoms are due to a disorder of the vestibular system or nonvestibular systems.

Anatomy

Dizziness or vertigo is frequently caused by a disorder of the vestibular system. The vestibular system is organized into peripheral and central components.

Peripheral Vestibular System

The peripheral vestibular system is composed of bilateral sensory organs, their afferent fibers, and brainstem efferent fibers that innervate the sensory organs. Figure 8.1 shows the location of the vestibular sensory organs within the inner ear. They are located in the bony labyrinth, which is a series of hollow channels connecting into a round chamber, called the vestibule, within the petrous portion of the temporal bone. The sensory organs within the bony labyrinth are three semicircular canals, the utricle, and the saccule, together constituting the membranous labyrinth. The semicircular canals are ring-shaped tubes aligned at

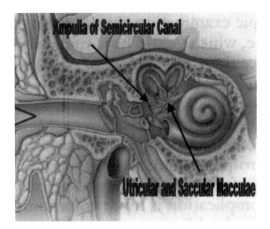

Figure 8.1. Coronal section of the ear illustrating the vestibular sensory organs. (Adapted with permission from *NEJM.* 2001:345;26:1901–8.)

right angles to each other, one in the horizontal plane (horizontal) and the other two in the vertical plane orthogonal to each other (superior and posterior). Each of the semicircular canals is able to interpret angular acceleration of the head relative to the plane of that canal by changes within the crista ampullaris, a neuroepithelial receptor organ in the ampullated end of the canal that is adjacent to the vestibule. Hair cells within the cristae sense displacement of fluid within the canals during head acceleration and transduce the stimulus into a generator potential. The utricle and saccule, commonly referred to as otolithic organs, are saclike structures that communicate with each other and with the fluids of the cochlea. The utricle and saccule sense linear inertial forces (gravity) as well as linear head accelerations. They contain the maculae, receptor organs that consist of a gelatinous material containing calcium carbonate crystals (otoliths) overlying a membrane containing sensory hair cells. The hair cells sense displacement of the otolithic membrane during linear acceleration of the head and transduce the stimulus to a generator potential similar to that of the hair cells within the cristae.

The fluid within the membranous labyrinth that bathes the vestibular sensory organs is called endolymph. The membranous labyrinth is surrounded by a continuous space within the bony labyrinth containing a chemically distinct second fluid type called perilymph. The perilymph and the endolymph fluid compartments are continuous with those inside the cochlea, the auditory sensory organ. Perilymph chemically resembles extracellular fluid, having low potassium and high sodium concentrations. The endolymph is believed to be produced in specialized cells of the cochlea and vestibular labyrinth. The endolymph resembles intracellular fluid, having high potassium and low sodium.

The hair cells of the vestibular sensory organs are innervated by afferent bipolar cells of the vestibular ganglion (Scarpa's ganglion), located in the internal auditory canal of the petrous portion of the temporal bone. The central processes of these cells form the superior and inferior vestibular nerves, which occupy the posterior half of the internal auditory canal. Afferent fibers from the cochlea form the auditory nerve, which occupies the anteroinferior part of the internal auditory canal. The vestibular nerves and the auditory nerve emerge from the internal auditory canal and combine to constitute the eighth cranial nerve. Afferent vestibular axons enter the brainstem and synapse mostly in the vestibular nuclei, with a small component of fibers synapsing within the cerebellum directly. The blood supply of the vestibular sensory organs and the nerves within the internal auditory canal originates from the anterior inferior cerebellar artery (AICA), which arises from the basilar artery.

Central Vestibular System

The central vestibular system includes the vestibular nuclei and their central nervous system (CNS) connections. The major connections of the vestibular nuclei of clinical importance are those to the cerebellum, ocular motor nuclei, spinal cord, and reticular formation. Connections among these structures are commonly referred to as vestibular pathways. Each side of the cerebellum influences the vestibular nuclei bilaterally. The vestibular-cerebellar interactions are important in the maintenance of equilibrium and locomotion.

The vestibular nuclei, median longitudinal fasciculus (MLF), and ocular motor nuclei are part of the neuronal circuitry that underlies the vestibulo-ocular reflex (VOR). The VOR is primarily a response to brief, rapid head movements, automatically producing compensatory eye movements in the opposite direction, thereby maintaining stable retinal images. The vestibular nuclei send projections to the spinal cord by the lateral and medial vestibulospinal tracts. The lateral vestibulospinal tract originates primarily from the lateral vestibular nucleus; its main action is to produce contraction of extensor (antigravity) muscles and relaxation of flexor muscles of the limbs. The medial vestibulospinal tract arises mainly from the medial vestibular nucleus and provides direct inhibition of motor neurons of the neck and axial muscles. The vestibulospinal tracts are important in vestibular reflex reactions and in the maintenance of posture.

The blood supply of the central vestibular system originates primarily from the posterior circulation. The vestibular nuclei and the vestibulocerebellum are supplied by the vertebral arteries, which ascend along the ventrolateral aspects of the medulla and unite at the pontomedullary junction to form the basilar artery. The basilar artery runs along the ventral aspect of the pons and ends at the caudal midbrain. A posterior inferior cerebellar artery (PICA) arises from each vertebral artery approximately 1 cm inferior to the basilar artery and supplies the lateral surface of the medulla and part of the surface of the cerebellar hemisphere ipsilaterally.

History and Physical Examination

History

A carefully obtained history is critical in the evaluation of a patient's complaint of dizziness or vertigo. This is important diagnostically because vertigo usually results from vestibular system disorders, whereas nonvertiginous dizziness usually results from nonvestibular system disorders. Symptom description can also differentiate peripheral from central vestibular system disorders. Special attention is paid to the quality and time course of symptoms, associated symptoms, predisposing factors, precipitating factors, and exacerbating or mitigating factors. Table 8.1 lists general properties of dizziness in vestibular and nonvestibular system dysfunction. Table 8.2 lists properties of vertigo and associated symptoms due to peripheral and central vestibular system dysfunction.

Table 8.1. Properties of Dizziness Due to Vestibular and Nonvestibular System Dysfunction

Property	Vestibular	Nonvestibular
Description	Spinning, whirling, rotating, off-balance	Lightheaded, faint, dazed, floating
Time course	Episodic or constant	Episodic or constant
Associated symptoms	Nausea, vomiting, pallor, diaphoresis, hearing loss, tinnitus	Paresthesias, palpitations headache, syncope
Predisposing factors	Congenital inner ear anomaly, ototoxins, ear surgery	Syncope due to cardiovascular disease, psychiatric illness
Precipitating factors	Head or body position changes, ear infection or trauma	Body position changes, stress, fear, anxiety, hyperventilation

Symptom Quality. The patient should accurately describe the symptoms experienced in his or her own words so that the examiner has a firm impression of the symptom quality. This information can distinguish different types of dizziness from vertigo. If the patient's description of symptoms is not clear, the patient can be asked if the symptoms resemble nervousness, confusion, weakness, lightheadedness, faintness, imbalance, or a sensation of spinning or whirling. The patient should specify whether one symptom gave rise to another. Symptom intensity is graded as mild, moderate, or severe.

Symptom Time Course. Symptom onset is described as sudden or insidious. Symptom duration is estimated as lasting seconds, minutes, hours, days, or longer. Symptoms are described as episodic or constant. The time course of symptom intensity includes the time to peak intensity, peak intensity duration, and the time of decreasing intensity.

Table 8.2. Properties of Vertigo and Associated Symptoms Due to Peripheral and Central Vestibular System Dysfunction

Symptom	Vestibular System Dysfunction	
	Peripheral	Central
Vertigo		
Onset	Sudden	Insidious
Quality	Spinning, rotation	Disequilibrium
Intensity	Severe	Mild to moderate
Occurrence	Episodic	Constant
Duration	Seconds, minutes, hours, or days	Weeks or longer
Exacerbation by head movement	Moderate to severe	Mild
Nausea and vomiting	Severe	Mild
Imbalance	Mild	Moderate
Ear pressure or pain	Occasional	None
Hearing loss	Frequent	Rare
Tinnitus	Frequent	Rare
Neurologic symptoms	Rare	Frequent

Particular attention is directed to the neuro-otologic examination of patients with a suspected vestibular disorder.

Mental Status. The mental status of the patient is determined as alert, confused, lethargic, stuporous, or comatose. Typically, patients presenting to the ED with the complaint of dizziness or vertigo are alert. Some may have an abnormal mental status at the time of presentation, which can deteriorate depending on the nature of the disorder (e.g., CNS infection or mass lesion, toxic or metabolic encephalopathies).

Cranial Nerves. The cranial nerve examination is focused and thorough including ophthalmoscopy, visual acuity evaluation, visual field evaluation, pupil size, and pupil deviation. Ocular alignment and the range of ocular movements are assessed carefully. A skew deviation, or vertical misalignment of the eyes, and head tilt can be seen in patients with the complaint of vertical diplopia. This can be due to a fourth cranial nerve palsy or an otolith disorder involving peripheral or central vestibular pathways. Smooth pursuit movements are tested with the patient visually following a slowly moving finger. Abnormalities of pursuit can indicate central disorders (e.g., impaired downward tracking in cerebellar degeneration or craniocervical junction anomalies). Saccadic breakdown of pursuit movements becomes extremely common with advancing age. Saccades are rapid eye movements associated with changes in ocular fixation or eye position within the orbit. Dysmetria, or undershooting or overshooting of saccadic eye movements, is pathological if it persists with repeated testing (e.g., hypermetria with a midline cerebellar lesion).

The evaluation of nystagmus is extremely important in the evaluation of a patient with a possible vestibular system disorder. Nystagmus is an involuntary rhythmic pattern of eye movements consisting of slow and fast components occurring in opposite directions. It is caused by physiological activation of the VOR, or by pathology in the peripheral or central vestibular system, and generally cannot be compensated by orbital eye movements. When the nystagmus is not particularly intense, it may be suppressed by gaze fixation. By convention, the direction of the fast component designates the direction of nystagmus. Physiological nystagmus occurs in healthy individuals and can be induced by head rotation, caloric irrigations, and rapidly moving (optokinetic) stimuli in the visual field. Two to three beats of "end point nystagmus" is a normal finding when the eye position is moved eccentrically in the orbit to the extremes of ocular range of motion. Pathological nystagmus suggests an underlying abnormality and can be characterized as one of several types: spontaneous (eyes in primary position), gaze-evoked (induced by changes in gaze position), positional (not present in seated position but present in some other head positions), and rapid positioning (appears only with sudden changes in body position).

In testing for pathological nystagmus, the eyes are examined in primary position and during horizontal and vertical gaze. Spontaneous nystagmus that is inhibited with visual fixation can be demonstrated by ophthalmoscopic visualization of the fundus of one eye while the patient covers the other eye. Another method of assessing spontaneous nystagmus involves the use of Frenzel glasses, which consist of 20-diopter magnifying lenses and an internal light source so that the examiner can easily visualize the patient's eyes. Gaze-evoked nystagmus

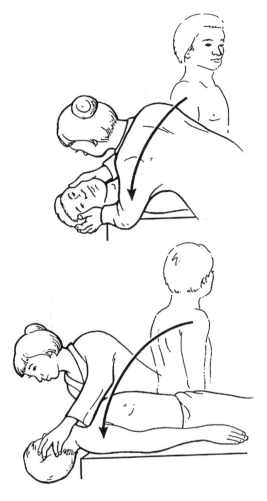

Figure 8.2. Illustrations of the technique for the Hallpike maneuver, for right side (top) and left side (bottom). Note the patient's eyes are open and fixated on the examiner. (Reprinted with permission from: *Practical Management of the Balance Disorder Patient*, Shepard and Telian, 1996, Singular Publishing Group, San Diego.)

can be assessed by having the patient change eye position by fixating on a target 30 degrees to the left, right, up, and down, and holding the eye position for 20 seconds. Positional nystagmus can be identified by placing the patient into right ear down and left ear down positions to see if nystagmus appears. Rapid positioning nystagmus can be induced by the Hallpike (Fig. 8.2) or Nylen-Barany maneuver. These are relatively synonymous eponyms for a series of maneuvers that produce rapid changes in head position relative to gravity. Classically, the patient is taken rapidly from sitting erect to a supine position, with the head extended and hanging over the edge of the table by 45° in the center position. This position is maintained for 30 seconds, after which the patient is rapidly brought back to sitting erect. The maneuver is repeated with an additional 45-degree rotation of the head to the left and repeated again with head rotation to the right. The patient is observed for nystagmus in the head-hanging and sitting positions. In clinical use, it is best to ask the patient which of these positions is most likely to produce vertigo and perform that maneuver first. If nystagmus is observed, the movement is repeated to determine whether the response is fatigable, that is, less intense on the repeat trial. Table 8.3 lists properties of spontaneous, gaze-evoked, and rapid positioning nystagmus due to peripheral and central vestibular system dysfunction.

Table 8.3. Properties of Nystagmus Due to Peripheral and Central Vestibular System Dysfunction

| Nystagmus | Vestibular System Dysfunction | |
	Peripheral	Central
Spontaneous		
Quality	Horizontal or combined torsional	Vertical, horizontal, torsional
Fixation	Inhibits,unless severe	Little effect
Direction	Unidirectional	May change direction
Gaze-evoked		
Type	None, although gaze in direction of fast phase intensifies nystagmus	Symmetrical, asymmetrical, dysconjugate, rebound (disappears or reverses)
Rapid positioning		
Quality	Torsional, never vertical	Horizontal or vertical
Latency	2–20 seconds	None
Duration	<30 seconds	>30 seconds
Direction	To downward ear	Up or variable, reversing
Fatigability	Usual	Unusual
Head position	One position	More than one position
Associated symptoms	Vertigo, nausea, vomiting	May have none

Bedside assessment of VORs can be done by the doll's eyes (oculocephalic) and cold caloric tests. These tests are most useful in the assessment of a comatose patient.

The corneal reflex tests the functional integrity of the trigeminal and facial nerves. A unilateral facial paralysis is due to an ipsilateral abnormality in the temporal bone, facial nerve, or brainstem.

Eighth cranial nerve function subserving hearing is evaluated by testing auditory threshold by presenting a minimal stimulus to each ear, such as the rubbing of fingers, a whispered word, or a watch tick. Tests using a tuning fork vibrating at 512 Hz can differentiate conductive from sensorineural hearing loss. In the Weber test, the vibrating tuning fork is applied to the middle of the forehead and the sound is normally heard in both ears. The sound is localized to the affected ear in conductive hearing loss and to the normal ear in sensorineural hearing loss. In the Rinne test, the vibrating fork is applied to the mastoid area until the sound extinguishes, and then it is held at the external auditory meatus. Air conduction is greater than bone conduction normally. In conductive hearing loss of the external or middle ear, bone conduction is greater than air conduction. In sensorineural hearing loss, the reverse is true, although air and bone conduction can be quantitatively reduced.

Palatal elevation and the gag reflex test the integrity of the glossopharyngeal and vagus nerves. The gag reflex is tested carefully to minimize the possibility of vomiting. Absent reflexes suggest impairment of the medulla. Tongue deviation with protrusion can be due to impairment of a cerebral hemisphere or a hypoglossal nerve lesion. Tongue deviation to the right suggests impaired function of the left cerebral hemisphere or the right hypoglossal nerve.

Motor System. Motor function is assessed initially by inspection of the patient. Tremor can be due to basal ganglial disease, cerebellar disease, or anxiety.

Carpopedal spasm is seen with hyperventilation. Atrophy, fasciculations, and decreased strength occur with lower motor neuron impairments. Increased resistance to passive manipulation of the joints and weakness suggest contralateral upper motor neuron impairment. Decreased resistance to passive manipulation is seen in cerebellar disease. Abnormal cerebellar tests in an appendage generally suggest ipsilateral cerebellar hemisphere impairment, although unilateral dysmetria can be a sign of an acute ipsilateral disturbance of peripheral vestibular function. Abnormalities of station and gait not related to weakness can localize impairments to the midline cerebellum or to the vestibular system.

Sensory System. Sensory function impairments such as paresthesias or numbness can result in abnormal responses to testing by light touch or pinprick. Paresthesia or numbness that is generalized or occurs in the distal extremities bilaterally and around the mouth suggests hyperventilation. A "stocking glove" distribution pattern suggests a peripheral neuropathy. When unilateral, these abnormalities can suggest an ipsilateral mononeuropathy, radiculopathy or plexopathy, or contralateral cerebral hemisphere impairments. Impaired proprioception and vibration sense can suggest posterior column disease. Impaired proprioception can be tested with the Romberg test, which assesses the patient's ability to maintain balance with the feet together and the eyes closed. Significant swaying or inability to maintain the posture is a positive test sign. Repeated falling to one side can be seen with a severe acute unilateral labyrinthine disorder, although most patients with isolated unilateral vestibular disorders can perform the Romberg test without difficulty.

Deep Tendon Reflexes. Deep tendon reflex testing can reveal decreased reflexes (e.g., Achilles tendon reflex) in peripheral neuropathy. Increased reflexes can be seen in contralateral upper motor neuron impairment. Pendular reflexes can be seen in cerebellar disease.

Provocative Tests

Hyperventilation. Hyperventilation is frequently the cause of presyncopal dizziness. When hyperventilation is suspected from the patient's history, the patient is asked to hyperventilate for 1–3 minutes. Breathing should be rapid and deep, and encouragement is offered to promote a good effort by the patient. Following hyperventilation, the patient is asked to describe the way he or she feels, and to judge whether any unusual sensations resemble the previously experienced dizziness.

Carotid Sinus Massage. The carotid sinus is sensitive to stretch, and massage of a hypersensitive carotid sinus can cause bradycardia or decreased arterial pressure resulting in dizziness or syncope. The carotid sinus is located at the bulb of the carotid bifurcation. It is localized by palpating the carotid bulb below the angle of the mandible anterior to the sternocleidomastoid muscle. The patient is seated, and each carotid sinus is massaged alternately for 15 seconds without significant compression of the carotid artery. Blood pressure and pulse are recorded, and the patient is asked if he or she has experienced any symptoms. A modest drop in blood pressure and pulse without associated symptoms is normal. Carotid sinus massage is contraindicated in patients with known cardiovascular disease.

Valsalva Maneuvers. The Valsalva maneuver is performed by having the patient forcibly exhale against a closed glottis, causing decreased cardiac output and cerebral hypoxia. The Valsalva maneuver can result in dizziness or syncope, vertigo can worsen with a perilymph fistula or a craniocervical junction anomaly (e.g., Arnold-Chiari malformation).

Fistula Test. A perilymph fistula can result from otological trauma, barotrauma (e.g., SCUBA diving incidents), or stapedectomy surgery. Fistulas produce disordered fluid mechanics within the inner ear and can lead to vertigo or disequilibrium, with or without hearing loss. In cases where a perilymph fistula is suspected, pneumatic otoscopy is performed as described earlier by applying positive and negative pressures to the tympanic membrane. The applied pressure can stimulate one of the semicircular canal cristae, resulting in a transient burst of nystagmus and vertigo. The nystagmus can occur toward or away from the involved ear. A false-positive fistula test can be seen in Meniere's disease or otosyphilis.

Head Shaking. Patients with compensated vestibular disorders can develop nystagmus after quickly shaking the head for 10 cycles in the horizontal plane. Unilateral peripheral lesions are in the direction of the slow phase of the nystagmus.

Fukuda Stepping Test. When a patient is able to perform the eyes-closed Romberg test, the Fukuda stepping test can identify and help to lateralize an acute or chronically uncompensated peripheral vestibular lesion. In this test, the patient extends the arms, closes the eyes, and marches in place. The examiner stands close by to ensure safety and to assist the patient's stability when necessary. Any rotation beyond 90 degrees within 50 steps suggests a paretic lesion on the side to which the patient turned or, less typically, an irritative lesion on the opposite side. The test sensitivity improves when head shaking is performed between eye closure and the initiation of marching in place. It is important to perform the testing in a relatively quiet room so that the patient cannot use auditory cues for orientation.

Differential Diagnosis

The differential diagnosis of dizziness or vertigo can be approached by determining whether the disorder is due to an abnormality of the vestibular system or of nonvestibular systems. Table 8.4 lists categories and common examples of nonvestibular system disorders. Table 8.5 lists vestibular system disorders and some nonvestibular disorders that can affect the vestibular system secondarily by virtue of anatomical or physiological involvement. Disorders common to Tables 8.4 and 8.5 suggest that a disorder may variably affect vestibular and nonvestibular systems. Vestibular system disorders of particular importance to ED management are described.

Benign Positional Vertigo

Benign paroxysmal positional vertigo (BPPV; also known as benign positional vertigo) is a condition characterized by brief periods of vertigo induced by position changes of the head. Onset is usually in middle age; it is the most common cause

Table 8.4. Differential Diagnosis of Dizziness or Vertigo: Nonvestibular System Disorders

Systematic disorders
Cardiovascular presyncope
    Hypovolemia
    Postural hypotension
    Vasovagal
    Carotid sinus
    Postmicturition
    Posttussive
    Vasodilators
    Autonomic nervous system dysfunction
    Addison's disease
    Brady/tachyarrhythmias
    Heart block
    Congestive heart failure
    Valvular heart disease
Medications
Hyperventilation
Chronic obstructive pulmonary disease
Infection
Hypoglycemia
Hyperglycemia
    Anemia
    Alcohol
    Street drugs
Ophthalmological disorders
    Glaucoma
    Lens implant
    Refractive errors
    New prescription lenses
    Acute ocular muscle paralysis
Neurological disorders
    Headache
        Sinus
        Muscle contraction
        Migraine
    Concussion
    Complex partial seizures
    Dementia
    Peripheral neuropathy
    Paraneoplastic cerebellar dysfunction
Psychiatric disorders
    Anxiety
    Panic attack
    Depression
    Psychogenic seizure
    Conversion reaction
    Malingering

Table 8.5. Differential Diagnosis of
Dizziness or Vertigo: Vestibular System
Disorders

Peripheral causes
 Middle ear
  Infection
   Viral
   Bacterial
  Otosclerosis
  Cholesteatoma
  Tumors
   Glomus tympanicum or jugulare
   Squamous cell carcinoma
 Inner ear
  Benign positional vertigo
  Vestibular neuronitis
  Meniere's disease
  Labyrinthitis
   Infection
   Autoimmune disorder
  Vascular disorders
   Vertebrobasilar insufficiency
    Labyrinthine
     Anterior inferior cerebellar artery
   Hemorrhage
    Labyrinthine
    Bleeding diathesis
  Systemic disorders
   Diabetes
   Uremia
  Trauma
   Perilymph fistula
  Ototoxins
   Alcohol
   Salicylates
   Antiepileptics
   Aminoglycosides
   Loop diuretics
   Cinchona alkaloids
    Quinidine
    Quinine
   Heavy metals
    Cisplatin
 Cranial nerve
  Infection
  Collagen vascular disease
  Tumor
   Schwannoma
   Neurofibroma
   Meningioma
   Metastasis

Central causes
   Cerebrovascular disorders
      Vertebrobasilar insufficiency
         Posterior fossa
         Basilar artery
         Posterior inferior cerebellar artery
      Hemorrhage
         Cerebellar
      Basilar migraine
      Vascular loop
   Mass lesions
      Tumor
         Brainstem
            Glioma
         Cerebellum
            Medulloblastoma
      Abscess
Metabolic disorders
   Alcoholic cerebellar degeneration
Infection
   Meningitis
   Encephalitis
Developmental disorders
   Malformations of the inner ear
   Craniocervical junction
      Arnold-Chiari malformation
Hereditary disorders
   Friedreich's ataxia
   Refsum's disease
   Olivopontocerebellar atrophy
Complex partial seizures
Demyelinating disease
Trauma

of vertigo assessed in clinical practice. Vertigo is often precipitated by rolling over in bed, getting in or out of bed, bending over, or extending the neck. It typically lasts for only a few seconds, always less than 1 minute. The patient may recognize a critical head position that reproduces the vertigo. Following the first attack or a flurry of episodes, lightheadedness and nausea may persist for hours to days.

It is likely that dislodgement of calcium carbonate crystals from the otolithic membrane in the utricle results in gravity-sensitive particles settling onto the cupula (cupulolithiasis) or floating freely in the membranous portion (canalolithiasis) of the posterior semicircular canal. BPPV can be the sequela of head injury, degeneration due to aging, viral labyrinthitis, vestibular neuronitis, vascular disease of the inner ear, or any cause of peripheral vertigo.

Diagnosis is based on history and supported by a positive rapid positioning test (Hallpike maneuver). The patient with classic BPPV demonstrates torsional rotatory nystagmus, with a fast horizontal component that beats toward the ear that is placed downward. The nystagmus has the following additional features to support the diagnosis of BPPV: (1) it is latent, beginning 2–5 seconds after assuming the provocative position; (2) it is transient, disappearing within 20–30 seconds; (3) it has a crescendo and decrescendo in intensity; and (4) it fatigues with repeat trials, usually with complete resolution by the fourth repetition of the

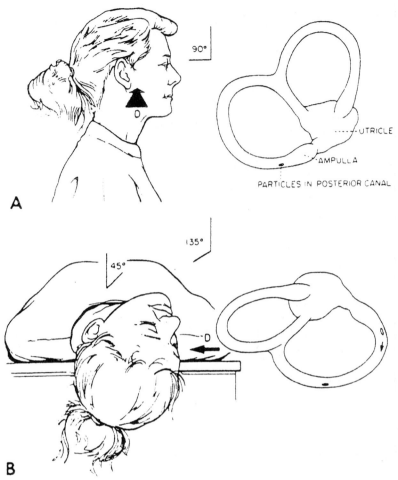

Figure 8.3. Particle repositioning maneuver for the right ear (A–D). The left side of each drawing shows the position of the patient. The arrow (D) represents the direction of view of the labyrinth depicted on the right side showing the relative position of the labyrinth and the movement of particles (dark oval, new position; open oval, previous position) in the posterior semicircular canal. (A) Patient sitting lengthwise on table. (B) Patient in Hallpike position placing the undermost (affected) ear in the earth-vertical axis. Nystagmus is exhibited in this position, possibly associated with vertigo. This position is maintained until the nystagmus is resolved. (C) Head is rotated to the left with the head turned 45 degrees downward. (D) Head and body are rotated until facing downward 135 degrees from the supine position and maintained for 1–2 minutes before the patient sits up. During B–D, particles gravitate in the posterior semicircular canal through the common crus and into the utricle. (Reprinted with permission from Parnes LS, Price-Jones RG. Particle repositioning maneuver for benign paroxysmal vertigo. *Ann Otol Rhinol Laryngol.* 1993;102:325–31.)

Hallpike maneuver. The dependent ear generally causes the symptoms, although bilateral disease can occur. Most patients with BPPV note resolution of symptoms without treatment. Although vestibular suppressants can provide temporary relief of associated nausea and lightheadedness, they usually do not prevent the motion-provoked spells of vertigo. Therefore, proper management includes discouraging the long-term use of such medications. Conventional

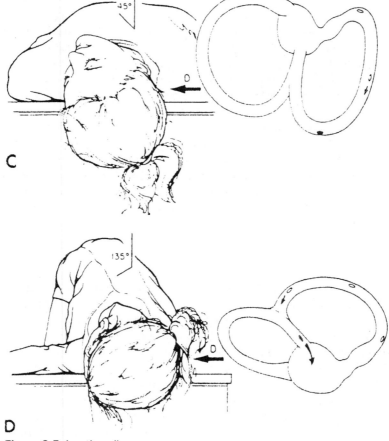

Figure 8.3 *(continued)*

vestibular rehabilitation training exercises are effective in treating this condition. A unique therapeutic procedure that can provide immediate relief of BPPV,
the particle repositioning maneuver, has been developed (Fig. 8.3). The procedure involves slowly bringing the patient's head through a series of movements
designed to permit the removal of the offending particulate material from the posterior semicircular canal. The rare patient who does not respond to conservative
therapy is a candidate for surgical therapy.

Vestibular Neuronitis

Vestibular neuronitis (also known as acute vestibulopathy, acute vestibular neuritis, and vestibular neurolabyrinthitis) is a condition typically characterized by
sudden, severe vertigo associated with nausea and vomiting in the absence of
auditory symptoms. Symptoms usually peak within 24 hours, and patients can remain relatively immobile because symptoms often worsen with head movement.
There can be truncal unsteadiness, imbalance, and difficulty focusing vision.
Symptoms subside in several days and resolve within several weeks to 3 months.
Recovery from any acute peripheral lesion depends on the process of vestibular
compensation within the CNS. During the compensation process, patients can

have a sense of disequilibrium that is aggravated by rapid head movements. In general, vestibular neuronitis is a benign condition characterized by one episode of symptoms. However, 20–30% of patients have at least one recurrent attack of vertigo. Several other more serious conditions can mimic vestibular neuronitis.

Vestibular neuronitis is a diagnosis of exclusion, based on a compatible history, signs of an acute unilateral vestibular loss (vertigo and spontaneous nystagmus, usually with the fast phase away from the abnormal ear), and the absence of any central findings on the neurological examination, imaging studies, or on electronystagmograpy. Management includes the short-term use of antihistamines or anticholinergics, an antiemetic, and/or a benzodiazepine for tranquilization as needed. Corticosteroids appear to reduce the intensity and duration of acute symptoms when administered early in the disease. The patient is encouraged to avoid prolonged immobility. Vestibular training exercises are undertaken and vestibular suppressant medication is discontinued as soon as the severe initial symptoms have improved.

Labyrinthitis

Labyrinthitis is a condition characterized by inflammation or infection of the labyrinthine system. The symptoms of acute labyrinthitis are identical to those of vestibular neuronitis, except that hearing loss accompanies the vertigo. Labyrinthitis can be caused by numerous agents including viruses, bacteria, spirochetes, and fungi and by possible involvement of systemic allergic or autoimmune diseases.

Viral labyrinthitis (viral neurolabyrinthitis) can occur with a systemic viral illness such as mumps, measles, influenza, or infectious mononucleosis. It can present with severe hearing loss that progresses over hours ("sudden deafness"), accompanied by tinnitus and ear fullness, acute vertigo, or some combination of auditory and vestibular symptoms. Management consists of vestibular suppressants, antiemetics, and vestibular training exercises as indicated.

Toxic labyrinthitis is a nonspecific disturbance of labyrinthine function that results from the products of inflammation entering the confines of the bony labyrinth. This occurs in response to acute or chronic otitis media and is not associated with frank suppuration in the labyrinth. Inner ear function frequently returns to normal following treatment of the underlying infection and symptomatic management of the labyrinthine symptoms.

Bacterial labyrinthitis is a more serious infection, with actual suppuration of the labyrinth itself. This condition usually presents with a fulminant course of severe vertigo, nausea, vomiting, and profound hearing loss. There can be associated fever, headache, or pain. Unilateral cases of bacterial labyrinthitis typically originate from infection in the pneumatized spaces of the temporal bone (acute or chronic otitis media, mastoiditis); bilateral cases can result from bacterial meningitis. Diagnosis is commonly based on clinical information. Treatment consists of aggressive parenteral antibiotic therapy with agents that provide adequate penetration of the blood–brain barrier. Surgery can be required for treatment of middle ear or mastoid infection, and to drain the resulting abscess within the labyrinth in the critically ill patient with unilateral suppurative labyrinthitis.

Syphilitic labyrinthitis occurs as a late manifestation of either congenital or acquired syphilis. It begins with deteriorating inner ear function and, when untreated, progresses slowly to profound bilateral loss of auditory and vestibular function. This course is punctuated with episodic fluctuating and progressive sensorineural hearing loss and vertigo. The peak incidence of congenital syphilitic labyrinthitis is in the fourth or fifth decade of life. The acquired form peaks in the fifth or sixth decade. Pathological changes consist of an inflammatory infiltration of the labyrinth and osteitis of the otic capsule (osseous boundary of the labyrinth). This condition can occur despite prior treatment of syphilis and may not be accompanied by neurosyphilis. Diagnosis is based on a history of unexplained vertigo, a course of fluctuating hearing loss, which is often bilateral, and a positive fluorescent treponemal antibody (FTA) test. Penicillin is the treatment of choice. Corticosteroid therapy may provide additional benefit, albeit often temporary, in some cases.

Meniere's Disease

Meniere's disease (endolymphatic hydrops) is characterized by fluctuating hearing loss, tinnitus, and episodic vertigo. Onset of the syndrome is usually in the third or fourth decade of life. The patient typically becomes symptomatic in one ear, with the development of a sensation of fullness or pressure, hearing loss, and tinnitus. Episodes of spontaneous, intense vertigo that peak within minutes and subside over several hours usually follow these symptoms but can precede them. Nausea, vomiting, diaphoresis, and pallor usually occur. Following an acute attack of vertigo, the patient can feel unsteady for several days. The syndrome follows a remittent course, with relapses having variable severity and periodicity. Tinnitus can resolve or decrease between episodes. When persistent, the tinnitus typically increases in intensity immediately prior to or during a recurrent attack. Hearing loss is reversible in the early stages of the disease, but a gradually worsening residual hearing loss occurs with repeated attacks. Approximately one-third of patients experience symptoms in both ears. The paroxysmal episodes cease spontaneously late in the course of the disease.

The characteristic histopathological finding in Meniere's disease is a distension of the entire endolymphatic system. The increased volume of endolymph likely results from retention of sodium in the endolymphatic compartment and possibly impaired resorption of endolymph due to dysfunction of the endolymphatic duct and sac. The mechanism responsible for the fluctuating course of severe symptoms is not known completely, but may be due to episodic ruptures of the delicate membranes separating endolymph and perilymph, such as Reissner's membrane, located between the scala media and the scala vestibuli in the cochlea. This would result in an admixture of the two fluid compartments and a potassium intoxication of the neural processes that lead to the afferent fibers of the eighth nerve until the fluid balance is restored. Several diseases can result in Meniere's disease, including temporal bone trauma, otological surgery such as stapedectomy, and viral, toxic, bacterial, or syphilitic labyrinthitis. However, the cause is idiopathic in most cases.

Diagnosis is based on a characteristic history and documentation of fluctuating hearing by audiometry. Electronystagmography (ENG) can show a peripheral spontaneous nystagmus acutely and vestibular paresis on caloric testing in chronic cases. Acute management is largely empirical and involves the use of vestibular suppressants and antiemetics. A low-salt diet and diuretic use is recommended for maintenance therapy. Surgical options in refractory cases include endolymphatic shunts and ablative procedures, with the latter providing more reliable results.

Perilymph Fistulas

Perilymph fistulas are defects of the otic capsule or its oval or round windows. These defects allow leakage of perilymph from the inner ear into the middle ear space. Perilymph fistulas can occur secondary to congenital defects of the inner ear; following stapedectomy surgery for otosclerosis; following pressure changes in the middle ear associated with nose blowing, sneezing, or barotrauma as in SCUBA diving; or with sudden increases in cerebrospinal fluid (CSF) pressure associated with lifting, coughing, or straining.

Perilymph fistulas are commonly experienced as an audible "pop" in the ear followed by hearing loss and vertigo. Diagnosis is made from the history and supported by a positive fistula test or Valsalva maneuver. Management is conservative except in cases of penetrating otologic trauma because most perilymph fistulas heal spontaneously. Bed rest, sedation, head elevation, and the avoidance of straining are recommended. Surgical exploration and repair can be indicated with persistent auditory and vestibular symptoms.

Cerebellopontine Angle Tumors

Tumors of the cerebellopontine angle (CPA) typically begin in the internal auditory canal and slowly grow into the CPA, compressing the seventh and eighth cranial nerves. The most common CPA tumor is the vestibular schwannoma (acoustic neuroma), which usually arises from schwann cells of the vestibular nerve but can also arise from the facial, acoustic, or trigeminal nerves. Vestibular schwannomas account for over 90% of tumors of the CPA. Unilateral hearing loss and tinnitus are the most frequently experienced symptoms. A progressive unilateral hearing loss in a patient with dizziness is considered diagnostic of an acoustic neuroma until proven otherwise by magnetic resonance imaging (MRI), which is extremely sensitive in identification of acoustic tumors. With few exceptions, such as small tumors in the elderly, treatment is surgical removal.

Vascular Disease

The vertebrobasilar circulation supplies blood to the labyrinth, eighth cranial nerve, and brainstem. Hypoperfusion of the vertebrobasilar system, or vertebrobasilar insufficiency (VBI), can lead to widespread or focal ischemia and/or stroke of the vestibular system. VBI is a common cause of vertigo that has an abrupt onset, lasts for minutes, and can occur with nausea and vomiting. Other associated symptoms include diplopia, visual field defects, and headache. The common cause of VBI is atherosclerosis of the subclavian, vertebral, and basilar arteries. Occasionally, VBI can be precipitated by postural hypotension or by decreased cardiac output. VBI due to compression of the vertebral arteries by bony cervical spine spurs is a rare occurrence.

There are several clinical syndromes of abnormalities of the vertebral and basilar arteries and their branches. Certain syndromes are of particular importance in the ED evaluation of vertigo. Occlusion of the AICA can result in labyrinthine ischemia or infarction. There is usually a sudden profound loss of auditory and vestibular function. Ipsilateral facial numbness and weakness, ipsilateral Horner's syndrome, ipsilateral cerebellar signs, paresis of lateral gaze, and nystagmus can occur. Occlusion of the PICA, known as the lateral medullary or Wallenberg's syndrome, results in infarction of the lateral medulla. There is usually a sudden onset of vertigo, nystagmus, diplopia, dysphagia, nausea, and vomiting. Ipsilateral abnormalities include Horner's syndrome, palatal paralysis, loss of pain and temperature sensation of the face, facial and lateral rectus weakness, and cerebellar signs. There is contralateral loss of pain and temperature sensation of the body.

Acute management of vertigo due to vascular disease is usually directed at correcting the underlying disorder, whenever possible. General medical stabilization includes oxygenation, control of blood pressure, and fluid balance regulation.

Laboratory Studies

Ordering of laboratory studies in the ED for a patient with dizziness or vertigo is guided by information obtained from the history and physical examination. Routine hematological and chemical tests to be considered include a complete blood count with white blood cell differential counts, serum electrolytes, glucose, blood urea nitrogen, and creatinine. Other studies include FTA, cardiac enzymes, carboxyhemoglobin, and ethanol levels. Urine can be obtained for routine and microscopic tests and for a toxicology screen. Arterial blood gases, pulse oximetry, chest radiograph, or electrocardiogram may be required.

Imaging Studies

Imaging studies of the skull and brain may be indicated in the evaluation of a patient with dizziness or vertigo. The two most important imaging techniques used for this purpose are computerized tomography (CT) and MRI. In the emergency setting, CT is useful to rule out a suspected infarct or hemorrhage. Definitive diagnostic imaging is usually performed later with gadolinium-enhanced MRI as the ideal study for neoplasm, thin cut CT without contrast for temporal bone lesions, and magnetic resonance angiography (MRA) for vascular pathology.

Other diagnostic studies can be performed in the evaluation of the patient with vertigo either in the hospital or on an outpatient basis. Frequently utilized tests include audiometry and brainstem auditory evoked potentials.

Management

Initial Stabilization

A patient who presents to the ED acutely ill with vertigo accompanied by severe nausea and vomiting requires immediate stabilization. These symptoms can cause the patient to be extremely frightened and can compromise the emergency physician's ability to obtain an adequate history and physical examination. The patient is given calm verbal reassurance and is allowed to assume a body position that minimizes symptoms. All unnecessary external stimuli (e.g., excessive light, noise) are removed from the examination room. When tolerated by a vomiting patient, a semiprone position can provide some airway protection against aspiration of gastric contents. Oxygen can be administered by nasal cannulae, and a peripheral intravenous line is established. Oropharyngeal suctioning can be performed when necessary. Any trauma associated with the patient's presentation is treated as a high priority.

Pharmacological Treatment

See Table 8.6.

Vestibular Suppressants. The main categories of vestibular suppressants are antihistamines, anticholinergics, benzodiazepines, and monoaminergics. These medications are commonly used to suppress vertigo associated with peripheral vestibular disorders. In experimental studies, these medications alter and usually suppress the level of tonic activity in vestibular neurons. Antihistamines suppress vestibular end organs and inhibit central cholinergic pathways. The macular end organs (utricle and saccule) are typically more suppressed than the semicircular canals. Therefore, antihistamines are often more effective in treating motion sickness than acute, severe vertigo. The side effects of antihistamines include dry mouth, drowsiness, blurred vision, and urine retention but are generally well tolerated by patients. Anticholinergics inhibit activation of central cholinergic pathways and are similar to the antihistamines with regard to effectiveness in treating motion sickness and side effects. Benzodiazepines suppress central and peripheral vestibular pathways, provide tranquilization, and are often beneficial when antihistamines and anticholinergics are ineffective. Benzodiazepines can cause confusion, drowsiness, and ataxia and are used judiciously because of abuse potential. Monoaminergics suppress activity within vestibular neurons and can cause hypertension, nervousness, palpitations, and insomnia.

The use of vestibular suppressants is guarded because of their ability to retard CNS compensatory mechanisms needed to restore vestibular balance. The CNS must recognize abnormal vestibular inputs in order for it to initiate adaptive changes. Recognition of a vestibular deficit by the CNS results from the integration of visual, proprioceptive, and vestibular sensory feedback information produced when the patient attempts to use his or her vestibular reflexes. Research in animals and humans suggests that compensation can be affected directly by the experience of the animal or patient immediately after loss of function. Therefore, suppression of vestibular symptoms by medications or immobilization can limit the potential of the CNS to establish, modify, and maintain the compensatory mechanisms necessary for full recovery.

Antiemetics. The main categories of antiemetic medications are the phenothiazines, butyrophenones, and benzamides. These medications are effective in treating nausea and vomiting by antagonism of dopamine receptors in the chemoreceptor trigger zone of the vomiting center in the lateral reticular formation of the medulla. Phenothiazines can also suppress vestibular nuclei and central vestibular pathways, likely due to their antihistaminic or anticholinergic activity. Side effects include sedation, hypotension, and extrapyramidal symptoms.

Table 8.6. Symptomatic Treatment of Vestibular Disorders: Medications, Dosing, and Routes of Administration

Vestibular suppressants
  Antihistamines
    Meclizine (Antivert) 12.5–25 mg PO q4–6h
    Dimenhydrinate (Dramamine) 50 mg PO, IM q4–6h
    Promethazine (Phenergan) 25–50 mg PO, PR, IM q4–6h
    Cyclizine (Marezine) 50 mg PO, IM q4–6h
    Diphenhydramine (Benadryl) 25–50 mg PO, IM, IV q4–6h
    Astemizole (Hismanal) 10 mg PO qd
  Anticholinergics
    Scopolamine (Transderm Scop) 1 disc delivers 0.5 mg q3d
  Benzodiazepines
    Diazepam (Valium) 5–10 mg PO, IM, IV q4–6h
  Monoaminergics
    Ephedrine 25 mg PO, IM q4–6h
Antiemetics
  Phenothiazines
    Prochlorperazine (Compazine) 5–10 mg PO, IM q6h or 25 mg PR q12h
    Thiethylperazine (Torecan) 10 mg PO, PR, IM q8–24h
    Promethazine (Phenergan) 12.5–25 mg PO, PR, IM, IV q4–6h
  Butyrophenones
    Droperidol (Inapsine) 2.5–5 mg IM, IV
  Benzamides
    Trimethobenzamide (Tigan) 250 mg PO q6–8h or 200 mg PR, IM q6–8h
Psychotherapeutic agents
  Benzodiazepines
    Alprazolam (Xanax) 0.25–0.50 mg PO q8h
    Chlordiazepoxide (Librium) 25–50 mg PO q6–8h
    Diazepam (Valium) 2–10 mg PO q6–12h
    Lorazepam (Ativan) 2–3 mg PO q8–12h
  Tricyclic antidepressants
    Amitriptyline (Elavil) 50–100 mg PO qd
    Imipramine (Tofranil) 50–150 mg PO qd
    Nortriptyline (Pamelor) 25 mg PO q6–8h

Notes: Recommended pharmacological regimen for the vertiginous patient to provide acute and short-term vestibular suppression, control of nausea and vomiting, and sedation:
Diazepam 2–10 mg PO, IM, IV q4–6h
Promethazine 12.5–25 mg PO, PR, IM, IV q4–6h
Dosing and route of administration are determined by body weight, severity of symptoms, and response to therapy. Therapy is intended to provide prompt control, continued relief, and convenience at the lowest effective dose to allow for vestibular compensation.

Psychotherapeutic Agents. Psychotherapeutic medications include benzodiazepines and tricyclic antidepressants. Benzodiazepines can be used acutely in the ED to treat moderately severe anxiety syndromes that cause dizziness. However, continued outpatient use of these medications is under the supervision of the patient's physician because of abuse potential. Tricyclic antidepressant medication can be instituted in the ED in consultation with the patient's family physician or psychiatrist to treat major depression that causes dizziness. The side effects of these medications are orthostatic hypotension and anticholinergic symptoms.

Pathophysiological treatment of vertigo is performed under the direction of an otolarynglogist, otologist, or neurologist. Such treatment can involve the use of diuretics, vasodilators, corticosteroids, or antibiotics, depending on the final diagnosis.

Surgical treatment is indicated for some patients with vertigo who do not respond adequately to conservative management. The best surgical candidates are those who have unstable labyrinthine disease that leads to fluctuating or progressively deteriorating inner ear function.

Emergency Treatment of the SCUBA Diver with Vertigo

Transient vertigo during SCUBA diving that resolves with equalization of pressure in the middle ear cleft is known as alternobaric vertigo and requires no treatment except to avoid diving when eustachian tube function may be impaired. Distinguishing between inner ear barotrauma, perilymphatic fistula, and inner ear decompression sickness can be complex and is best done by an otolaryngologist in consultation with a diving medicine expert.

Vestibular Rehabilitation

Vestibular rehabilitation is an exercise-based physical therapy program designed to facilitate CNS compensatory mechanisms in patients with vestibular pathology. Rehabilitative therapy can be beneficial for patients with acute or chronic symptoms of vestibular dysfunction. Patient assessment and the development of a training program are usually done by a properly trained physical or occupational therapist, who designs a customized program tailored to the needs of the individual patient.

PEARLS AND PITFALLS

- Carefully obtained clinical information can determine whether dizziness is caused by a disorder of the peripheral or central vestibular system or nonvestibular systems.
- Vertigo usually suggests a vestibular system disorder but cannot reliably localize it.
- The neuro-otologic examination is important in assessing a patient with dizziness or vertigo.
- The Hallpike maneuver can diagnose benign paroxysmal positional vertigo; the particle repositioning maneuver can treat it.
- Symptomatic treatment of severe vertigo in the ED usually includes vestibular suppressant and antiemetic medications.
- Unexplained dizziness or vertigo may require referral of the patient to an otolaryngologist or neurologist.
- Vestibular rehabilitation is exercise-based physical therapy designed to facilitate CNS compensatory mechanisms in patients with vestibular pathology; prolonged bed rest, inactivity, or use of vestibular suppressant medication can result in poor vestibular compensation and a less-than-desired clinical outcome.

SELECTED BIBLIOGRAPHY

Epley JM. The canalith repositioning procedure for treatment of benign paroxysmal positional vertigo. *Otolaryngol Head Neck Surg.* 1992;107:399–404.

Parnes LS, Price-Jones RG. Particle repositioning maneuver for treatment of benign paroxysmal vertigo. *Ann Otol Rhinol Laryngol.* 1993;102:325–31.

Shepard NT, Telian SA. Programmatic vestibular rehabilitation. *Otolaryngol Head Neck Surg.* 1995;112:173–82.

Smith DB. Dizziness: a clinical perspective. In: Kaufman AI, Smith DB, eds. *Neurologic Clinics: Diagnostic Neurotology.* Philadelphia, Pa: WB Saunders; 1990: 8.

Victor M, Ropper AH. *Adams and Victor's Principles of Neurology*, 7th ed. New York, NY: McGraw-Hill; 2001.

9 Seizures

Kevin M. Kelly and Nick E. Colovos

INTRODUCTION

There are an estimated 10,000 to 15,000 new cases of epilepsy per year in the United States with prevalence rates of 4–10 per 1,000 persons. These data, combined with the large number of patients who have seizures from nonepileptic causes, indicate that seizure occurrence is relatively frequent and can result from diverse causes. Although many patients who have a seizure do not need emergency department (ED) care, some present to the ED critically ill and require immediate, definitive management. Advances in the understanding of seizure types and use of new antiepileptic drugs (AEDs) have enhanced the emergency physician's ability to diagnose the cause of a patient's seizures accurately and to treat both the underlying abnormality and the seizures in a rational and systematic fashion.

Epileptic Seizures

There are various types of seizures, epilepsies, and epileptic syndromes. The International Classification of Epileptic Seizures (Table 9.1) is based on clinical and electrophysiological properties of the ictal event that categorize it as one of two fundamental groups of seizure: partial or generalized. A partial seizure has clinical or electroencephalogram (EEG) evidence indicating a focal onset in one cerebral hemisphere. A generalized seizure has no evidence of focal onset and therefore appears to begin simultaneously from both cerebral hemispheres. Epilepsies with partial seizures are distinguished from epilepsies with generalized seizures. Additionally, epilepsies of unknown cause, or idiopathic (primary), are distinguished from those of known etiology, or symptomatic (secondary), and those that are cryptogenic (i.e., the cause is not known but the epilepsy is presumed to be symptomatic). Idiopathic epilepsies and syndromes are considered to have a possible hereditary predisposition, whereas symptomatic epilepsies and syndromes are considered a consequence of a known or suspected disorder of the central nervous system (CNS). Many of the different types of idiopathic and symptomatic epilepsies are listed in the differential diagnosis of seizures (Table 9.2). A basic

---

Table 9.1. International Classification of Epileptic Seizures

I. Partial (focal, local) seizures
  A. Simple partial seizures
    1. With motor signs
    2. With somatosensory or special sensory symptoms
    3. With autonomic symptoms or signs
    4. With psychic symptoms
  B. Complex partial seizures
    1. Simple partial onset followed by impairment of consciousness
    2. With impairment of consciousness at onset
  C. Partial seizures evolving to secondarily generalized seizures
    1. Simple partial seizures evolving to generalized seizures
    2. Complex partial seizures evolving to generalized seizures
    3. Simple partial seizures evolving to complex partial seizures
      evolving to generalized seizures
II. Generalized seizures (convulsive or nonconvulsive)
  A. Absence seizures
    1. Typical absences
    2. Atypical absences
  B. Myoclonic seizures
  C. Clonic seizures
  D. Tonic seizures
  E. Tonic–clonic seizures
  F. Atonic seizures (astatic seizures)
III. Unclassified epileptic seizures

---

understanding of the types of partial and generalized seizures is important for the evaluation and treatment of seizures in the ED.

Partial Seizures

Partial seizures are divided into simple (without impairment of consciousness) and complex (with impairment of consciousness). Simple partial seizures are classified by the type of symptom experienced by the patient. These include motor, sensory, autonomic, and psychic events. The EEG shows a restricted area of electrical discharge over the contralateral cerebral cortex corresponding to the body area involved. A simple partial seizure with motor signs is a focal motor seizure that can occur in any body area (e.g., clonic activity of digits). If the abnormal electrical discharge causing the seizure spreads to contiguous cortical areas, a sequential involvement of body parts occurs in a "march" (e.g., clonic activity of digits spreading to the wrist and then to the elbow). This type of seizure is known as a Jacksonian seizure. When focal motor seizures are continuous, the condition is known as epilepsia partialis continua, a form of status epilepticus (SE), which is a condition characterized by a seizure that lasts longer than 30 minutes or when a patient has two or more consecutive seizures without regaining consciousness. A simple partial seizure with somatosensory symptoms is a focal sensory seizure, usually consisting of paresthesias (tingling, pins-and-needles sensations) or numbness. These symptoms may also undergo a progression, or march, as in focal motor seizures. A simple partial seizure with special sensory symptoms includes elaborate visual or auditory experiences, olfactory

Table 9.2. Idiopathic and Symptomatic Epileptic Disorders and Causes of Provoked Seizures

Idiopathic epileptic disorders
    Benign neonatal familial convulsions
    Benign myoclonic epilepsy in infancy
    Childhood and juvenile absence epilepsy
    Juvenile myoclonic epilepsy
    Epilepsy with grand mal seizures on awakening
Symptomatic epileptic disorders
    Genetic disorders
    Metabolic disorders
      Amino acid and protein
        Phenylketonuria
        Porphyria
      Lipid
        Gangliosidoses
          Tay-Sachs disease
          Gaucher's disease
        Ceroid lipofuscinoses
      Vitamin
        Pyridoxine deficiency
    Myelin disorders
      Krabbe's disease
      Adrenoleukodystrophy
    Phakomatoses
      Tuberous sclerosis
      Neurofibromatosis
      Sturge-Weber syndrome
    Progressive myoclonic epilepsies
      Lafora body disease
      Unverricht-Lundborg syndrome
    Acquired disorders
      Brain anoxia
        Perinatal
        All ages
        Stroke
    Brain trauma
      Perinatal
        Subdural hematoma
        Subarachnoid hemorrhage
        Intraventricular hemorrhage
      All ages
        Contusions
        Lacerations
        Hematomas
    Brain tumors
    CNS infections
      Prenatal and perinatal
        Toxoplasmosis
        Rubella
        Herpes
        Syphilis
        Cytomegalovirus
        Meningitis

Older
  Meningitis
  Encephalitis
  Abscess
  Syphilis
  HIV
Degenerative disorders
  Alzheimer's disease
  Multiple sclerosis
Malformations
  Arteriovenous malformation
Causes of provoked seizures
  Metabolic disorders
    Uremia
    Hepatic insufficiency
  Hypoglycemia
Electrolyte disorders
Acid–base disorders
Connective tissue and inflammatory disorders
  Systemic lupus erythematosis
  Rheumatic fever
  Vasculitis
Endocrine disorders
  Infections
  Meningitis
Vascular
  Ischemic stroke
  Subarachnoid hemorrhage
  Intracerebral hemorrhage
Toxic disorders
  Substances of abuse
  Medications
  Environmental toxins
Head trauma
  Contusion
  Hematoma
Pregnancy

Source: Adapted from Engel J Jr. *Seizures and Epilepsy*. Philadelphia, Pa: FA Davis; 1989.

sensations (e.g., unpleasant odor), or gustatory sensations (e.g., metallic taste). A simple partial seizure with autonomic symptoms can include pallor, flushing, diaphoresis, piloerection, and pupil dilatation. A simple partial seizure with psychic symptoms is a disturbance of higher cerebral function usually occurring with impairment of consciousness (i.e., complex partial seizures). The psychic symptoms include distorted memories such as déja vu (the sensation that the present situation has already been experienced) and jamais vu (a familiar visual experience is not recognized). Other symptoms include dreamy states, intense fear or terror, illusions, and structured hallucinations.

The word *aura* has been used traditionally to describe the sensory, autonomic, or psychic symptoms perceived by the patient before the onset of impaired consciousness and/or a motor seizure. Actually, an aura is itself a simple partial seizure that may or may not progress to another seizure type. Prodromal symptoms of prolonged mood changes, uneasiness, or premonitions are usually not auras. Postictal paralysis (Todd's paralysis) or weakness can occur in muscles involved in a seizure. The paralysis usually resolves within 48 hours, although it may persist for much longer periods. Less commonly, focal sensory seizures that have associated paresthesias may be followed by postictal numbness in the same body distribution. The numbness is the sensory equivalent of a postictal paralysis. The cause of these postictal phenomena is thought to be transient, reversible biochemical alterations in the neurons involved in the seizure activity.

A simple partial seizure may progress to a complex partial seizure, which also can occur spontaneously. A complex partial seizure includes impairment of consciousness, which refers to the patient's abnormal awareness and responsiveness to environmental stimuli. The initial features of the seizure include an arrest reaction or motionless stare usually followed by automatisms, which are relatively coordinated motor activities occurring during the period of impaired consciousness. The automatism may be a continuation of motor activity that was present at the time of seizure onset (e.g., continuing to drive a car) or an apparently purposeful activity such as scratching, lip smacking, or fumbling with clothing. The seizure is usually brief, lasting from seconds to minutes, and there is a period of postictal confusion. Complex partial SE is a series of complex partial seizures without intervening return to full responsiveness. A partial seizure, simple or complex, can evolve into a generalized tonic–clonic seizure and is then referred to as a "partial seizure secondarily generalized."

Generalized Seizures

Generalized seizures are divided into convulsive (major motor) or nonconvulsive (brief loss of consciousness or minor motor) types. Generalized convulsive seizures include tonic, clonic, and tonic–clonic types. Generalized tonic seizures typically occur in childhood and typically include impaired consciousness, muscle contraction of the face and trunk, flexion of the upper extremities, flexion or extension of the lower extremities, and postictal confusion. Generalized clonic seizures usually begin in childhood and include impaired consciousness, bilateral limb jerking, and postictal confusion. Generalized tonic–clonic seizures, commonly referred to as grand mal seizures, are characterized by a sudden loss of consciousness and tonic and clonic phases. The tonic phase lasts 10–20 seconds and begins with brief flexion, eyelid opening, upward movement of the eyes, and elevation and external rotation of the arms. More prolonged extension follows involving the back and neck, a cry may occur, the arms extend, and the legs extend and rotate externally. At this point, the patient becomes apneic. The clonic phase lasts about 30 seconds and begins by brief, repetitive relaxations of the tonic rigidity, creating pronounced flexor spasms of the face, trunk, and limbs. This clonic jerking gradually decreases in rate until it ceases. Following this, there is muscular flaccidity, respirations resume, and there may be incontinence. Consciousness returns gradually and the patient awakens in a confused state. Fatigue and headache are common.

Generalized nonconvulsive seizures include absence, myoclonic, tonic, and atonic types. Generalized absence seizures, commonly referred to as petit mal seizures, typically are 5- to 10-second episodes of loss of consciousness characterized by staring and unresponsiveness. Clonic movements, changes in postural tone, automatisms, and autonomic phenomena commonly accompany absence seizures. The patient quickly resumes normal consciousness, has no postical confusion, and is generally unaware of the episode. Continuous absence seizures are known as absence SE. Generalized myoclonic seizures are bilaterally synchronous jerks that can be single or repeated in trains. The muscles involved may be few and restricted to a body part (e.g., the face) or extensive, involving all limbs. Most myoclonic seizures occur with no impairment of consciousness. Generalized tonic seizures that are brief are considered nonconvulsive, in contrast to the longer generalized tonic seizures, which are classified as convulsive. Generalized atonic seizures, commonly referred to as drop attacks, consist of a sudden loss of tone in postural muscles, often resulting in a fall. There is brief, mild impairment of consciousness and little postictal confusion.

Prehospital Care

Most seizures that occur in an out-of-hospital setting do not result in the patient going to the ED for evaluation. This is because most seizures occur in patients with epilepsy who recognize that their seizures are usually self-limited and do not require immediate evaluation. However, some seizures are severe or life-threatening and require immediate evaluation and management. Management of airway, breathing, and circulation is addressed first. Management of SE by EMS personnel essentially follows the same guidelines as in the ED. When EMS personnel are called for a patient who has had a seizure, information obtained in the field is frequently important for establishing a diagnosis and a treatment plan. The patient is usually transported to the ED for evaluation, and the emergency physician is updated as needed. Conditions that can require transport to the hospital include seizures that last for several minutes without evidence of abatement, failure to regain consciousness after a seizure, serial seizures, seizures resulting in significant injury, new or severe seizures in pregnancy, medical conditions such as diabetes, or seizures occurring at the extremes of age.

ED Evaluation

History. Patients assessed in the ED can be postictal, or experiencing a recurrent seizure. It is the responsibility of the emergency physician to evaluate the seizure by obtaining pertinent information regarding the patient's medical, surgical, neurological, and psychiatric history. This information is obtained from all available sources including patient, family, friends, witnesses to the seizure, EMS personnel, the patient's physician, and hospital records. A history of a seizure disorder is especially important and ideally provides information regarding the patient's age at seizure onset, the cause and type of the seizure(s), the frequency of seizures, the last known seizure occurrence, and the use of AEDs. When little information is available about the patient, descriptions of the seizure and the circumstances of its occurrence are extremely important in determining the cerebral localization of the epileptogenic lesion, the seizure type, and its likely cause; however, the seizure may not have been witnessed, and the patient may be unable to provide information. Important information includes the occurrence of a prodrome or aura, the features of the clinical seizure (e.g., autonomic changes, alteration of consciousness, arrested body movements, automatisms, the temporal sequence of tonic and/or clonic movements affecting one or both sides of the body, tongue biting, incontinence), and postictal symptoms. When AEDs are used, recent drug or dosage changes and the patient's compliance with medication taking should be determined. Associated factors that may be important include chronic disease states, intercurrent illness, stress, sleep deprivation, menses, pregnancy, the use of other medications, alcohol or drug ingestion, or withdrawal.

General Physical Examination. A careful general physical examination is performed to assess the condition of the patient and to find physical signs that may be related to the underlying cause of the seizure and to possible resultant trauma. Vital signs can give evidence of infection, hypotension or hypertension, arrhythmias, and respiratory or metabolic disturbances. The skin may reveal decreased turgor with dehydration, a rash with infection or connective tissue disorders, cyanosis with hypoxemia, hirsutism with chronic phenytoin therapy, contusions, lacerations, scarring from seizure-related injury, characteristic abnormalities of the phakomatoses, or congenital ectodermal disorders. These include axillary freckling, café-au-lait spots, and neurofibromas associated with neurofibromatosis; facial sebaceous adenoma, ash leaf spots, and shagreen patches associated with tuberous sclerosis; and port wine stain of the face associated with Sturge-Weber syndrome. The head may reveal microcephaly, macrocephaly, or facial asymmetry, suggesting abnormal cerebral development or injury. A tense fontanelle can be seen in infection or hydrocephalus. There may be evidence of trauma or previous neurological surgery such as craniectomy for tumor or arterio-venous malformation (AVM) removal or aneurysm clipping, or placement of a ventriculoperitoneal shunt for hydrocephalus. The sinuses may be tender to tap and the tympanic membranes or oropharynx may be red – findings associated with infection. The mouth may reveal gingival hypertrophy with chronic phenytoin therapy, lacerations or scarring of the tongue and buccal mucosa, or a smell of alcohol. The neck may be stiff, and a positive Brudzinski or Kernig sign suggests meningeal irritation from infection or subarachnoid hemorrhage. The limbs may be asymmetrical, suggesting lateralized cerebral injury. Auscultation of the heart may reveal arrhythmia or murmurs of acquired heart disease underlying inadequate cerebral perfusion and hypoxia or embolism. Auscultation of the lungs may reveal decreased ventilation in several disease states including exacerbations of chronic obstructive pulmonary disease and asthma resulting in cerebral hypoxia, infection resulting in cerebral abscess, and tumor resulting in cerebral metastasis. The abdomen may be rigid with infection or hemorrhage, resulting in hypotension or shock. Hepatomegaly may be associated with liver insufficiency and an encephalopathic state. There may be urinary or fecal incontinence.

Neurological Examination. A focused neurological examination assesses mental status, functioning of the cranial nerves, motor and sensory systems, and deep tendon reflexes. Abnormal findings may be from ictal or postictal states of complex partial or generalized seizures, the patient's interictal condition, toxic or metabolic encephalopathies, or intracranial injury. Prolonged bizarre behavior with alteration of consciousness may represent complex partial SE and not delirium or a psychotic event. Prolonged lethargy and decreased mental status may represent absence SE rather than a postictal state. Reversible memory impairment occurs frequently with complex partial and generalized convulsive seizures.

Cranial nerve examination is focused. The optic nerve may show papilledema, suggesting increased intracranial pressure. Abnormalities of pupil size may suggest focal impairments (e.g., a nonreactive dilated pupil in transtentorial herniation) or generalized effects (e.g., bilateral miosis or mydriasis from drug effect). Tonic deviation of the eyes may represent an ictal event and can localize the abnormality (e.g., a right-hemisphere seizure tonically drives the eyes to the left). Nystagmus may be due to AED intoxication. A central facial paresis is caused by a contralateral cerebral hemisphere abnormality and may represent a postictal paralysis.

Motor function should be assessed initially by inspection of the patient. An abducted lower extremity suggests focal weakness that may be related to stroke in the contralateral cerebral hemisphere or to postictal paralysis. Tremors may be related to alcohol withdrawal states, and fasciculations can occur in severe dehydration. Myoclonus may be caused by toxic, metabolic, or infectious disturbances. Tonic rigidity or clonic movements occur with ongoing seizure activity.

Sensory function impairments such as paresthesias or numbness may result in abnormal responses to testing by light touch or pinprick. When focal, these abnormalities suggest ipsilateral mononeuropathy, plexopathy, radiculopathy, or contralateral brain impairment, including ongoing simple partial seizure activity or a postictal equivalent.

Muscle stretch reflexes may be decreased in postictal paralysis or increased because of contralateral upper motoneuron impairment, which also underlies a plantar extensor response. A decreased rate of reflex relaxation (a "hung-up" reflex) suggests hypothyroidism.

Differential Diagnosis

Epileptic Seizures

The ED evaluation of a seizure is directed toward determining whether the seizure is due to epilepsy or nonepileptic causes. When a seizure has the characteristics of a partial or generalized seizure, represents a chronic condition, and has no identifiable cause or a cause that cannot be cured by specific treatment, the seizure is caused by epilepsy. This distinguishes provoked seizures, due to a transient reversible insult (e.g., minor head trauma), from recurrent provoked seizures, which can be cured by definitive therapy of an underlying disease state (e.g., resection of a brain tumor, hypoglycemia). The causes of epileptic seizures are diverse and numerous. Table 9.2 lists categories and representative types of idiopathic and symptomatic epileptic disorders and causes of provoked seizures.

Nonepileptic Paroxysmal Events

Paroxysmal events from nonepileptic causes are frequently confused with epileptic seizures, and their accurate identification is important for appropriate management. Nonepileptic paroxysmal events that cannot be distinguished from epileptic seizures on clinical features alone are studied by appropriate tests, including EEG. Nonepileptic paroxysmal events have been classified as being inducible by systemic, neurological, or psychiatric disorders. Examples of these disorders, which occur commonly in the ED, are listed in Table 9.3 and described next.

Table 9.3. Nonepileptic Paroxysmal Events

Systemic disorders
  Syncope
    With decreased cardiac output
    Reflex syncope
    With decreased systemic vascular resistance
    With arrhythmias
  Breath holding
  Hyperventilation
  Toxic and metabolic disturbances
    Alcohol and drug withdrawal
    Hepatic and renal failure
Neurologic disorders
Cerebrovascular disorders
    Transient ischemic attacks
    Stroke
    Migraine
      Classical
      Complicated
      Equivalent
  Transient global amnesia
  Narcolepsy
  Movement disorders
    Paroxysmal dyskinesias
    Hemifacial spasm
  Sensory disorders
    Trigeminal neuralgia
    Positional vertigo
    Acute labyrinthitis
    Meniere's disease
Psychiatric disorders
  Psychogenic seizures
  Intermittent explosive disorders
  Dissociative states
    Fugue states
    Psychogenic amnesia
    Depersonalization disorders

Source: Adapted with permission from Engel J Jr. *Seizures and Epilepsy.* Philadelphia, Pa: FA Davis; 1989 and Dohrmann ML, Cheitlin MD. Cardiogenic syncope: seizure versus syncope. *Neurol Clin.* 1986;4:549–62.

Systemic Disorders. Systemic disturbances include syncope, breath holding, hyperventilation, and toxic and metabolic disturbances. Syncope is a relatively frequent event and is related to a sudden decrease in cerebral blood flow. After a syncopal episode, the patient usually falls to the ground, can display tonic and clonic movements lasting only a few seconds, and has a prompt return to consciousness. These brief tonic and clonic movements reflect decerebrate rigidity and are commonly called syncopal seizures or convulsive syncope. They can occur with prodromal diaphoresis and vertigo, are frequently associated with stress (such as the death of a relative), and do not require treatment.

    Breath holding in infants and children can also result in syncope and is common between 6 and 18 months of age. It is often precipitated by frustration, fear, or surprise followed by autonomic phenomena and loss of consciousness. Brief syncopal seizures may follow and do not require treatment.

Hyperventilation occurs most frequently in adolescents and adults and is usually precipitated by anxiety or stress. Typical symptoms include shortness of breath, lightheadedness, and perioral and phalangeal tingling. Carpopedal spasm and loss of consciousness may occur. Seizures are infrequent but can occur in susceptible patients or those with a history of epilepsy. Treatment of hyperventilation consists of rebreathing expired air, calm reassurance of the patient, and sedation when indicated.

Toxic and metabolic disturbances can result in transient neurological dysfunction that may be difficult to distinguish from some features of seizure activity. Toxic disturbances that are frequently seen in the ED are caused by alcohol and psychomimetic drugs. Delirium tremens (DTs) occurs within 48 hours of cessation of drinking and is characterized by confusion, hallucinations, tremor, and autonomic changes. Psychomimetic drugs can cause altered awareness and responsiveness, hallucinations, and autonomic changes. Aspects of DTs and drug intoxication can resemble features of complex partial seizures. Metabolic disturbances such as hepatic and renal failure can create lethargy and confusion, which may be mistaken for ictal or postictal phenomena.

Neurological disturbances include cerebrovascular, sleep, movement, and sensory disorders. Cerebrovascular disorders include transient ischemic attacks (TIAs), stroke, migraine, and transient global amnesia. Stroke can be the reason for a provoked seizure (secondary to ischemia-related physiological derangement) and epileptic seizures (secondary to scar formation in the area of stroke). Complicated migraine is migraine headache followed by prolonged neurological deficits including mental aberrations. These impairments can be difficult to distinguish from those related to partial seizures or TIAs. Transient global amnesia is an episode lasting approximately 20 minutes to several hours characterized by a sudden loss of memory and apparent confusion with repetitive questions. After the episode, there is permanent amnesia concerning the event. This constellation of symptoms can suggest a postictal state following a complex partial seizure.

Movement disorders that occur as paroxysmal events can resemble epileptic seizures. Paroxysmal dyskinesias include familial and acquired types. Hemifacial spasm consists of irregular contractions of one side of the face, including blinking, and is related to facial nerve pathology. Although hemifacial spasm may resemble a partial motor seizure clinically, the EEG is normal.

Sensory disorders with paroxysmal features include those that are characterized by pain (e.g., trigeminal neuralgia) and vertigo (e.g., positional vertigo, acute labyrinthitis, and Meniere's disease). The specific symptoms and precipitants of these sensory disorders generally distinguish them as nonepileptic paroxysmal events.

Psychiatric Disorders. Psychogenic disturbances include psychogenic seizure, intermittent explosive disorders, and dissociative states. Psychogenic seizures are nonepileptic behavioral events that can mimic different seizure types, usually convulsive. Intermittent explosive disorders (episodic dyscontrol) are episodic or impulsive violent behaviors resulting in personal assault or destruction of property without significant precipitating psychosocial stress. The directed aggression of these episodes distinguishes them from stereotyped, aggressive epileptic ictal behavior, which is relatively rare. Dissociative states include fugue states, psychogenic amnesia, and depersonalization disorders. Features of these disorders can resemble some of the cognitive features of complex partial SE, particularly memory loss. The specific nature of the abnormality seen in dissociative states generally distinguishes them from epileptic seizures. However, EEG may be required for definitive diagnosis.

Laboratory Studies and Procedures

Patients with a new-onset seizure are assessed for underlying systemic abnormalities that can cause or predispose to the occurrence of a seizure. Hematological testing is a complete blood count with white blood cell (WBC) differential counts. Chemistries include a capillary blood sugar level upon arrival in the ED, followed by serum sodium, potassium, chloride, bicarbonate, calcium, magnesium, and glucose levels. Blood urea nitrogen, creatinine, serum glutamic-oxaloacetic transaminase, alkaline phosphatase, total bilirubin, and ethanol levels can be helpful. When indicated, urine is obtained for routine and microscopic tests and for a toxicology screen. An electrocardiogram can be helpful with cardiac disease, and a chest radiograph can be obtained when infection is suspected. Patients with known seizure disorders who have had an isolated seizure followed by rapid and complete recovery and a normal neurological examination may not require laboratory studies other than serum AED levels, especially when medication noncompliance is suspected.

Computerized tomography (CT) of the brain is available in most hospitals, and its judicious use is important in seizures associated with neurodegenerative disease, major brain malformations, intracranial hemorrhage, space-occupying lesions, or head trauma. CT scanning with bone windows can be indicated to assess for penetrating wounds or depressed skull fractures and has largely replaced the need for skull radiographs. Magnetic resonance imaging (MRI) of the brain is available in many hospitals and has greater sensitivity than CT in demonstrating certain types of abnormalities (e.g., temporal lobe abnormalities in patients with partial seizure disorders). The use of MRI is usually not helpful during the ED evaluation of a seizure. The EEG is the single most useful study in assessing the cause of seizures. Although its use is also limited in the ED, it should be considered in patients with an unexplained and prolonged impaired level of consciousness.

Lumbar puncture is performed when CNS infection is suspected and there are no signs of increased intracranial pressure. An opening pressure is recorded, and CSF is obtained for blood counts, including a WBC differential count, protein, glucose, Gram stain, acid-fast bacilli, cryptococcal antigen, Venereal Disease Research Laboratory (VDRL) test, bacterial cultures, and counterimmunoelectrophoresis or agglutination assays for bacterial antigens. Treatment of suspected meningitis or encephalitis is instituted immediately. It is important to note that the CSF may reveal pleocytosis after a single simple or complex partial seizure, a generalized tonic–clonic seizure, or SE. Treatment of suspected CNS infection is not withheld because of the possibility that the observed pleocytosis is simply due to seizure occurrence.

Management

The ED management of a patient with a seizure is commonly determined by the cause, type, severity, and frequency of the seizure. At times, treatment of the

Table 9.4. Antiepileptic Drugs, Clinical Indications, Adult Dosing Requirements, and Therapeutic Serum Concentrations

Drug	Seizure Types	Daily Dosing	Therapeutic Levels
Phenytoin	Partial, tonic–clonic	4–7 mg/kg	10–20 µg/ml
Carbamazepine	Partial, tonic–clonic	8–20 mg/kg	4–12 µg/ml
Phenobarbital	Tonic–clonic, partial	1–3 mg/kg	15–40 µg/ml
Primidone	Tonic–clonic, partial	750–2,000 mg	5–12 µg/ml
Valproic acid	Tonic–clonic, myoclonic absence, partial	15–60 mg/kg	50–100 µg/ml
Ethosuximide	Absence	500–1,500 mg	40–100 µg/ml
Clonazepam	Partial; generalized (Lennox-Gastaut)	2–20 mg	20–80 ng/ml
Felbamate	Partial; generalized (Lennox-Gastaut)	1,200–3,600 mg	Not defined
Gabapentin	Partial	900–4,800 mg	Not defined
Lamotrigine	Partial, tonic–clonic, absence, myoclonic, generalized seizures in Lennox-Gastaut	300–500 mg (with EI-AED[a]) 100–400 mg (with VPA[b])	3–14 µg/ml
Topiramate	Partial, tonic–clonic, generalized seizures in Lennox-Gastaut	200–600 mg	Not defined
Tiagabine	Partial	32–56 mg	Not defined
Levetiracetam	Partial	1–3 g	3–14 µg/ml
Oxcarbazepine	Partial, tonic–clonic	1,200–2,400 mg	12–30 µg/ml (MHD[c])
Zonisamide	Partial, tonic, myoclonic	200–600 mg	10–30 µg/ml

[a] EI-AED (enzyme-inducing AED).
[b] VPA (valproic acid).
[c] MHD (10-hydroxycarbazepine; active metabolite).
Source: Adapted from Fischer JH, Patel T. Guide to antiepileptic agents 2002. *CNS News.* 2001;3:101–7.

seizure precedes diagnosis of its cause. When identified, the underlying cause of seizures is treated, and AEDs are used when indicated. AEDs are chosen on the basis of their clinical effectiveness in treating specific epileptic syndromes or seizure types. Commonly prescribed AEDs and their associated clinical indications, dosing requirements, and therapeutic serum concentrations are given in Table 9.4.

Status Epilepticus

SE can be nonconvulsive or convulsive. Nonconvulsive SE includes absence SE, simple partial SE, and complex partial SE. These conditions are encountered relatively infrequently in the ED and are not as immediately serious as convulsive (generalized tonic–clonic) SE. The diagnosis of nonconvulsive SE is often difficult to make unless the patient has a history of such episodes. EEG may be necessary to confirm the diagnosis. Absence SE is treated with diazepam, 0.3 mg/kg given intravenously (<5 mg per minute), followed by an initial dose of ethosuximide or valproic acid, 20 mg/kg per day, in three divided doses. Simple partial SE and complex partial SE can be treated with the same AED regimens as in convulsive SE, but aggressive treatment is usually not necessary or warranted.

Table 9.5. Treatment Protocol for Convulsive Status Epilepticus in Adults

Time (minutes)	Management
0	Place patient on left side to prevent aspiration. Establish airway and administer oxygen. Obtain blood pressure and begin ECG monitoring. Establish a peripheral intravenous line with isotonic saline in right arm. Place a nasogastric tube for persistent vomiting. Obtain EEG where available.
5	Obtain blood for laboratory tests including a capillary blood glucose level. Consider thiamine, 100 mg IV, followed by glucose, 50 g IV.
10	Give diazepam, not to exceed 2 mg/min IV, until seizures cease or a total dose of 20 mg. OR Give lorazepam, not to exceed 2 mg/min IV, until seizures cease or a total dose of 8 mg.
25	If seizures continue, give phenytoin 20 mg/kg IV (<50 mg/min), with continuous monitoring of blood pressure and ECG. OR Give fosphenytoin, 20 mg PE/kg IV (150 mg PE/min), with continuous monitoring of blood pressure and ECG. If seizures continue, give an additional dose of phenytoin 5 mg/kg (fosphenytoin 5 mg PE/kg) and, if necessary, repeat the dose to a maximum of 30 mg/kg (fosphenytoin 30 mg PE/kg).
60	If seizures continue, perform endotracheal intubation and give phenobarbital, 20 mg/kg (<100 mg/min), with continuous monitoring of vital signs, until seizures cease. OR Induce general anesthesia with pentobarbital, 5–15 mg/kg IV, given slowly to achieve suppression of all EEG epileptiform activity, followed by 0.5–5.0 mg/kg per hour to maintain suppression. The rate of pentobarbital infusion should be lowered every 2–4 hours to determine if seizure activity has ended. If unable to suppress all epileptiform activity, give propofol, 1 mg/kg IV given over 5 minutes, then 2–4 mg/kg per hour; adjust to 1–15 mg/kg per hour. OR Give midazolam 0.2 mg/kg IV bolus, then 0.05–0.5 mg/kg per hour.

Convulsive SE is a medical emergency requiring prompt and focused treatment. Treatment of convulsive SE must be aimed at controlling the seizures while proceeding with the evaluation to establish their cause. Failure to stop the seizures of convulsive SE can cause significant morbidity or mortality, which is directly related to the duration of ongoing seizure activity. Descriptive details of management of convulsive SE follow and are summarized in Table 9.5. Management of convulsive SE begins by placing the patient in a left lateral decubitus position in the middle of a gurney. The head is supported and protected from injury during convulsions. An adequate airway is established immediately. When the teeth are not clenched, the oropharynx is suctioned and an oral airway inserted. Insertion of other hard objects between the teeth, including a padded tongue blade, is not advised because of potential dislodgement and local trauma. Oxygen can be administered by nasal cannula or face mask. A nasogastric tube can be placed for continuous vomiting. Endotracheal intubation is considered when there is evidence of compromised ventilation despite implementation of these procedures. Endotracheal intubation can be performed by the orotracheal route when the patient's teeth are not clenched and there is little movement or resistance by the patient. When the patient is having generalized tonic–clonic seizures, endotracheal intubation can be performed by the nasotracheal route to provide controlled ventilation and airway protection. When nasotracheal intubation fails, rapid sequence intubation is performed (see Chapter 28, "Traumatic Brain Injury").

While the patient's airway is being secured, blood pressure is measured and electrocardiogram (EKG) monitoring begun. A peripheral intravenous line is established with plastic catheters and is protected against movement and subcutaneous infiltration during clonic motor activity. Blood is drawn for a capillary blood sugar, complete blood count; serum electrolytes including Na^+, Ca^{2+}, and Mg^{2+}; serum glucose, urea nitrogen, and creatinine; serum AEDs or other potentially neuroactive medications; and a toxicology screen. After blood drawing is complete, the intravenous line is kept open with isotonic saline. Thiamine, 100 mg by intravenous push, is given to protect patients with thiamine deficiency against a possible exacerbation of Wernicke's encephalopathy precipitated by administration of glucose. Wernicke's encephalopathy occurs in chronic alcoholics or patients with chronic malnutrition and is relatively common among patients with SE. Glucose, 50 g (50 ml of 50% dextrose in water) by intravenous push, can be given for treatment of potential hypoglycemia. Only rarely does hypoglycemia cause SE. Administration of thiamine and glucose does not pose a risk to patients who are not deficient in them.

Use of Medications in Status Epilepticus

A benzodiazepine is the first class of drug to be administered in treating SE. The available benzodiazepines for initial intravenous treatment of SE are diazepam and lorazepam. Selection of a particular benzodiazepine is usually determined by its availability and the practitioner's familiarity with its use. Sedation, hypotension, and respiratory depression can occur with their use. Midazolam can be used in cases of refractory SE. Mild to moderate hypotension can be associated with its use and can be treated with fluid or pressors as needed.

Phenytoin or fosphenytoin (see later) is administered after the use of diazepam or lorazepam. Phenytoin is given by intravenous push with continuous monitoring of electrocardiogram (ECG) and blood pressure because of the potential for cardiac arrhythmias and hypotension, respectively. Cardiac arrhythmias and hypotension occur largely due to the effects on the atrioventricular conduction system by propylene glycol, the diluent for phenytoin. Therefore, the use of phenytoin is relatively contraindicated in patients with known cardiac conduction abnormalities; fosphenytoin should be used instead when available. Cardiac arrhythmias and hypotension can often be corrected by decreasing the rate of phenytoin infusion. Phenytoin usually can be given safely to patients who have been on maintenance phenytoin therapy before a serum phenytoin level is available.

Fosphenytoin is a phosphorylated pro-drug of phenytoin, which is cleaved by tissue phosphatases into phenytoin. Fosphenytoin is water soluble and, therefore, does not need to be diluted with propylene glycol. Rates of infusion of the drug can be approximately three times faster than that of phenytoin. Therefore, it takes approximately 10 minutes to infuse 1,500 mg of fosphenytoin (expressed as 1,500 mg of phenytoin equivalents (PE) when ordering fosphenytoin) at a rate of 150 mg PE per minute. However, it takes approximately 10–15 minutes for the full in vivo conversion of fosphenytoin to phenytoin. Comparing this to the expected 30 minute loading time for 1,500 mg of phenytoin given intravenously at 50 mg per minute, there is marginal savings in time with use of fosphenytoin. However, phenytoin is frequently given more slowly than 50 mg per minute, thus increasing the time saved by using fosphenytoin.

Phenobarbital, a barbiturate, can be given when phenytoin or fosphenytoin has not been effective after 25–30 minutes. Severe respiratory depression and hypotension can occur with high doses of phenobarbital, requiring continuous monitoring of vital signs. When seizures have not stopped after the use of phenobarbital, pentobarbital can be used to induce coma. This step involves EEG monitoring to assess the desired aim of burst suppression or EEG silence. The patient can be kept in an EEG burst suppression pattern for days, when necessary, and the rate of pentobarbital infusion lowered every 2–4 hours to determine when seizure activity has ended. The major side effect of pentobarbital is hypotension, which can be reversed with saline infusion or pressors.

Propofol is a relatively new anesthetic compound that has been used increasingly in the treatment of refractory SE. As with other anesthetics used in treating SE, the dose is titrated using EEG monitoring to ensure suppression of all ictal activity and maintenance of a burst suppression pattern. Propofol has the advantage of a very short half-life, and patients can recover more quickly from prolonged intravenous infusions than with benzodiazepines or barbiturates.

Alcohol Withdrawal Seizures

Alcohol withdrawal seizures are generalized tonic–clonic convulsions that usually occur within 48 hours after cessation of ethanol ingestion, with a peak incidence between 13 and 24 hours. The seizures are usually brief, occur as a single episode or in bursts of two or more, and can evolve into SE. These seizures typically occur in chronic alcoholics or after episodes of binge drinking. Other causes of generalized seizures that may occur during alcohol withdrawal include head trauma, subdural hematoma, meningitis, and metabolic derangements and should be evaluated as indicated. Partial seizures that occur during the withdrawal period suggest focal brain injury – old or new – and require evaluation.

The standard treatment of alcohol withdrawal seizures is based on the principle of providing a medication with cross-tolerance to alcohol. Because these seizures are usually brief and limited in number, a benzodiazepine such as chlordiazepoxide (Librium), 50–100 mg given intravenously, or diazepam, 5–10 mg given intravenously, can be administered to treat an ongoing seizure. These medications can be repeated at regular intervals (chlordiazepoxide every 1–2 hours orally or intravenously, diazepam every 15–20 minutes orally or intravenously) as indicated to suppress other withdrawal symptoms and continued for several days on a tapering schedule. Patients are assessed carefully for hypotension and respiratory depression. Patients who have a history of epileptic seizures should have serum levels obtained for their prescribed AEDs and supplemented as needed to achieve therapeutic serum concentrations. Patients with seizures refractory to benzodiazepine treatment or those with a history of epileptic seizures not currently treated can be given a loading dose of phenytoin, 15–18 mg/kg given intravenously (50 mg per minute with EKG monitoring) or orally (2–3 split doses over 6 hours), respectively. Alcohol withdrawal seizures that evolve into SE should be treated as described previously.

Disposition of Patients Following a Seizure

The disposition of a patient who has experienced a seizure is largely based on the cause and the severity of the seizure. New-onset seizures may or may not require treatment with an AED. A decision to treat with an AED is best made after discussing the patient's case with his or her primary care physician or a neurologist. Usually, patients can be discharged safely when the seizure is brief, nonfocal, and uncomplicated; the neurological examination is normal; and the diagnostic evaluation is unremarkable. Patients are admitted to the hospital for further evaluation and management when there has been SE, trauma-induced seizures, identification of a space-occupying CNS lesion or infection, anoxia, or a serious toxic or metabolic derangement. Typically, patients admitted to the hospital are started and maintained on an AED during their hospitalization.

Medicolegal Issues

A patient who has experienced a seizure must be informed of the cause of the seizure, the determined need for AEDs and their potential side effects, reasonable restrictions on activities of daily living, and the state's law regarding restriction of driving privileges. This information is documented clearly in the medical record for potential medicolegal issues.

For patients with seizures, there are no uniform restrictions on activities of daily living that might be of potential harm to them or others. The range of activities must be determined for each patient based on the type of seizures experienced, the associated functional impairment, and the degree of seizure control achieved with AEDs. In general, patients with seizures are encouraged to lead full and active lives. They are advised to develop regular routines for sleeping, eating, working, and medication taking and to avoid excessive exertion, sleep deprivation, excessive use of alcohol and caffeine, and undue stress. Excessive use of alcohol can increase the risk of seizure recurrence during a withdrawal period. Excessive use of caffeine can make seizures more difficult to control. Common sense and good judgment should dictate avoidance of certain activities that may pose substantial risk to the patient or others. These include driving, swimming, bathing, and working at heights or with heavy machinery or power tools. Patients with seizures may be able to swim but should never swim alone. High-risk sports such as sky diving, hang gliding, or rock climbing should probably be avoided.

The laws for restriction of driving privileges after a seizure with impairment of consciousness vary among different states. It is important that the emergency physician know the laws of the state so that the patient can be informed accurately. Generally, patients who experience a seizure are not permitted to drive for 6–12 months. Most neurologists consider a patient capable of driving without serious risk posed to the patient or others when the patient is seizure-free for 1 year and compliant with the prescribed AEDs. In patients with seizures who have no history of seizures associated with impairment in consciousness or significant motor dysfunction (e.g., simple partial seizures), driving may be considered safe when the patient can drive without difficulty during a seizure. Patients experiencing only nocturnal seizures may not need to have their licenses suspended. When seizures have been well controlled on an AED regimen and drug withdrawal is undertaken, it is reasonable to recommend against driving during the withdrawal period or for 6 months, whichever is longer.

Some states require that the physician responsible for treating the seizures report that information to the agency responsible for issuing drivers' licenses. Most states hold the patient responsible for providing information about his or her condition to the appropriate authority when applying for a driver's license. Specific infromation regarding drivers' license restriction can be obtained from each state's department of motor vehicles.

Documentation on the ED medical record of the patient who has had a seizure includes common side effects of AEDs, informing the patient of the state laws regarding driving restrictions, and potential risks. When an AED is not initiated in the ED, or is delayed, the reasons are documented. For example, when the seizure has been a single, isolated event, treatment with an AED may not be initiated. This decision is made with the patient's physician, and appropriate follow-up determined.

PEARLS AND PITFALLS

■ Patients evaluated in the ED following a seizure may be postictal, normal, or experiencing a recurrent seizure.

■ Patients who appear confused or postictal may be experiencing absence or complex partial SE.

■ Convulsive SE is a medical emergency associated with high morbidity and mortality.

■ Although used infrequently in the ED, an EEG can diagnosis ongoing seizure activity in a patient with a prolonged period of impaired consciousness.

■ Syncope can be difficult to distinguish from seizure.

■ The diagnosis of psychogenic seizures is made cautiously after a thorough neurological examination and focused diagnostic evaluation are normal; many patients with psychogenic seizures have epilepsy.

■ Alcoholics can have epilepsy; patients with epilepsy can drink alcohol.

■ It is important that the emergency physician knows the state's law regarding restriction of driving privileges for patients who have experienced a seizure.

SELECTED BIBLIOGRAPHY

Adams RD, Victor M, Ropper AH. *Principles of Neurology*, 7th ed. New York, NY: McGraw-Hill; 2001.

Dohrmann ML, Cheitlin MD. Cardiogenic syncope: seizure versus syncope. *Neurol Clin*. 1986;4:549–62.

Engel J Jr. *Seizures and Epilepsy*. Philadelphia, Pa: FA Davis; 1989.

Fisher JH, Patel T. Guide to antiepileptic agents 2002. *CNS News*. 2001;3:101–7.

Wylie E, ed. *The Treatment of Epilepsy: Principles and Practice*, 3rd ed. Philadelphia, Pa: Lippincott, Williams & Wilkins, 2001.

10 Gait Disturbances

Jon Brillman

INTRODUCTION

Abnormalities of gait are commonly seen in the emergency department (ED) and commonly reflect some disorder of the nervous system. Station and gait is unique to each individual and reflects gender, age, body habitus, mood, and even culture. The goal of evaluation is to determine what part(s) of the nervous system are involved by the type of gait observed. Different types of gait disturbance are described with regard to neuroanatomical localization and specific neurological disorders (Figure 10.1).

ED Evaluation and Management

Senescent Gait (Early Gait Apraxia)

Senescent gait is observed commonly in patients of advanced age and is characterized by small uncertain steps. Generally the foot is planted flat without springing from the heel to the ball of the foot, and there is reduced associated arm movement. This is seen in cerebral atrophy but also reflects loss of joint mobility, tightness of the hamstrings, and loss of proprioception.

Advanced Senescent Gait (Late Gait Apraxia)

Patients with advanced senescent gait are usually demented. They may have Alzheimer's disease or cerebral atrophy from other causes or subcortical involvement from multiple strokes. Communicating hydrocephalus (normal pressure hydrocephalus) may produce this type of gait, but under those circumstances, the degree of cognitive dysfunction is variable. Steps are extremely small and hesitant and the feet tend to be "magnetized" to the floor. Patients may be tipped over easily forward or backward.

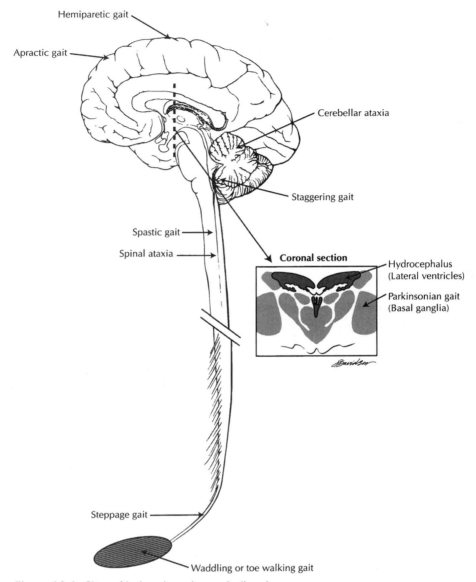

Figure 10.1. Sites of lesions in various gait disorders.

Parkinson's Disease and Parkinsonian Conditions

The gait of patients with Parkinson's disease and related disorders is stereotyped but may be confused with senescent gait. There is usually a flexion of all limbs and trunk and a tendency to lean forward and accelerate with walking, a disturbance referred to as festination. Tremor commonly accompanies the gait disturbance. As with patients with gait apraxia, they are easily tipped in one direction or another. Characteristically, patients may get stuck in doorways or with other obstacles. Turning is accomplished with very small steps and is segmented. An associated tremor and the state of universal flexion help to distinguish this gait from gait apraxia.

Hemiparetic Gait

The most frequent cause of hemiparetic gait is cerebral infarction, and it may represent a chronic problem. The arm may be adducted and fingers and wrist flexed with hyperextension and plantar inversion of the foot. To avoid tripping, the patient swings the affected leg out in a circumducting fashion.

Spastic Gait

Patients with spastic gait have problems involving the spinal cord. Children diagnosed with cerebral palsy may also have a spastic gait. Under these circumstances, the characteristic gait is "wooden-legged" or stiff. Chronic spasticity, which may be associated with congenital abnormalities or long-standing problems, can be characterized by "scissoring" of gait with the thighs rubbing together during walking.

Ataxic Gait

Ataxia is a disordered balance not associated with specific neuroanatomical localization. Frequently it is seen in cerebellar disease, but it may also be seen with spinal cord disease and frequently coexists with spasticity. Ataxic gait refers to a wide base of gait that the patient requires to maintain balance. Severe peripheral neuropathies with large fiber involvement and loss of proprioception may be associated with ataxic gait because the feet have difficulty with spatial organization. Ataxic gait is seen with dorsal column disease and pancerebellar disease. Midline (vermian) cerebellar disorders are seen in patients with drug intoxication or alcoholism and may be associated with difficulty with tandem walking. The Romberg sign refers to the patient's ability to maintain balance with upright stance until the eyes are closed when the patient begins to sway back and forth. This is due to loss of position sense caused by abnormalities of large peripheral nerve fibers or dorsal columns as seen in Vitamin B_{12} deficiency.

Staggering Gait

Staggering gait is observed commonly in EDs and is characteristic of alcoholic intoxication and patients who have taken sedative drugs. It can be distinguished from a cerebellar ataxic gait because it is wide-based and associated with pitching and reeling to one side, loss of balance, and a need to grasp and hold onto objects. Associated features of intoxication are frequently present.

Steppage Gait

Steppage gait is observed in patients who have foot drop due to peripheral neurologic disorders. It is usually unilateral and caused by an injury to the common peroneal nerve at the level of the fibular head in the lateral portion of the knee. Injury to this nerve can be due to direct trauma and is commonly seen in cachectic bedridden patients. Other causes of peripheral neuropathy are mononeuritis multiplex, which may cause a foot drop and steppage gait. The steps are normal but the advancing foot cannot be dorsiflexed and has to be elevated by excessive flexion of the hip and knees so the foot can clear the ground, curbsides, or steps. The affected foot will slap the ground and make an audible noise. Occasionally, foot drop results from an L5 radiculopathy due to a herniated disc at the L4–5 level, and bilateral foot drops suggest a more severe disease process such as Charcot-Marie Tooth, amyotrophic lateral sclerosis, or polio.

Waddling Gait

Waddling gait is characteristic of patients who have hip girdle weakness. It is seen in hip dislocations usually in adults and is characteristic of polymyositis and muscular dystrophy. Patients with waddling gait shift their weight from side to side in an exaggerated fashion. When the leg is planted on the ground, the opposite hip rises. The trunk tends to incline to the side of the patient's step. The alteration in trunk movement results in the waddling feature.

Hysterical Gait

Hysterical gait is a gait abnormality that cannot be explained satisfactorily by a specific neuroanatomical localization or disease process. As is the case with other hysterical disorders, associated features of emotional disturbance can be elicited in a nonthreatening manner by the examiner. Gait may be bizarre, pitching and starting to one side or the other, wavering suddenly from left to right, or with twirling motions with the arms outstretched and flopping about (astasia–abasia). Frequently, patients suddenly topple or fall into a position where they may take a step and push the other leg. In hysterical hemiparesis, there is absence of circumducting gait, hyperactive deep tendon reflexes, and a Babinski sign. A diagnosis of hysterical gait is not made when there is objective evidence of nervous system dysfunction.

Antalgic Gait

Antalgic gait results from a shortened stance phase or a painful limb. Osteoarthritis is a common cause. Sometimes called coxalgic gait, it commonly refers to hip disease and the compensatory gait of decreased stride length and stance phase that minimizes discomfort in the hip joint.

PEARLS AND PITFALLS

■ Advanced senescent gait may be similar to that seen in normal pressure hydrocephalus where cognitive dysfunction is variable.

■ Universal flexion is typically associated with the gait of Parkinson's disease.

■ Circumduction is a characteristic of hemiparetic gait.

■ Chronic spasticity of both lower extremities can result in "scissoring" of gait.

■ Sensory ataxias are caused by dorsal column and peripheral nerve disease.

■ Steppage gait is caused by foot drop.

■ Hysterical gait cannot be diagnosed in the presence of nervous system dysfunction.

11 Central Nervous System Infections in Adults

Oliver W. Hayes, Earl J. Reisdorff, Paul Blackburn, and Anthony Briningstool

INTRODUCTION

Central nervous system (CNS) infections range from rapidly fatal bacterial meningitis to slowly progressive infectious processes from mycobacterial, fungal, or viral agents. Viral and bacterial meningitis are the most frequent CNS infections encountered in the emergency department (ED) (see Table 11.1). History of the course of illness, exposures to infectious agents, and factors that increase susceptibility to CNS infections is required because of varying clinical presentations (see Table 11.2). The examination is focused on the identification of systemic infection and localization of neurological dysfunction. Clinical assessment is supplemented by cerebrospinal fluid (CSF) analysis and neuroimaging studies. Empirical antibiotic therapy and supportive care should be initiated promptly while awaiting definitive diagnosis. Seizures occur in 30% of adults with meningitis.

Bacterial Meningitis

Of all bacterial meningitis cases, 30% occur in adults, and approximately 70–85% of cases are caused by *Hemophilus influenzae*, *Neisseria meningitidis*, or *Streptococcus pneumonia*. Although the overall incidence of CNS infections has declined in the United States, the incidence in the geriatric population has increased. Infection with multiple organisms occurs in 1% of patients and is usually secondary to paranasal sinus and ear infections, skull fractures, neurosurgery, and immunosuppression.

Typical presentation of meningitis includes fever, headache, nuchal rigidity, and altered mental status, but 15% of patients do not have these findings. Symptoms such as nausea, vomiting, sweating, myalgias, weakness, and photophobia are frequently present. Approximately 33% of patients with meningitis have dermatological findings. Diffuse maculopapular eruptions progressing to petechiae and purpura occur with *N. meningitidis* infection. Focal neurological findings complicate meningitis in 5% of cases. Signs of acutely increased intracranial pressure (ICP; sluggishly reactive, dilated pupils, or ophthalmoplegia) can be present (see Chapter 23, "Increased Intracranial Pressure and Iternation Syndromes").

113

Table 11.1. Central Nervous System
Infections in Adults

1. Meningitis
   a. Aseptic
   b. Bacterial
   c. Chronic or recurrent
   d. Fungal
   e. Rickettsial
   f. Tuberculous
2. Abscess, empyema, and effusion
   a. Intraparenchymal
   b. Extraparenchymal
3. Encephalitis
   a. Viral encephalitis
4. Other conditions
   a. HIV-related CNS infections
   b. Lyme disease
   c. Neurosyphilis
      (1) Syphilis of the brain
      (2) Syphilis of the spinal cord
   d. Sarcoidosis
   e. Tetanus
   f. Cerebral brucellosis
   g. Protozoan infections
   h. Psittacosis and lymphogranuloma venereum

Papilledema suggests brain abscess, subdural empyema, tertiary syphilis, or venous sinus thrombosis. The level of consciousness correlates with clinical outcome and is closely monitored. Patients with focal seizures have a poor prognosis.

Diagnosis. The diagnosis of acute bacterial meningitis is made by the examination of CSF. CSF in bacterial meningitis is characterized by a polymorphonuclear (PMN) pleocytosis, depressed glucose level, elevated protein level, and elevated pressure (normal range 80–200 mm of H_2O). Table 11.3 lists typical CSF findings in patients with meningitis.

Table 11.2. Conditions Associated with Increased Risk of Meningitis

Underlying immunocompromise state secondary to:
HIV infection
Malignancy
Alcoholism
Sickle cell disease
Organ transplantation
Splenectomy
High-dose corticosteroid therapy
Neurosurgical procedures
Head trauma
Chronic renal failure and those on hemodialysis
Presence of a CNS shunt accompanying contiguous focus of infection such as
   sinusitis, otitis media
Anatomic factors such as presence of CSF leak or fistula

Table 11.3. Characteristic Findings in Cerebrospinal Fluid with Meningitis

	Normal	Bacterial	Viral	Fungal/TB	Abscess
Glucose (mg/dl)	45–65	<40	45–65	30–45	45–65
Protein (mg/dl)	<50	>150	>50	>100	>50
Leukocytes (WBC/ml)	0–5	>1,000	100–1,000	100–500	10–1,000
Type	Mononuclear	PMN	Mononuclear	Mononuclear	Indeterminate
CSF : blood glucose ratio	0.6	<0.4	0.6	<0.4	0.6

Note: CSF: cerebrospinal fluid; PMNs: polymorphonuclear neutrophils.

Antibiotics received earlier may complicate the diagnostic interpretation of CSF analysis. Patients treated with oral antibiotics have a reduced number of neutrophils, a decreased protein concentration in the CSF, and a reduced yield on Gram stain and culture results. Organisms are detected on CSF Gram stain in 60–90% of untreated patients and 40–60% of patients treated with antibiotics. Antigen detection testing by counterimmunoelectrophoresis, coagglutination, or latex agglutination is more sensitive and specific than organisms identified on Gram stain.

Presence of mental status changes, focal neurological findings, or seizures requires a prior brain computerized tomography (CT) scan to exclude increased ICP. When lumbar puncture (LP) is delayed in order to obtain neuroimaging studies, antibiotics are administered promptly after obtaining blood cultures. Patients with suspected meningitis should receive parenteral antibiotic therapy within 30–60 minutes of arrival because earlier antibiotic therapy is known to improve survival rate and reduce adverse neurological sequeli (Table 11.4). In patients with immunosuppression, or those with recent neurosurgical procedure, CSF leak or ventriculoperitoneal shunts, therapy is directed at *Staphylococcus aureus* and gram-negative bacilli. A third-generation cephalosporins, often accompanied by ampicillin, are the initial therapies of choice.

Table 11.4. Initial Antibiotic Therapy for Acute Bacterial Meningitis in Adults

S. pneumoniae	Cefotaxime, ampicillin, penicillin G (plus vancomycin with/without rifampin)
N. meningitidis	Penicillin G, ampicillin, cefotaxime, chloramphenicol
H. influenzae	Cefotaxime, ceftriaxone, ampicillin
S. aureus (methicillin-sensitive)	Nafcillin, oxacillin
S. aureus (methicillin-resistant)	Vancomycin plus rifampin
L. monocytogenes	Ampicillin
Streptococci (group A, B, etc.)	Penicillin G, ampicillin
Gram-negative bacilli	Ceftriaxone, cefotaxime, trimethoprim-sulfamethoxazole
P. aeruginosa	Ceftazidime
Anaerobes	Cefotaxime plus metronidazole plus rifampin

Adapted from Ashwal S. Neurologic evaluation of the patient with acute bacterial meningitis. *Neurol Clin.* 1995;13(3):549–77.

For patients with meningococcal meningitis, penicillin remains the drug of choice, and treatment is initiated with parenteral ampicillin (200 mg/kg per day) or penicillin G (200 mg/kg per day). When *Staphylococcal* infection is suspected, Nafcillin or oxacillin is usually effective, although in cases of methicillin resistance, vancomycin plus rifampin or metronidazole is indicated. For *S. pneumoniae* meningitis, cefotaxime, ceftriaxone, and penicillin are the drugs of choice. Strains of pneumococci resistant to third-generation cephalosporins have been reported, requiring therapy with cefotaxime or ceftriaxone plus vancomycin.

The emergence of beta-lactamase production in *H. influenzae* type B and chloramphenicol-resistant strains of *H. influenzae* (1%) has led to the use of cefotaxime or ceftriaxone as the initial agents of choice. Similarly, ceftriaxone has proven effective against gram-negative meningitis in adults. The effectiveness of corticosteroids as adjunctive therapy remains unproven.

Currently chemoprophylaxis is recommended for household contacts of patients with meningococcal or *Hemophilus meningitis*. Antimicrobial agents for chemoprophylaxis include rifampin (10 mg/kg – up to 600 mg – every 12 hours for 4 days), ceftriaxone (250 mg given intramuscularly in adults, 125 mg in children), ciprofloxacin (one dose of 500 mg or 750 mg), or ofloxacin (one dose of 400 mg).

Brain Abscess

Brain abscess is a suppurative infection involving brain parenchyma through (1) seeding from the bloodstream or hematogenous spread, (2) direct extension from an adjacent infectious focus, and (3) implantation during trauma or surgery.

The onset of clinical findings of brain abscess is often subacute, resulting in delay of diagnosis. The size and location of the abscess, general health of the patient, duration of the illness, and prior treatment lead to a variety of clinical presentations. Headache is the most common symptom and is often located on the same side as the abscess. Fever is present in approximately 50% of patients with brain abscesses, and focal neurological signs develop days to weeks after the headache. Specific neurological deficits depend on the site of abscess (Table 11.5). The triad of fever, headache, and focal neurological findings is present in less than 50% of patients. A high clinical index of suspicion is a critical factor in the assessment of a patient with suspected brain abscess. A comprehensive search is directed toward identifying occult sources of infectious foci. Due to the possibility of brain herniation, lumbar puncture is contraindicated when brain abscess is suspected.

The diagnostic studies of choice are CT or magnetic resonance imaging (MRI) of the brain, with contrast enhancement. During the earlier stages of abscess formation, un-enhanced CT images can be normal. MRI provides more diagnostic information. Contrast enhancement of the lesion demonstrates the classic "ring" appearance of the mature encapsulated abscess, with lesions less than 0.5 mm in diameter appearing homogeneous without ring-enhancing. HIV-infected patients with ring-enhancing lesions are presumed to have toxoplasmosis.

Management and Disposition. Prompt neurosurgical evaluation is necessary for possible surgical drainage of a brain abscess. Surgery is indicated for relief of elevated ICP due to space occupation; biopsy, for diagnostic confirmation.

Table 11.5. Anatomic Location of Brain Abscess and Related Neurological Findings

Location	Signs
Temporal lobe	Wernicke's aphasia, homonymous superior quadranopsia, contralateral facial weakness
Frontal lobe	Mental status change, seizures, positive grasp, suck and snuff reflexes, contralateral hemiparesis (large abscess)
Parietal lobe	Impaired position sense, two point discrimination and stereognosis focal sensory and motor seizures, homonymous hemianopsia, impaired opticokinetic nystagmus
Cerebellum	Ataxia, nystagmus, ipsilateral arm and leg incoordination with intention tremor
Brainstem	Facial weakness, dysphagia, multiple cranial nerve palsies, contralateral hemiparesis

Adapted from Hoeprich PD, Jordan MC, Ronald AR, eds. *Infectious Diseases: A Treatise of Infectious Processes*, 5th ed. Philadelphia, Pa: Lippincott; 1994.

The choice of antibiotic therapy depends on the culture and sensitivity reports of the tissue. Current recommendations for empirical treatment while awaiting culture results are a combination of intravenous penicillin G in high dosages (320,000–480,000 units, or 200–300 mg/kg per day) and metronidazole (20–30 mg/kg per day). When staphylococcal infection is suspected, a penicillinase-resistant penicillin or vancomycin (50–60 mg/kg per day) is used. Dexamethasone in a loading dose of 10 mg may help reduce the edema surrounding the lesion. The use of prophylactic anticonvulsants are recommended.

HIV-Related Central Nervous System Infections

Although the CNS infections most commonly associated with HIV infection are toxoplasmosis and cytomegalovirus (CMV), such patients are susceptible to many other infections including aseptic meningitis, neurosyphilis, and *M. tuberculosis*.

HIV can directly cause *HIV encephalitis* (multinucleated giant cell encephalitis) and *HIV leukoencephalopathy* (progressive diffuse leukoencephalopathy). HIV encephalitis is characterized by dementia, weakness, and spasticity. Of those who die of AIDS, 10% demonstrate evidence of HIV encephalopathy at autopsy. Other forms of viral encephalitis are seen in another 22% of patients. HIV encephalitis may eventually become the most common viral CNS infection worldwide.

Toxoplasma encephalitis can cause both focal neurological and general complaints including headache (49%), fever greater than 38°C (40%) and abulia or generalized behavioral slowing (37%), focal hemiparesis or hemiplegia (49%), generalized seizures (24%), and cranial nerve palsies (17%). A contrast-enhanced brain CT frequently shows multiple hypodense, ring-enhancing lesions in the cerebral hemispheres. CSF analysis reveals a mild mononuclear pleocytosis.

Because confirmation of the diagnosis of CNS toxoplasmosis is difficult; empirical therapy of pyrimethamine (200 mg on day 1, then 50–75 mg per day) and sulfadiazine (4–6 g per day) or clindamycin (2.4–3.6 g per day for 6 weeks) is promptly initiated. Common side effects of therapy include leukopenia, thrombocytopenia, and anemia. Adverse drug reactions are common and were reported in 62% of patients receiving therapy in one study.

Cytomegalovirus infection commonly displays end organ damage of the gastrointestinal system (esophagitis, gastritis, and colitis), the eye (chorioretinitis), and the neurological system (meningoencephalitis, ventriculitis, and ascending polyradiculopathy). CMV encephalitis can present as a chronic, indolent process with psychomotor slowing, chronic cephalgia, or progressive ataxia, or as an acute process with encephalopathy, generalized or focal seizures, or hallucinations. The diagnosis depends on CSF analysis. Radiological studies are often inconclusive. The definitive diagnosis of CMV encephalitis often is made only with surgical specimens obtained at autopsy.

The decision to initiate treatment for CMV encephalitis is based on high clinical suspicion (ganciclovir, 5 mg/kg every 12 hours is given intravenously). The addition of foscarnet (given intravenously in doses of 60 mg/kg every 8 hours), an inhibitor of DNA polymerase, is effective, especially against ganciclovir-resistant strains.

Aseptic Meningitis

The term *aseptic meningitis* has been used to describe conditions of acute meningeal irritation that prove to be benign and self-limiting; however, the term *aseptic meningitis* is a misnomer because up to 70–80% of the cases are caused by viruses (see viral encephalitis). Other causes include tuberculosis, syphilis, Lyme disease, and the fungal meningitis syndromes. Moreover, certain medications can create a similar clinical picture including nonsteroidal anti-inflammatory agents (especially ibuprofen, sulindac, tolmetin, and naproxen), antibiotics (trimethoprim-sulfamethoxazole, metronidazole, ciprofloxacin, penicillin, and isoniazid), and intravenous immunoglobulin therapy. Additional causes are intrathecal injections of air, radiological dyes, isotopes, antibiotics, chemotherapeutic agents, steroids, neurosurgical procedures (particularly those involving the posterior fossa), connective tissue diseases, and certain CNS tumors, which can present with acute or recurrent episodes of aseptic meningitis.

Tuberculous Meningitis

The incidence of tuberculosis (TB) is on the rise, due to an increase in numbers of HIV-infected persons, numbers of homeless individuals, and immigrants from developing countries. CNS tubercular infection accounts for 15% of extrapulmonary cases and is divided into three categories: (1) meningoencephalitis, (2) intracranial tuberculoma, and (3) spinal tuberculous arachnoiditis. Tuberculous meningitis (TBM), the result of bacteremia, is insidious, with a vague prodrome of constitutional symptoms (malaise, low-grade fever, and intermittent headache) that can be accompanied by personality changes. Cranial nerve palsies and upper motor neuron lesions can accompany protracted headache, meningismus, vomiting, and confusion. Factors that predispose to TBM are extremes of age, immunosuppression, lymphoma, alcoholism, HIV infection, family history of tuberculosis, and recent exposure to others with active TB.

The diagnosis of TBM is confirmed by CSF analysis. Typical CSF findings are elevated protein level (100–500 mg/dl), diminished glucose level (<45 mg/dl), and a mononuclear pleocytosis with a total white blood cell (WBC) count of 100–500 cells/ml. The confirmation of TBM depends on culturing mycobacteria in the CSF. Acid fast bacilli (AFB) are readily demonstrated on a smear of the clot or sediment. The highest yield of AFB will be in the last drops of CSF removed by lumbar puncture (LP). CT imaging of the brain demonstrates basilar arachnoiditis, cerebral edema, infarction, ring-enhancing lesions, or hydrocephalus. Hydrocephalus appears to be the most common CT finding in the HIV-infected patient with TBM, followed by meningeal enhancement and parenchymal involvement.

Isoniazid remains the drug of choice, initiated at 10 mg/kg per day in both adults and children. Pyridoxine in a dose of 50 mg per day is administered concomitantly to avoid isoniazid-induced neurological complications.

Fungal Meningitis

Individuals with impaired cellular immunity are susceptible to fungal meningitis. *Cryptococcus neoformans*, a common fungal pathogen, commonly affects HIV-infected patients. *Coccidioides immitis*, endemic to the southwest United States, Central America, and portions of South America, can cause meningitis, particularly in patients with disseminated HIV infection. Less common fungal infections include *Candida albicans* in patients who have undergone neurosurgical procedures, and in those treated for bacterial meningitis. Aspergillosis is common in organ transplants.

The clinical presentation of fungal meningitis is highly variable, in part because the majority of patients harbor significant underlying diseases. Headache, although nonspecific, is present in most patients. Alteration of mental status can manifest as confusion, lethargy, or even coma. Seizures can be generalized or focal. Isolated or combined cranial nerve abnormalities or focal motor deficits can also be present.

CT imaging or MRI of the brain with contrast enhancement help provide the diagnosis. The imagings studies rarely result in a specific diagnosis because fungal lesions appear similar to many other diverse conditions.

CSF pleocytosis is predominantly lymphocytic, although CSF can be acellular in the severely immunocompromised patient. Protein levels are increased, and glucose levels diminished. Identification of the organism by Gram stain or silver stain of CSF sediment is usually not successful. CSF eosinophilia is a nonspecific but frequent finding in *C. immitis* meningitis. The diagnosis of Cryptococcus or Coccidioides is made from serological tests. Cryptococcal antigen is detected in 90% of cases and is the single most useful diagnostic test for this condition. The diagnostic yield of serological testing for Cryptococcus is up to 95% in patients with AIDS. Complement fixation tests for Coccidioides in CSF are positive in up to 95% of patients. *Cryptococcus neoformans* can be detected with India ink preparation in about 50% of cases. The optimal volume of CSF required for fungal cultures is about 40–50 ml. Multiple LPs are required to obtain the necessary volume of CSF.

The use of amphotericin B is recommended for most fungal meningitides. The use of flucytosine as a sole agent or with other antifungal agents has had variable results. The CSF penetration by flucytosine is better than that of amphotericin B, and the combination of flucytosine and amphotericin B has some synergistic effect. Fluconazole penetrates the CSF and has proven efficacious in treating Cryptococcal meningitis.

Neurosyphilis

Clinical neurosyphilis typically is divided into four syndromes: meningeal, meningovascular, parenchymatous, and gummatous syphilis.

Acute meningeal syphilis presents with findings of headache, confusion, nausea, vomiting, nuchal rigidity, and cranial nerve involvement, particularly CN VII and CN VIII. Sensorineural deafness occurs in up to 20% of patients, but normal hearing usually returns following therapy. CSF abnormalities such as pleocytosis, elevated protein (>45 mg/dl), and mild diminution of CSF glucose levels (glucose <50 mg/dl) are frequent.

Meningovascular syphilis is a result of focal arteritis leading to thrombosis and infarction. Neurological deficits include hemiparesis, hemiplegia, aphasia, and seizures, which can occur due to vessel occlusion (stroke). The middle cerebral artery is most involved commonly, followed by the basilar artery. CSF in meningovascular neurosyphilis is uniformly abnormal. Paretic neurosyphilis and tabes dorsalis presents with subtle loss of cognitive function and behavioral changes. The images are commonly mistaken for a psychiatric disturbance. The progression of the disease leads to hypotonia, dementia, seizures, and, finally, general paresis. Sensory loss caused by posterior column destruction leads to Charcot's joints and trophic ulcerations. The classical Argyll Robertson pupil, a small, irregular pupil that accommodates but fails to react to light, occurs in up to 48% of patients.

Gummatous neurosyphilis is the least common syndrome. Gummas, a manifestation of late-stage syphilis, are masses of necrotic tissue surrounded by dense connective tissue with marked vascularity. The clinical presentation is that of an intracranial mass lesion. No single laboratory assay is sufficiently sensitive and specific to serve as a definitive test for CNS syphilis. Serological testing has emerged as the standard for confirming the diagnosis of neurosyphilis. More specific laboratory tests such as the CSF Venereal Disease Research Laboratory (VDRL) test or the fluorescent treponemal antibody–antibody absorption (FTA-ABS) test, combined with nonspecific parameters (CSF pleocytosis, greater than 9 WBCs per high power field, elevated CSF protein, and depressed glucose levels) in the context of history and physical examination are required to diagnose neurosyphilis accurately. Unless CSF is contaminated with seropositive blood during the LP, a reactive CSF VDRL indicates past or present neurosyphilis.

The treatment of neurosyphilis for both immunocompetent and immunocompromised patients is penicillin G, 12–24 million units per day for 10 days intravenously, given as 2–4 million units every 4 hours.

CNS Manifestations of Lyme Disease (Neuroborreliosis)

Lyme disease whose etiological agent is *Borrelia burgdorferi*, a tick-borne spirochete, is characterized by three clinical stages. The first stage is erythema chronicum migrans (ECM), an erythematous eruption at the location of the bite. The second stage occurs when the disease disseminates, producing rheumatologic, cardiac, and neurologic manifestations. The third stage is characterized by ocular and joint findings. The neurological syndromes can occur during any of the three stages but are generally categorized into those seen early in the infection cycle and those that complicate the late stage of the disease. The three syndromes that characterize early infection are meningoencephalomyelitis, cranial nerve palsies, and radiculoneuritis. The three syndromes that occur during late-stage infection are encephalopathy, polyradiculoneuropathy, and meningoencephalomyelitis.

Early in the disease course, *B. burgdorferi* seeds the meninges, producing fluctuating headache, neck stiffness, and fevers. Examination of CSF reveals mononuclear pleocytosis of less than 200 cells/ml. CSF protein is usually less than 100 mg/dl, and CSF glucose levels are rarely depressed. Lyme antibodies are found in 73–92% of patients. In some patients, the disease progresses to produce cognitive changes and mood and sleep disturbances suggestive of encephalitis. Cranial nerve involvement with meningitis is highly suggestive of Lyme disease. The facial nerve is involved in 11% of clinical infections, and 33% of these have bilateral facial nerve involvement. The optic nerve is the second most frequently involved, producing optic neuritis or disc edema. All cranial nerves reportedly have been involved with Lyme disease. Radiculoneuritis, an uncommon complication of Lyme's disease referred to as Bannworth's syndrome, typically causes lancinating extremity pain in a dermatomal distribution. Syndromes of late-stage infection include encephalopathy, polyneuropathy, and meningoencephalomyelitis. Encephalopathy is characterized by malaise with memory and concentration impairment. Polyneuropathy manifests as distal limb paresthesias and asymmetrical radicular pain. Median nerve involvement at the carpal tunnel has been reported in 25% of late-stage infections. Involvement of brain or spinal cord parenchyma is an uncommon late-stage infectious syndrome. Continued or recurrent meningeal involvement is also uncommon.

The number of CSF organisms in Lyme disease is scant and often tissue-bound; therefore, serological testing is the mainstay of diagnosis. Examination of CSF can be normal with peripheral nervous system involvement and in those with encephalopathy. Polymerase chain reaction (PCR) studies on CSF and serum are likely to be available in the future. Neuroimaging studies are abnormal in 25% of patients with neuroborreliosis, but no unique pattern is noted.

The treatment for most neurological syndromes associated with Lyme disease is parenteral administration of ceftriaxone, given 2 grams intravenously every day for a minimum of 2 weeks. Alternative intravenous regimens include ampicillin, cefotaxime, chloramphenicol, doxycycline, and penicillin G. A Jarisch-Herxheimer reaction, which occurs in 10–20% of patients within the first 24–48 hours of treatment, generally responds to antipyretics and anti-inflammatory agents. Antibiotics are not discontinued during a Jarisch-Herxheimer reaction. Patients who have mild peripheral syndromes with normal CSF analysis are treated with oral antibiotics for 30 days. Preferred agents include amoxicillin, 500–1,000 mg three times per day (50 mg/kg per day), and doxycycline, 100 mg three times per day or 200 mg two times per day. The chronic sequelae of Lyme disease (headache, fatigue, myalgias, cognitive deficits) are treated symptomatically.

Viral Encephalitis

Viral encephalitis is an infectious and inflammatory process involving the brain. It is associated with an altered state of consciousness, impaired cognitive abilities, and a CSF pleocytosis. Encephalitis is differentiated from meningitis primarily on a clinical basis. Patients who have encephalitis are encephalopathic, while patients with meningeal inflammation have meningitis. Patients with

Table 11.6. Viral Causes of Encephalitis

Togavirus (arbovirus)
   Eastern equine encephalitis
   Western equine encephalitis
   Venezuelan equine encephalitis
Flavivirus
   St. Louis encephalitis
   Japanese encephalitis
   Powassan
   West Nile Virus (WNV)
Bunyavirus (arbovirus)
   California (LaCrosse) encephalitis
Arenatirus
   Lymphocytic choriomeningitis
Reovirus
   California tick fever
Rhabdovirus
   Rabies
Herpes virus
   Herpes simplex I and II
   Herpes varicella zoster
   Ebstein-Barr
   Cytomegalovirus
Picornovirus
   Polioviruses 1–3
   Coxsackieviruses A2, 5, 6, 7, 9
   Coxsackieviruses B1–6
   Enteroviruses (70 and 71)
   Echoviruses 2–4, 6, 7, 9, 11, 14, 16, 18, 19, 30
Paramyxovirus
   Measles virus
   Mumps virus
Adenovirus
   Adenovirus
Retrovirus
   Human immunodeficiency virus

characteristics of both have meningoencephalitis. In the United States, 1,000–2,000 cases of viral encephalitis are reported each year. In general, the overall mortality of viral encephalitis is 5–10% with certain forms approaching 70–80%.

The central nervous system is commonly exposed to viral pathogens through hematogenous spread. Direct neuronal migration can occur with rabies encephalitis and probably with certain strains of the herpes virus. Herpes simplex virus (HSV) encephalitis preferentially affects the frontal and temporal lobes of the brain. Eastern equine encephalitis (EEE) has a predilection for the hippocampus. Cerebellar involvement with resultant ataxia can occur with herpes varicella zoster (HVZ) virus. Rabies has a proclivity for the brainstem and cortical gray matter. Localized cerebritis (aseptic meningitis) can occur with other viruses including the mumps virus, Epstein-Barr virus (EBV), poliovirus, coxsackievirus, echovirus, enterovirus, and measles virus.

Viral infections cause most cases of encephalitis. (Table 11.6). In about 50% of cases of encephalitis, the cause is nonviral or no etiology is discovered. Encephalitis caused by nonviral pathogens includes infection by bacteria

Table 11.7. Differential Diagnosis of Viral Encephalitis

Infectious	Lead encephalopathy
Nonviral encephalitis	Substances of abuse
Mycobacterium tuberculosis	Sedative-hypnotic agents
Mycoplasma pneumoniae	Narcotics–opiates
Rickettsia rickettsii	Anticholinergic toxicity
Lyme disease *(Borrelia burgdorferi)*	Alcohols
Leptospirosis	Mushroom poisoning (amatoxins,
Treponema pallidum	monomethylhydrazine)
Coccidioides immitis	Valproate toxicity
Naegleria fowleri	Other causses
Toxoplasma gondii[a]	Tumors
Cryptococcus neoformans[a]	Leukemia
Listeria monocytogenes	Lymphoma
Meningitis	Cerebral vascular event
Viral	Hydrocephalus with shunt
Bacterial (including mycoplasma,	malfunction
mycobacterium, rickettsia)	Postictal state
Fungal	Infantile botulism
Protozoa	Reye's syndrome
Brain abscess	Cat scratch disease
Subdural–epidural empyema	SIADH
Sepsis	Hypoglycemia
Trauma	Hypoglycemia hyperosmolar coma
Epidural hematoma	Uremic encephalopathy
Subdural hematoma	Collagen vascular disease
Subarachnoid hemorrhage	Alcohol withdrawal syndrome
Concussion – closed head injury	Hyperammonemia
Toxins	Chronic encephalitis (Rasmussen's
Carbon monoxide	syndrome)

[a] Seen more frequently in immunodeficient patients.

(e.g., *Mycobacterium tuberculosis, Mycoplasma pneumoniae*), fungi (e.g., *Coccidioides immitis, Cryptococcus neoformans*), and protozoa (e.g., *Naegleria fowleri, Toxoplasma gondii*).

The differential diagnosis for viral encephalitis is extensive (Table 11.7).

Herpes Virus Encephalitis

Herpes simplex virus type-2 (HSV-2), genital herpes, typically causes a perinatal infection. The constellation of encephalitis, hepatitis, and pneumonitis strongly suggests HSV-2 infection. HSV-1 is the most common cause of encephalitis from the group of herpes viruses. HSV-1 encephalitis accounts for 10–20% of all cases of encephalitis. With HSV-1, there is no gender predominance or seasonal pattern of outbreak.

HSV-1 encephalitis is a progressive disease, with a succession from lethargy to deep coma. It is commonly characterized by an altered state of consciousness, abnormal behavior, seizures, olfactory or gustatory hallucinations, memory loss, and anosmia. Focal neurological deficits occur in at least 60% of patients. Temporal lobe involvement (e.g., speech difficulties and olfactory hallucinations) strongly suggests HSV-1 encephalitis. The mortality rate approaches 70% in untreated patients. Determinants of the outcome include the age of the patient, the duration of illness, and the level of consciousness at the start of therapy. Therefore, prompt initiation of antiviral therapy is essential.

Herpes varicella zoster virus, predominantly known for "chickenpox" and "shingles" can cause an encephalitis, but this is rare and occurs largely in immunocompromised patients. When HVZ encephalitis occurs, the symptoms appear 1–3 weeks after the onset of the exanthem with cerebellar ataxia being a common associated finding. The mortality rate of HVZ encephalitis is 15–35%, with up to 30% of survivors having long-term sequelae.

Arbovirus Encephalitis

The term "arbovirus" is no longer an official taxonomic term. It refers to over 450 RNA viruses that are arthropod-borne (mosquitoes, ticks), hence the prefix *arbo*-. These viruses cause eastern equine encephalitis, western equine encephalitis (WEE), St. Louis encephalitis (SLE), Japanese B encephalitis, yellow fever, and California encephalitis (including La Crosse strain). Although arboviruses account for about 10–15% of all cases of encephalitis, in an epidemic year they can cause up to 50% of all cases.

West Nile Virus (WNV) Encephalitis

Mosquitoes transmit West Nile Virus (WNV), a member of the Flaviviridae, a family of single-stranded RNA viruses. The majority of infections are clinically silent. Symptoms typically include fever, headache, myalgias, lymphadenopathy, pharyngitis, conjunctivitis, and diarrhea. A nonpruritic roseolar or maculopapular rash on the chest, back, and arms reportedly develops in about half of patients. Encephalitis or meningitis is rare, probably occurring in less than 1% of the cases.

The findings that raise the suspicion of WNV encephalitis include:

➤ Mosquito season
➤ Unexplained bird or horse deaths
➤ Age > 50 years
➤ Muscle weakness and/or paralysis
➤ Hyporeflexia
➤ Lymphocytopenia
➤ MRI showing enhancement of leptomeninges and/or periventricular area

Eastern Equine Encephalitis

EEE is fatal in over 55% of cases. EEE occurs sporadically along the east coast of the United States, especially near freshwater marshes (e.g., cranberry bogs). An abrupt onset of a high fever, headache, and vomiting is followed by a progressive stupor. EEE can produce focal neurological signs, mimicking HSV-1.

Western Equine Encephalitis

WEE occurs sporadically in rural areas of the western two-thirds of the United States. Infants younger than 1 year of age are particularly prone to infection. The infant with WEE appears "septic" with a bulging fontanelle. Older children have "flu-like" symptoms. Seizures and long-term neurologic sequelae are common in infected infants.

St. Louis Encephalitis

During epidemic years, SLE is typically the prevalent arbovirus disease in the United States. In nonepidemic years, California encephalitis (CE; LaCrosse strain) is the most common type of viral encephalitis. SLE most commonly occurs in regions bordering the Ohio and Mississippi Rivers.

California Encephalitis

The term *California encephalitis* is used to describe most cases of bunyavirus disease. The virus that causes CE most frequently is the LaCrosse strain. CE is most common in the upper Mississippi valley. Children (5–9 years) are most often affected. Symptoms tend to abate after 3–5 days, and most children recover without neurological sequelae.

Other Viral Causes

Enteroviral encephalitis occurs primarily in children typically during the summer and fall months. Although enteroviruses cause 30–50% of all cases of viral meningitis, they account for less than 5% of all cases of encephalitis. Most patients recover without sequelae.

Measles (rubeola) can cause encephalitis. Measles encephalitis has occurred as a consequence of measles immunization; the incidence is about 1 case per 1 million doses. Symptoms begin 1–8 days after the appearance of a rash, but it can be delayed for up to 3 weeks. The patient is usually recovering from the primary measles infection when the encephalitis abruptly occurs. Seizures occur in 50% of patients, and neurological morbidity (mental retardation, epilepsy, behavioral changes, paralysis) occurs in 20–50% of patients. Mortality is estimated at 10%.

Mumps encephalitis is usually mild, typified by fever, headache, nausea, vomiting, nuchal rigidity, and lethargy. The prognosis is favorable.

The rabies virus causes encephalitis that is almost always fatal. It is characterized by headache, fever, and dysesthesia at the inoculation site. Rabies encephalitis causes progressive agitation with painful muscular spasms. Ultimately, seizures, coma, apnea, and death occur.

Lymphocytic choriomeningitis (LCM) virus infection is caused by exposure to rodents and typically resembles influenza. LCM encephalitis is usually mild, although it can be associated with arthritis, orchitis, parotitis, and cerebellar incoordination. Death or neurological sequelae is rare.

Evaluation and Differential Diagnosis of Viral Encephalitis

Viral encephalitis can present as a headache with mild mental status changes or as a fulminant neurologic disease leading to death. The incubation period varies for different pathogens. Viral encephalitis is often preceded by a 1–4 day prodrome of fever, chills, headache, pharyngitis, conjunctivitis, myalgias, and malaise. Once encephalitis is apparent clinically, vomiting and impaired cognition occur. Ataxia, tremor, confusion, speech difficulties, stupor, delirium, seizures, and coma can follow. Rapid clinical deterioration suggests HSV-1 or EEE infection. Bizarre behavior, memory loss, olfactory or gustatory hallucinations, personality changes, and anosmia are associated with HSV-1. In addition, gross motor aberrations and cranial nerve palsies are common with HSV-1. Focal localized neurological disturbances occur in 80% of patients with HSV-1 and 20% of patients with CE. SLE and EEE have higher rates of infection among children. Some encephalitides have a seasonal predilection. For example, arbovirus encephalitides (SLE, CE, WEE, EEE) occur most often in the summer months. Enteroviral encephalitis peaks during the summer and fall months. Varicella encephalitis usually begins in the winter, peaks in the spring, and is lowest during summer and fall. Mumps and HSV-1 encephalitis occur year-round.

LCM can be accompanied by arthritis, orchitis, or parotitis. One should inspect the skin for evidence of trauma, rash, or needle marks. Abnormal pupil size suggests drug or toxin exposure. Funduscopy identifies papilledema (suggesting encephalitis) and retinal hemorrhages (suggesting alternative diagnoses).

Rarely diagnosed in the ED, the definitive diagnosis of viral encephalitis rests on antibody testing, recovery of viral DNA from the CSF, or brain biopsy with viral culture. Presumptive evidence for encephalitis is obtained through LP, neuroradiological imaging, and common laboratory studies.

CSF Findings. Viral encephalitis is characterized by CSF pleocytosis with a lymphocytic or mononuclear cell predominance. This pattern can also occur with cryptococcal or mycobacterial infection. Early in the disease process, the CSF can have a neutrophilic predominance. The CSF protein levels are usually modestly elevated and the glucose level is normal. PCR studies for HSV DNA are performed when HSV-1 is suspected.

HSV-1. A CSF pleocytosis, with a WBC count over 100 (cells/ml) is usually evident. Red blood cells in the CSF due to necrotizing frontotemporal lesions are characteristic (75–85% of cases).

Arboviruses. SLE usually has a CSF lymphocytic pleocytosis (50–500 cells/ml) and a protein concentration of 50–100 mg/dl. The CSF glucose is usually normal. EEE typically causes an elevated CSF pressure and 200–2,000 cells/ml, 50% of which are neutrophils. The peripheral WBC count with EEE can be as high as 66,000 cells/ml. WEE has a mixture of neutrophils and lymphocytes in the CSF; later only lymphocytes may be observed. CE shows primarily lymphocytic pleocytosis (usually about 50–200 cells/ml).

Detection of viruses in the CSF is variable. Enteroviruses, mumps, adenoviruses, HVZ virus, and CMV can be detected in the CSF. Viral antigens or antibodies can be detected in the CSF by enzyme-linked immunosorbent assays. In addition, HSV immunoglobulin G and immunoglobulin A detection by enzyme-linked immunosorbent assay allows for the diagnosis of HSV encephalitis. This method has had limited success. New assays using PCR technology can detect HSV-1 in the CSF. This technique can detect HSV-1 in the CSF early in the course of the illness, even as early as 24 hours after the onset of symptoms. At this time, PCR is the most specific, rapid, and sensitive available assay for the detection of HSV-1.

Neuroradiology. Most cases of viral encephalitis have no pathognomonic CT or MRI findings. Cerebral edema, obstructive hydrocephalus, and multifocal or disseminated lesions are consistent with viral encephalitis. Conversely, HSV-1

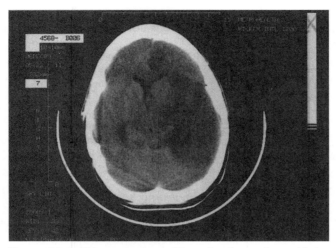

Figure 11.1. This noncontrast CT study of a patient with herpes simplex encephalitis demonstrates a large low-density area in the left temporoparietal region with mass effect (courtesy of Judith E. Simon, MD, Department of Radiology, Metro-Health Medical Center, Cleveland, Ohio).

encephalitis frequently is associated with CT abnormalities such as edema, mass effect, or hemorrhage. There are frequently hypodense, enhancing lesions in the temporal or frontal lobes (Fig. 11.1). MRI is more sensitive for evaluating suspected viral encephalitis. In patients with HSV-1 encephalitis, the electroencephalogram (EEG) often reveals temporal lobe epileptiform activity.

Brain Biopsy. Brain biopsy is the definitive test for diagnosing HSV encephalitis. Biopsy can confirm HSV encephalitis and establish alternative diagnoses for other conditions in almost 50% of patients.

Management

Management of viral encephalitis is symptom-specific and supportive. Specific interventions include airway protection, intracranial pressure regulation, and seizure control. Although use of dexamethasone in meningitis is increasing, its use in viral encephalitis remains controversial. Seizures are controlled with benzodiazepines initially, followed by phosphenytoin loading. Until bacterial meningitis can be excluded, empirical treatment with a third-generation cephalosporin and corticosteroids (e.g. ceftriaxone 50–100 mg/kg IV) and dexamethasone 0.15mg/kg IV) is appropriate.

Antiviral Therapy. Most viruses causing encephalitis have no specific treatment. HSV-1 encephalitis is the notable exception. Acyclovir (10 mg/kg IV) every 8 hours for 10–14 days is the treatment of choice. Among untreated patients, 30–70% die, and few regain normal neurological function. When treated with acyclovir, patients younger than 3 years have a mortality rate of 6%. Acyclovir also significantly improves the outcome of surviving patients. Relapse occurs in up to 27% of children. Acyclovir is indicated in the treatment of HVZ encephalitis and has in vitro activity against EBV, CMV, and human herpes virus type 6. The regimen of acyclovir for HVZ encephalitis is the same as that for HSV-1. The success of acyclovir therapy is contingent upon the patient's condition at the start of therapy. Alert patients are most likely to recover. Most patients who are diagnosed early can be expected to survive and resume nearly normal neurological function. Other antiviral agents can improve the course of certain viral CNS infections (e.g., Gancyclovir for CMV). All patients with a presumptive diagnosis of viral encephalitis are admitted to the hospital.

PEARLS AND PITFALLS

■ A common pitfall in the emergency department is not to consider CNS infection in the differential diagnosis of many nonspecific and apparently nonurgent clinical conditions. The evolution of CNS infection can be very rapid.

■ For many patients with CNS infections, the examination results are deceptively benign. Physical examination can help localize mass lesions and reveal papilledema, nuchal rigidity, or coinfections.

■ CT scanning and MRI can be very sensitive but nonspecific for CNS infections.

■ CSF studies in certain conditions can be difficult to interpret. In the severely immuno-compromised patient, CSF can appear acellular or inappropriately consistent with aseptic meningitis. A nonspecific lymphocytic pleocytosis can be observed with a variety of conditions, including partially treated bacterial meningitis.

■ Neuroimaging precedes LP in patients with altered mental status, a focal neurological examination, or frequent seizures. Bleeding diatheses and coagulopathies are corrected prior to the diagnostic LP.

■ The absence of red blood cells in the CNS does not exclude the diagnosis of HSV-1 encephalitis.

■ A "negative" LP does not exclude a viral CNS infection.

■ LP should be repeated when a patient is sent home from the ED and returns more than 24–48 hours later with a progression of symptoms.

■ Tuberculous meningitis is considered in the differential diagnosis of HSV encephalitis.

SELECTED BIBLIOGRAPHY

Alzeer AH, FitzGerald JM. Corticosteroids and tuberculosis: risks and adjunct therapy. *Tuber Lung Dis.* 1993;74:6–11.

Anderson M. Management of cerebral infection. *J Neurol Neurosurg Psychiatry.* 1993;56:1243–58.

Arndt CA, Walsh TJ, McCully CL, et al. Fluconazole penetration into cerebrospinal fluid: implications for treating fungal infections of the central nervous system. *J Infect Dis.* 1988;157:178–80.

Ashwal S. Neurologic evaluation of the patient with acute bacterial meningitis. *Neurol Clin.* 1995;13:549–77.

Berenguer J, Moreno S, Laguna F, et al. Tuberculous meningitis in patients infected with the human immunodeficiency virus. *N Engl J Med.* 1992;1326:668–72.

Castro C, Barros N, Campos Z, et al. CT scans of cranial tuberculosis. *Radiol Clin North Am.* 1995;33:753–69.

Centers for Disease Control. Bacterial meningitis & meningococcemia. United States, 1978. *MMWR.* 1979;28:277.

The choice of antibacterial drugs. *Med Lett Drugs Ther.* 1994;36:53–60.

Chuck SL, Sande MA. Infections with cryptococcus neoforms in the acquired immunodeficiency syndrome. *N Engl J Med.* 1989;321:794–9.

Connolly KJ, Hammer SM. The acute aseptic meningitis syndrome. *Infect Dis Clin North Am.* 1990;4:599–619.

Corson AP, Chretien JH. Metronidazole-associated aspetic meningitis. *Clin Infect Dis.* 1994;19:974.

Coyle PK, Deng Z, Schutzer SE, et al. Detection of borrelia burgdorferi antigens in cerebrospinal fluid. *Neurology.* 1993;43:1093.

Davis LE, Schmitt JW. Clinical significance of cerebrospinal fluid tests for neurosyphilis. *Ann Neurol.* 1989;25:50–5.

Dismukes WE. Cryptococcal meningitis in patients with AIDS. *J Infect Dis.* 1988;157:624–8.

Drug-resistant Streptococcus pneumoniae – Kentucky and Tennessee, 1993. *MMWR.* 1994;43:23–31.

Duttwyler RJ, Volkman DJ, Conaty SM, et al. Amoxicillin plus probenecid versus doxycycline for treatment of erythema migrans borreliosis. *Lancet.* 1990;336: 1404.

Feldman HA. Epidemiology of toxoplasma infections. *Epidemiol Rev.* 1982;4: 204–13.

Grant IH, Gold JWM, Rosenblum M, et al. 1990. Toxoplasma gondii serology in HIV infected patients: the development of central nervous system toxoplasmosis in AIDS. *AIDS.* 1990;4:519–21.

Greelee JE. Approach to diagnosis of meningitis: cerebrospinal fluid evaluation. *Infect Dis Clin North Am.* 1990;4:583–95.

Halperin JJ, Volkman DJ, Luft BJ, et al. CTS in Lyme borreliosis. *Muscle Nerve.* 1989;12:397.

Hasso AN. Current status of enhanced magnetic resonance imaging in neuroradiology. *Invest Radiol.* 1993;28(suppl 1):S3–S20.

Hoeprich PD, Jordan MC, Ronald AR, eds. *Infectious Diseases: A Treatise of Infectious Processes,* 5th ed. Philadelphia, Pa: Lippincott; 1994.

Kovacs JA, Kovacs AA, Polis M, et al. Cryptococcosis in the acquired immunodeficiency syndrome. *Ann Intern Med.* 1985;103:533–8.

Lamonte M, Silberstein SD, Marcelis JF. Headache associated with aseptic meningitis. *Headache.* 1995;35:520–6.

Larsen RA, Bozzette SA, Jones BE, Haghigh D. Fluconazole combined with flucytosine for treatment of cryptococcal meningitis in patients with AIDS. *Clin Infect Dis.* 1994;19:714–5.

Larsen RA, Bozzette S, McCutchan JA. Persistent cryptococcus neoformans infection of the prostate after successful treatment of meningitis. *Ann Intern Med.* 1989;111: 125–8.

Leonard JM, Des Perez R. Tuberculous meningitis. *Infect Dis Clin North Am.* 1990;4: 769–87.

Marinac JS. Drug and chemical-induced aseptic meningitis: a review of the literature. *Ann Pharmacother.* 1992;26:813–22.

Mischel PS, Vinters HV. Coccidioidomycosis of the central nervous system: neuropathological and vasculopathic manifestations and clinical correlates. *Clin Infect Dis.* 1995;2:400–5.

Nguyen NM, Yu VL. Meningitis caused by candidal species: an emerging problem in neurosurgical patients. *Clin Infect Dis.* 1995;21:323–7.

Peters M, Timm U, Schurmann D, et al. Combined and alternating gangcyclovir and foscarnet in acute and maintenance therapy of human immunodeficiency virus-related cytomegalovirus encephalitis refractory to gangyclovir alone. *Clin Invest Med.* 1992;70:456–8.

Porter SB, Sande MA. Toxoplasmosis of the central nervous system in the acquired immunodeficiency syndrome. *N Engl J Med.* 1992;327:1643–8.

Ragland AS, Arsura E, Ismail Y, Johnson R. Eosinophilic pleocytosis in coccidioidal meningitis: frequency and significance. *Am J Med.* 1993;95:254–7.

Rousseaux M, Lesoin F, Destee A, Jomin M, Petit H. Developments in the treatment and prognosis of multiple brain abscesses. *Neurosurgery.* 1985;16:304–8.

Saag MS, Powderly WG, Cloud GA, et al. Comparison of amphotericin B with fluconazole in the treatment of acute AIDS-associated cryptococcal meningitis. *N Engl J Med.* 1992;326:88–9.

Schenk DN, Hood EW. Neurosyphilis. *Infect Dis Clin North Am.* 1994;8:769–95.

Scribner CL, Kapti RM, Phillips ET, Rickles NM. Aseptic Meningitis and intravenous immunoglobulin therapy. *Ann Intern Med.* 1994;121:305–6.

Schroth G, Kretzschmar K, Gawehn J, Voigt K. Advantage of magnetic resonance imaging in the diagnosis of cerebral infections. *Neuroradiology.* 1987;29:120–6.

Segreti J, Harris AA. Acute bacterial meningitis. *Infect Dis Clin North Am.* 1996;10:797–809.

Sekul EA, Cupler EJ, Daladas MC. Aseptic meningitis associated with high-dose intravenous immunoglobulin therapy: frequency and risk factors. *Ann Intern Med.* 1994;121:259–62.

Simon RP. Neurosyphilis. *Arch Neurol.* 1985;42:606–13.

Torre-Cisneros J, Lopez OL, Kusne S, et al. CNS aspergillosis in organ transplantation: a clinicopathologic study. *J Neurol Neurosurg Psychiatry.* 1993;56:188–93.

Tunkel AR, Wispelwey B, Scheld WM. Pathogenesis and pathophysiology of meningitis. *Infect Dis Clin North Am.* 1990;4:555–75.

Villoria MF, de la Torre J, Fortea F, et al. Intracranial tuberculosis in AIDS: CT and MRI findings. *Neuroradiology.* 1992;34:11–14.

Vincent T, Galgiani JN, Huppert M, Salkin D. The natural history of coccidioidal meningitis: VA-armed forced cooperative studies, 1955–1958. *Clin Infect Dis.* 1993;16:247–54.

Zuger A, Louie E, Holzman RS, Simberkoff MS, Rahal JJ. Cryptococcal disease in patients with the acquired immunodeficiency syndrome. Diagnostic features and outcome of treatment. *Ann Intern Med.* 1986;104:234–40.

12 Cerebrovascular Disease

Michael R. Frankel, Marc Chimowitz, Sam Josvai,
Rashmi U. Kothari, and Sid M. Shah

INTRODUCTION

Cerebrovascular disease is the leading cause of adult disability and the third leading cause of death in the United States. Approximately 700,000 individuals experience a stroke each year, with an estimated cost of $30 billion. Symptoms generally begin abruptly and can include unilateral weakness or numbness, difficulty speaking, loss of vision, inability to walk, or severe headache. With the development of acute stroke therapies, rapid recognition and triage of these patients has become more important than ever before.

Pathophysiology

Cerebrovascular disease encountered in the emergency department (ED) includes transient ischemic attacks (TIAs) and infarcts (strokes). TIAs are defined as episodes of reversible brain ischemia caused by thrombosis or embolism and the corresponding neurological symptoms that last less than 24 hours. In fact, most TIAs last less than 15 minutes; fewer last for several hours. Reversal of neurological deficits is due to spontaneous reperfusion of the ischemic brain region, possibly associated with dissolution of the responsible thrombus. Frequently, a patient's symptoms may have resolved by the time of ED evaluation. Patients who experience a stroke due to atherosclerotic disease have a history of a TIA 50% of the time, whereas those with lacunar stroke or cardioembolism have a neurological warning only 25% and 5% of the time, respectively.

Strokes are classified as ischemic or hemorrhagic. Approximately 85% of strokes are ischemic and result from cardioembolic, lacunar, or atherosclerotic causes. The remaining 15% of strokes are hemorrhagic and include both intracerebral hemorrhages (ICH) and subarachnoid hemorrhages (SAH).

Ischemic strokes are further categorized as either anterior circulation strokes or posterior circulation strokes depending on the vessel involved. Anterior circulation strokes involving the internal carotid artery or its large branches (the middle and anterior cerebral arteries) result from either atherosclerotic narrowing of the vessels with subsequent thrombosis or occlusive emboli from

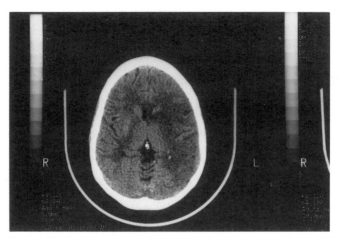

Figure 12.1. CT scan showing early ischemic changes in the left hemisphere (blurring of basal ganglia, sulcal effacement, mild hypodensity in the left hemisphere). CT scan done approximately 12 hours from symptom onset (right hemiplegia, global aphasia).

the heart (Figures 12.1 and 12.2). In both instances, distal hypoperfusion results in syndromes of contralateral arm and leg weakness. This may be accompanied by aphasia (if the dominant hemisphere is involved) or neglect (involvement of the nondominant hemisphere). If the occlusion involves the first branch of the internal carotid (the ophthalmic branch), amaurosis fugax (transient monocular blindness) may result. Selected uncommon stroke syndromes are listed in Table 12.1.

Lacunar infarcts most commonly occur in the internal capsule and result from changes in the small, penetrating arteries that supply it. Chronic hypertension or diabetes can lead to the deposition of lipid and hyaline material in the vessel walls. In situ thrombosis can subsequently occur, and the resulting occlusion produces classic "lacunar syndromes" such as a pure motor deficit without accompanying sensory loss, aphasia, or neglect.

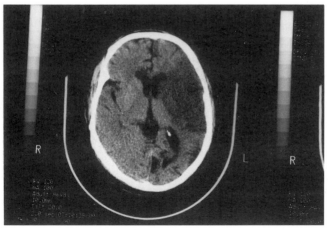

Figure 12.2. CT scan of left middle cerebral artery distribution infarct 24 hours from symptom onset. (Not the same patient as in Figure 12.1.)

Table 12.1. Selected Uncommon Clinical Stroke Syndromes

Syndrome	Arterial Occlusion Site	Clinical Manifestations
Lateral medullary syndrome (Wallenberg syndrome)	Posterior inferior cerebellar art (often a lesion in vertebral art)	(a) Ipsilateral limb ataxia, (b) ipsilateral loss of facial cutaneous sensation, (c) hiccup, (d) ipsilateral Horner syndrome, (e) nausea, vomiting, nystagmus, (f) contralateral loss of pain and temperature, (g) dysphagia, (h) hoarseness with ipsilateral vocal cord paralysis, (i) loss of ipsilateral pharyngeal reflex
Lateral inferior pontine syndrome	Anterior inferior cerebellar artery	(a–f) above and, in addition, ipsilateral facial paralysis, hearing loss and/or tinnitus, and ipsilateral gaze paralysis
Lateral midpontine syndrome	Short circumferential artery	(a–f) above and, in addition, trigeminal nerve impairment: chewing difficulty (bilateral lesions) or ipsilateral jaw deviation with mouth opened (unilateral lesions)
Lateral superior pontine syndrome	Superior cerebellar artery	(a–f) above and absence of specific cranial nerve involvement findings
Medial medullary syndrome	Paramedial branches of basilar artery	(a) Contralateral hemiparesis, (b) contralateral loss of proprioception
Median inferior pontine syndrome	Paramedian branches of basilar artery	(a–c) above plus ipsilateral gaze paralysis, ipsilateral lateral rectus paralysis, and gaze-evoked nystagmus
Median superior pontine syndrome	Paramedian branches of the basilar artery	(a) Contralateral hemiparesis, (b) contralateral supranuclear facial paresis, (c) ipsilateral oculomotor nerve palsy
Central midbrain syndrome (tegmental syndrome)	Paramedian branches of basilar artery	(a) Ipsilateral oculomotor nerve palsy, (b) hemichorea of contralateral limbs, (c) contralateral loss of cutaneous sensation and proprioception
Dorsal midbrain syndrome (Perinaud's syndrome)	Usually caused by compression of extra axial lesion (pinealoma)	Paralysis of upward gaze
Locked-in syndrome	Basilar artery occlusion causing bilateral ventral pontine lesions	Complete quadriplegia, inability to speak, and loss of all facial movements despite normal level of consciousness: patients may communicate with eye or eyelid movements

Reproduced with permission from WB Saunders Co., Philadelphia. Thurman RJ, Jauch EC. Acute ischemic stroke: emergent evaluation and management. *Emerg Med Clin N Am.* 2002;20:609–30.

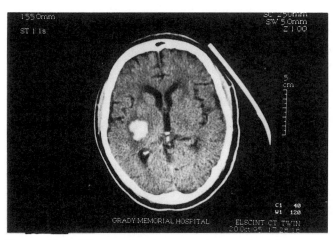

Figure 12.3. CT scan showing acute intracerebral hemorrhage in a patient with left hemisphere hemiplegia.

Posterior circulation stroke due to atherosclerosis can also occur and is becoming an increasingly recognized cause of stroke. Occlusion of the cerebellar arteries with subsequent infarction produces the combination of ipsilateral ataxia, disequilibrium, and vertigo. Brainstem strokes result in a crossed presentation with ipsilateral cranial nerve dysfunction and contralateral limb weakness. The locked-in syndrome results from basilar artery occlusion and consists of quadriparesis, facial paralysis, and the inability to speak, but preserves vertical gaze. Finally, occlusion of the small vessels, which supply the thalamus, produces a lacunar infarct with purely sensory findings affecting the contralateral side of the face or body.

Intracerebral hemorrhages (Figure 12.3) are most commonly the result of long-standing hypertension. Symptoms begin abruptly and typically worsen over a few minutes to hours. Patients complain of a severe headache, which may be accompanied by vomiting, hemiplegia, somnolence, and a decreased level of consciousness. Clinical findings associated with specific anatomic locations of ICH are listed in Table 12.2. ICH in the elderly can result from cerebral amyloid angiopathy. Amyloid is deposited in the blood vessels and is presumed to make them weaker and more susceptible to rupture. ICH in a younger patient is more commonly due to an arteriovenous malformation or cavernous angioma. ICH can precipitate a cascade of noxious events in addition to initial local parenchymal brain injury. Even a small ICH can lead to an increase in intracranial pressure with the loss of autoregulatory mechanisms of the brain. Hydrocephalus is a known complication of ICH and is an independent predictor of mortality after ICH. Obstructive hydrocephalus can result from compression of CSF pathways, particularly with posterior fossa and brainstem hemorrhages. Even a small brainstem ICH or ICH that extends into the ventricular system can potentially result in catastrophic obstructive hydrocephalus.

Subarachnoid hemorrhage (Figure 12.4) results from rupture of an intracranial aneurysm, typically located at the bifurcation of an artery. When rupture occurs, blood quickly leaks into the subarachnoid space, producing symptoms similar to those seen in an ICH, though unilateral weakness is much less common.

Table 12.2. Clinical Findings and Anatomic Location of ICH

Anatomic Area of Involvement	Clinical Findings
Lobar	
Frontal	Frontal headache, motor weakness arm > leg, behavioral abnormalities
Parietal	Unilateral headache, hemisensory deficits, spatial neglect (nondominant), visual field deficits
Temporal	Unilateral headache, aphasia (dominant), visual field defects
Occipital	Ipsilateral periorbital headache, visual field loss or blurring
Deep	
Putaminal	Unilateral motor, sensory and visual field loss, aphasia (dominant), neglect (nondominant), coma
Thalamic	Hemisensory deficit > hemiparesis. Gaze deviation, pupil asymmetry
Cerebellum*	Nausea, vomiting, ataxia, depressed level of consciousness, coma
Pontine	Coma, quadriplegia, decerebrate posturing, pinpoint pupils

* Cerebellar hemorrhage is a true emergency.

Adapted from Feldman E, ed., *Intracranial Hemorrhage*. Armonk, NY: Futura Publishing Company; 1994 and Panagos et al. *Emerg Med Clin N Am*. 2002;20:631–55.

Evaluation

The purpose of the initial evaluation is to determine whether there is evidence of a stroke, what part of the brain is affected, and whether the patient is a candidate for urgent intervention such as thrombolytic therapy. Brief questioning of the patient and family is essential to determine the onset of symptoms, relevant past medical history, and baseline functional status. A brief, focused neurological examination that enables accurate localization of the lesion can be performed in less than 10 minutes. Mental status is initially assessed by evaluating the patient's level of consciousness. Most patients with focal cerebral ischemia are awake or easily aroused to voice. Patients that are somnolent or comatose are more likely to have experienced a hemorrhagic or posterior circulation infarct.

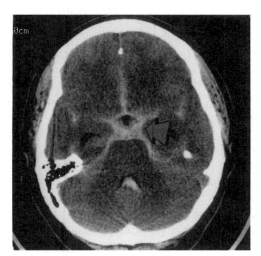

Figure 12.4. CT scan showing acute subarachnoid hemorrhage (arrow points to blood in the basal cisterns).

Aphasia is the inability to process language and occurs with injury to the dominant cerebral hemisphere (typically the left hemisphere in right-handed individuals). Aphasia may be receptive (i.e., inability to understand language), expressive (i.e., inability to express information), or a combination of both. Receptive aphasia is detected by asking the patient to follow simple commands such as "Place your right thumb on your left ear." The presence of an expressive aphasia can be detected by asking the patient to describe why he or she has come to the ED. Patients with expressive aphasia have difficulty producing free-flowing speech and are usually quite frustrated. Testing for naming ability helps detect even mild aphasia. Neologisms (altering the names of objects) are useful clues to the presence of aphasia.

Neglect can arise from nondominant parietal lobe dysfunction. Patients with frontal or parietal infarcts may deny their contralateral paralysis or even the existence of their contralateral limbs. In patients with subtle symptoms, the patient's lack of concern may cause the inexperienced examiner to misdiagnose the patient and thus delay critical interventions.

Brief cranial nerve examination includes the assessment of pupillary symmetry and reactivity, visual fields, and extraocular movements. Asking the patient to smile and to raise his eyebrows assesses facial symmetry. Unlike peripheral lesions (e.g., Bell's palsy), central deficits produce weakness of the lower face with relative sparing of the forehead. Dysarthria (slurred speech) should be evident upon discussing the patient's symptoms. Symmetry of palatal elevation and tongue protrusion can also be assessed quickly.

Examination of motor function can be performed in a quick and efficient manner. It is not necessary to examine every muscle in the extremities. Asking the patient to hold both arms up with the wrists extended for a count of 10 provides sufficient information. Asymmetrical downward drift usually implies significant weakness. Similarly, the patient can be asked to raise each leg for a count of 5 while the examiner looks for downward drift.

The sensory examination is performed by observing the response to pinprick using a safety pin or broken tongue blade on the patient's face, arm, trunk, and leg. The sensory exam need not be exhaustive and should not take more than one minute during the initial encounter.

Coordination is assessed by asking the patient to touch finger-to-nose and heel-to-shin to evaluate for ataxia. Testing the deep tendon reflexes is usually not helpful in acute stroke and can be skipped during the initial encounter. The plantar response is usually, but not always, extensor (Babinski sign) on the hemiparetic side.

Testing gait is necessary in all patients with suspected stroke, unless there is evidence of postural hypotension or obvious severe weakness. Gait ataxia may be the only sign of cerebellar infarct or hemorrhage.

Ancillary Testing

After completion of this focused history and brief examination, appropriate laboratory tests and neuroimaging can be obtained. A chemistry profile, complete blood count (CBC) with platelets, and coagulation profile are essential. An electrocardiogram (EKG) should be obtained to determine possible cardiac causes of the stroke. Cardiac enzymes may be obtained if evidence of an acute myocardial

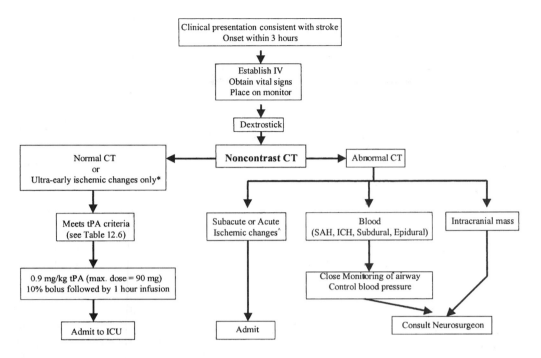

Figure 12.5. Management of patients with acute stroke.

infarction exists. A noncontrast computerized tomography (CT) scan of the head is currently considered the radiological study of choice and is virtually 100% sensitive for detecting acute intracerebral hemorrhage. CT is not as sensitive in detecting acute ischemic strokes or SAH. The abnormalities associated with ischemic strokes may not appear on CT for 3 hours or more after symptom onset. Similarly, CT will miss up to 5% of SAH when performed within 72 hours of symptom onset, with decreasing sensitivity as time progresses. If SAH is clinically suspected and a normal head CT is obtained, one should subsequently perform a lumbar puncture and assess for the presence of xanthrochromia. This is accomplished by centrifuging the cerebrospinal fluid and examining the supernatant for the presence of pink or yellow discoloration. Spectrophotometry is far more sensitive than direct visual inspection in identifying xanthrochromia.

General Management

The management of patients with acute stroke is outlined in Figure 12.5. Attention to adequate airway protection, oxygenation, and circulatory function is essential. Most patients with ischemic strokes do not require ventilatory support. However, patients with hemorrhagic infarcts can have a profound change in their level of consciousness and may require early intubation. Pretreatment with IV lidocaine is recommended prior to intubation, and hyperventilation should only be considered if impending herniation is suspected.

Cardiac arrhythmias can occur in patients with acute stroke, and continuous cardiac monitoring is recommended. Many patients with acute stroke are volume-depleted, which can exacerbate their cerebral ischemia. Gradually restoring an euvolemic state with isotonic fluids is recommended to minimize the extent of ischemic damage. Hypoglycemia can cause confusion and rarely hemiparesis and needs to be corrected immediately when present. The use of lorazepam is indicated for patients with generalized convulsions lasting longer than 2 minutes or for patients with more than one seizure in any given hour.

Hypertension is common in the setting of acute stroke. If the infarct is ischemic in nature, treatment is not automatically required and may actually worsen the patient's neurological deficits. In general, treatment is not recommended unless the patient is a candidate for thrombolytic therapy, and there is concomitant cardiovascular decompensation, suspected aortic dissection, or repeated blood pressure measurements of greater than 220/120. When hypertension does require treatment, IV labetalol is recommended, with immediate discontinuation should the patient's neurological status worsen (Table 12.3).

The management of elevated blood pressure in acute intracerebral hemorrhage is controversial. One common practice is to treat systolic blood pressures greater than 180 mmHg with a goal of lowering to prestroke values. The American Heart Association recommends blood pressure levels be maintained at less than a mean pressure of 130 mmHg in persons with hypertension. Cerebral perfusion pressure (requiring invasive intracranial pressure monitoring) is maintained at greater than 70 mmHg. In SAH, elevated blood pressure increases the risk of rebleeding and subsequent mortality. If SAH is diagnosed, the patient's blood pressure should be lowered to normotensive levels.

Antiplatelet Therapy

See Tables 12.4 and 12.5

Patients with TIAs not due to a cardioembolic event should be treated with antiplatelet agents while undergoing a full diagnostic evaluation. When a patient has not been treated previously with an antiplatelet agent, aspirin (81 mg or 325 mg) can be given acutely. For patients with a TIA while on aspirin, clopidogrel (75 mg) or extended-release dipyridamole and aspirin (Aggrenox) can be started. Maintenance dosing is based on the patient's history of antiplatelet use, the specifics of the clinical presentation, and relative contraindications and should be done in consultation with the patient's primary care provider and/or an attending neurologist.

Anticoagulation

See Tables 12.4 and 12.5.

The use of anticoagulants (heparin or low molecular heparins) remains the most controversial subject in the management of acute stroke. Even the widely accepted indication for anticoagulation (heparin given intravenously) in the acute ischemic stroke for the prevention of recurrent stroke in patients with an unequivocal cardiac source of embolus (e.g., atrial fibrillation or dilated cardiomyopathy) is now under scrutiny. The International Stroke Trial (IST) demonstrated a lack of significant improvement in the clinical outcome of stroke victims treated with heparin. Patients with large embolic stroke (e.g., global aphasia or neglect with

Table 12.3. Antihypertensive Therapy for Acute Ischemic Stroke

Blood Pressure*	Treatment
Not candidates for thrombolytic therapy	
1. DBP > 140 mmHg	Sodium nitroprusside (0.5 µg/kg per minute). Aim for 10 to 20% reduction in DBP.
2. SBP > 220, DBP > 120, or MAP > 130 mmHg	10–20 mg labetalol‡ IV push over 1–2 minutes. May repeat or double labetalol every 20 minutes to a maximum dose of 150 mg.
3. SBP < 220, DBP < 120, or MAP < 130 mmHg	Emergency antihypertensive therapy is deferred in the absence of aortic dissection, acute myocardial infarction, severe congestive heart failure, or hypertensive encephalopathy.
Thrombolytic candidates	
Pretreatment	
1. SBP > 185 or DBP > 110 mmHg	1–2 inches of nitropaste or one to two doses of 10–20 mg labetalol‡ IV push. If BP is not reduced and maintained to < 185/110 mmHg, the patient should not be treated with rtPA.
During and after treatment	
1. Monitor BP	BP is monitored every 15 minutes for 2 hours, then every 30 minutes for 6 hours, and then every hour for 16 hours.
2. DBP > 140 mmHg	Sodium nitroprusside (0.5 µg/kg per minute).
3. SBP > 230 mmHg or DBP 121 to 140 mmHg	(1) 10 mg labetalol‡ IV over 1–2 minutes. May repeat or double labetalol every 10 minutes to a maximum dose of 150 mg or give the initial labetalol bolus and then start a labetalol drip at 2–8 mg/min. (2) If BP not controlled by labetalol, consider sodium nitroprusside.
4. SBP 180 to 230 mmHg or DBP 105 to 120 mmHg	10 mg labetalol‡ IV. May repeat or double labetalol every 10–20 minutes to a maximum dose of 150 mg or give initial labetalol bolus and then start a labetalol drip at 2–8 mg/min.

DBP indicates diastolic blood pressure; SBP, systolic blood pressure; MAP, mean arterial pressure; BP, blood pressure; and rtPA, tissue plasminogen activator.

* All initial blood pressures should be verified before treatment by repeating reading in 5 minutes.

‡ Labetalol should be avoided in patients with asthma, cardiac failure, or severe abnormalities in cardiac conduction. For refractory hypertension, alternative therapy may be considered with sodium nitroprusside or enalapril.

hemiplegia and gaze deviation) can be particularly vulnerable to symptomatic hemorrhagic transformation related to heparin given intravenously in the first few days. At this time, there are no definitve studies confirming significant clinical improvement in victims of stroke treated with either heparin or low molecular weight heparin (LMWHs) except for the prophylaxis of deep venous thrombosis or pulmonary embolus.

Thrombolytics

Intravenous tissue Plasminogen Activator (tPA), given within 3 hours of symptom onset is the only Food and Drug Administration (FDA)-approved drug for

Table 12.4. American Stroke Association/American Academy of Neurology Scientific Statement

Anticoagulants and Antiplatelet Agents in Acute Ischemic Stroke: Report of the Joint Stroke Guideline Development Committee of the American Academy of Neurology and the American Stroke Association (a Division of the American Heart Association)

Recommendations: (see also Appendix A for levels of evidence and recommendation grade classification scheme)
1. Patients with acute ischemic stroke presenting within 48 hours of symptom onset should be given aspirin (160 to 325 mg/day) to reduce stroke mortality and decrease morbidity, provided contraindications such as allergy and gastrointestinal bleeding are absent, and the patient has or will not be treated with recombinant tissue-type plasminogen activator (Grade A). The data are insufficient at this time to recommend the use of any other platelet antiaggregant in the setting of acute ischemic stroke.

2. Subcutaneous unfractionated heparin, LMW heparins, and heparinoids may be considered for DVT prophylaxis in at-risk patients with acute ischemic stroke, recognizing that nonpharmacologic treatments for DVT prevention also exist (Grade A). A benefit in reducing the incidence of PE has not been demonstrated. The relative benefits of these agents must be weighed against the risk of systemic and intracerebral hemorrhage.

3. Although there is some evidence that fixed-dose, subcutaneous, unfractionated heparin reduces early recurrent ischemic stroke, this benefit is negated by a concomitant increase in the occurrence of hemorrhage. Therefore, use of subcutaneous unfractionated heparin is not recommended for decreasing the risk of death or stroke-related morbidity or for preventing early stroke recurrence (Grade A).

4(A). Dose-adjusted, unfractionated heparin is not recommended for reducing morbidity, mortality, or early recurrent stroke in patients with acute stroke (i.e., in the first 48 hours) because the evidence indicates it is not efficacious and may be associated with increased bleeding complications (Grade B).

4(B). High-dose LMW heparin/heparinoids have not been associated with either benefit or harm in reducing morbidity, mortality, or early recurrent stroke in patients with acute stroke and are, therefore, not recommended for these goals (Grade A).

5. IV, unfractionated heparin or high-dose LMW heparin/heparinoids are not recommended for any specific subgroup of patients with acute ischemic stroke that is based on any presumed stroke mechanism or location (e.g., cardioembolic, large vessel atherosclerotic, vertebrobasilar, or "progressing" stroke) because data are insufficient (Grade U). Although the LMW heparin, dalteparin, at high doses may be efficacious in patients with atrial fibrillation, it is not more efficacious than aspirin in this setting. Because aspirin is easier to administer, it, rather than dalteparin, is recommended for the various stroke subgroups (Grade A).

Appendix A

Levels of evidence and recommendation grade classification scheme.

Levels of evidence. Class I. Evidence provided by a prospective, randomized, controlled clinical trial with masked outcome assessment, in a representative population. The following are required:

Primary outcome(s) is/are clearly defined.
Exclusion/inclusion criteria are clearly defined.
Adequate accounting for dropouts and crossovers with numbers sufficiently low to
    have minimal potential for bias.

Relevant baseline characteristics are presented and substantially equivalent among treatment groups, or there is appropriate statistical adjustment for differences.

Class II. Evidence provided by a prospective, matched cohort study in a representative population with masked outcome assessment that meets all the above, OR a randomized, controlled trial in a representative population that lacks one of the above criteria.

Class III. Evidence provided by all other controlled trials (including well-defined natural history controls or patients serving as own controls) in a representative population, in which outcome assessment is independent of patient treatment.

Class IV. Evidence from uncontrolled studies, case series, case reports, or expert opinion.

Grades of Recommendation. Grade A. At least one convincing Class I study or at least two consistent, convincing Class II studies.

Grade B. At least one convincing Class II study or at least three convincing Class III studies.

Grade C. At least two convincing and consistent Class III studies.

Reproduced with permission from American Heart Association Inc. Coull BM, Williams LS, Goldstein LB, Meschia JF, Heitzman D, Chaturvedi S, Johnston KC, Starkman S, Morgenstern LB, Wilterdink JL, Levine SR, Saver JL. *Stroke.* 2002;33:1934.

the treatment of patients with acute ischemic stroke. Appropriate patients treated with intravenous tPA are 30–50% more likely to have minimal or no deficits at 3 months as compared to placebo. Though tPA-treated patients are at increased risk of ICH (6.4% tPA group versus 0.6% placebo group), there is no increase in mortality (17% tPA versus 21% placebo) or morbidity. tPA must be considered in all ischemic stroke patients presenting within 3 hours of symptom onset.

Patients must meet strict inclusion criteria to be considered for tPA therapy (Table 12.6). These include a noncontrast CT scan of the head with no evidence of hemorrhage and a time interval of 3 hours or less from the time of symptom onset to the initiation of tPA therapy. The latter criteria must be strictly adhered to, and the time of symptom onset must be verified by the patient and/or the patient's family members. Patients who awaken with stroke symptoms should be considered to have had symptom onset at the time they were last seen normal, not the time they awoke.

Patients must also meet strict exclusion criteria (Table 12.6). Patients with minor or rapidly improving symptoms should not be treated with tPA. A history of intracranial hemorrhage, recent major surgery, recent head trauma, or recent gastrointestinal bleed are also contraindications. Elevated systolic (>185) or diastolic (>110) blood pressures also prevent tPA therapy unless the blood pressure lowers spontaneously or can be brought under control with nonaggressive measures (Table 12.1).

If the decision is made to employ tPA therapy, it should be administered at a dose of 0.9 mg/kg (maximum dose 90 mg) with 10% given as an IV bolus over 60 seconds and the remainder slowly infused over 1 hour. Blood pressure should be closely monitored and kept below 180/105. IV labetalol or nitroprusside can be used for blood pressure control as needed (Table 12.3). No anticoagulants or antiplatelet agents should be used during the first 24 hours after tPA infusion.

Table 12.5. Anticoagulants and Antiplatelet Agents in Acute Ischemic Stroke: Summary of Results Platelet Antiaggregants and Anticoagulants Within 48 Hours of Acute Ischemic Stroke

Treatment	Benefit Data	Risk Data
Aspirin	Prevention of early recurrent ischemic stroke (CAST, IST)* Small benefit in reducing death and dependence (CAST, IST, MAST)	Small increase in intracerebral hemorrhage or hemorrhagic transformation (CAST, IST, MAST)* Small increase in transfused or fatal extracranial hemorrhage (IST, CAST)*
IV unfractionated heparin	Inadequate data	Inadequate data
SQ unfractionated heparin	Small benefit in reducing early recurrent stroke outweighed by small increase in CNS hemorrhage (IST)[†] No benefit in reducing morbidity, mortality (IST)[†] Reduces PE and DVT (IST[†], McCarthy and Turner[6])[‡]	Increase in symptomatic CNS hemorrhage (8/1000 treated, IST)[†] Increase in fatal or transfused systemic hemorrhage (9/1000 treated, IST)[†]
LMW heparins/ heparinoids	Benefit in reducing 6-month morbidity (nadroparin, Kay et al[5])[¶] No benefit in reducing 3-month morbidity (TOAST)[¶] Reduces DVT (TOAST)[¶]	Variable increase in systemic and CNS hemorrhage across studies (Kay et al., TOAST,[¶] Berge[§])

* Compared with placebo/no aspirin.
[†] Compared with no subcutaneous heparin (50% on ASA, 50% on no ASA).
[‡] Compared with no subcutaneous heparin.
[¶] Compared with placebo.
[§] Compared with aspirin.
CAST = The Chinese Acute Stroke Trial; IST = The International Stroke Trial; MAST = The Multicentre Acute Stroke Trial – Italy; PE = pulmonary emboli; DVT = deep vein thrombosis; LMW = low molecular weight; TOAST = Trial of the Heparinoid ORG 10172 in Acute Stroke.

From Report of the Joint Stroke Guideline Development Committee of the American Academy of Neurology and the American Stroke Association

Disposition

Patients with acute or hemorrhagic strokes need to be admitted to the hospital for further evaluation and management. Patients hospitalized with acute cerebral ischemia should be cared for by physicians with experience and expertise in this area. This is typically a neurologist or a primary physician with close consultation with neurology. A neurosurgeon should participate in the care of most patients with ICH and all patients with SAH.

Table 12.6. Thrombolytic Therapy for Ischemic Stroke: Inclusion/Exclusion Criteria

Inclusion Criteria (all YES boxes must be checked before treatment):

YES

☐ Age 18 years or older

☐ Clinical diagnosis of ischemic stroke causing a measurable neurological deficit

☐ Time of symptom onset well established to be less than 180 minutes before treatment would begin

Exclusion Criteria (all NO boxes must be checked before treatment):

NO

☐ Evidence of intracranial hemorrhage on noncontrast head CT

☐ Only minor or rapidly improving stroke symptoms

☐ High clinical suspicion of subarachnoid hemorrhage even with normal CT

☐ Active internal bleeding (e.g., gastrointestinal bleed or urinary bleeding within last 21 days)

☐ Known bleeding diathesis, including but not limited to
 • Platelet count <100{ths}000/mm^3
 • Patient has received heparin within 48 hours and had an elevated activated partial thromboplastin time (greater than upper limit of normal for laboratory)
 • Recent use of anticoagulant (e.g., warfarin sodium) and elevated INR > 1.5

☐ Within 3 months of intracranial surgery, serious head trauma, or previous stroke

☐ Within 14 days of major surgery or serious trauma

☐ Recent arterial puncture at noncompressible site

☐ Lumbar puncture within 7 days

☐ History of intracranial hemorrhage, arteriovenous malformation, or aneurysm

☐ Witnessed seizure at stroke onset

☐ Recent acute myocardial infarction

☐ On repeated measurements, systolic pressure >185 mmHg or diastolic pressure >110 mmHg at time of treatment, requiring aggressive treatment to reduce blood pressure to within these limits

PEARLS AND PITFALLS

■ Elevated blood pressure after acute ischemic stroke is common. Aggressively lowering blood pressure in this setting can worsen the ischemia and cause greater neurological injury.

■ Some strokes do not cause weakness. Common locations of stroke without paralysis include the occipital lobe (hemianopia), dominant temporal/parietal lobe (Wernicke's aphasia), nondominant temporal/parietal lobe (confusion, agitation, and hemianopia), and thalamus (confusion, somnolence, and hemianopia).

■ A psychogenic neurological deficit (e.g., hysterical paralysis) is often difficult to differentiate from organic brain injury. In general, the diagnosis is not made without neurological consultation.

■ A normal CT scan does not rule out SAH. Lumbar puncture is required in patients with normal imaging whose clinical presentation suggests SAH. After cerebrospinal is centrifuged, the supernatant may not become discolored for up to 12 hours after the onset of SAH.

SELECTED BIBLIOGRAPHY

A special Writing Group of the Stroke Council, American Heart Association Guidelines for Thrombolytic Therapy for acute stroke. A supplement to the guidelines for the management of patients with acute ischemic stroke. 1996;94:1167–74.

Albers GW, Bates VE, Clark WM, Bell R, Verro, Hamilton SA. Intravenous tissue-type plasminogen activator for treatment of acute stroke: the Standard Treatment with Altepase to Reverse Stroke (STARS) study. *JAMA*. 2000;283:1145–50.

Bath PMW, Lindenstrom E, Boysen G, et al. Tinzaparin in acute ischaemic stroke (TAIST): a randomized aspirin-controlled trial. *Lancet*. 2001;358:702–10.

Berge E, Abdelnoor M, Nakstad PH, Sandset PM. Low molecular-weight heparin versus aspirin in patients with acute ischaemic stroke and atrial fibrillation: a double-blind randomised study. HAEST Study Group Heparin in Acute Embolic Stroke Trial. *Lancet*. 2000;355:1205–10.

Broderick JP, et al. Guidelines for the management of spontaneous intracerebral hemorrhage: a statement for healthcare professionals from a special writing group of the Stroke Council, American Heart Association. *Stroke*. 1999;30:905–15.

CAST (Chinese Acute Stroke Trial) Collaboration Group. CAST: randomized placebo-controlled trial of early aspirin use in 20,000 patients with acute ischaemic stroke. *Lancet*. 1997;349:1641–9.

Chen ZM, Sandercock P, Pan HC, et al. Indications for early aspirin use in acute ischemic stroke: a combined analysis of 40,000 randomized patients from the Chinese acute stroke trial and the international stroke trial. On behalf of the CAST and IST collaborative groups. *Stroke*. 2000;31:1240–49.

Ciuffetti G, Aisa G, Mercuri M, et al. Effects of ticlopidine on the neurologic outcome and the hemorheologic pattern in the postacute phase of ischemic stroke: a pilot study. *Angiology*. 1990;41:505–11.

Clark WM, Wissman S, Albers GW, Jhamandas JH, Madden KP, Hamilton S. Recombinant tissue-type plasminogen activator (Altepase) for ischemic stroke 3 to 5 hours after symptom onset. The ATLANTIS study: a randomized controlled trial. Altepase Thrombolysis for Acute Noninterventional Therapy in Ischemic Stroke. *JAMA*. 1999;282:1504–9.

Counsell C, Sandercock P. Low-molecular-weight heparins or heparinoids versus standard unfractionated heparin for acute ischemic stroke. In: *The Cochrane Library*, Issue 1. Oxford, UK; 2000.

Diener HC, Ringelstein EB, von Kummer R, et al. Treatment of acute ischemic stroke with the low-molecular-weight heparin certoparin. Results of the TOPAS Trial. *Stroke*. 2001;32:22–9.

EAFT Study Group. Secondary prevention in non-rheumatic atrial fibrillation after transient ischaemic attack or minor stroke. *Lancet*. 1993;342:1255–62.

European Stroke Council, European Neurological Society and European Federation of Neurological Societies. European Stroke Initiative recommendations for stroke management. *Cerebrovasc Dis*. 2000;10:335–51.

Gubitz G, Counsell C, Sandercock P, et al. Anticoagulants for acute ischemic stroke (Cochrane Review). In: *The Cochrane Library*, Issue 1. Oxford, UK; 2000.

Gubitz G, Sandercock P, Counsell C. Antiplatelet therapy for acute ischemic stroke. In: The Cochrane Library, Issue 1. Oxford, UK; 2000.

International Stroke Trial Collaborative Group. The International Stroke Trial (IST): a randomized trial of aspirin, subcutaneous heparin, both, or neither among 19,435 patients with acute ischaemic stroke. *Lancet.* 1997;349:1569–81.

Kay R, Sing Wong K, Yu YL, et al. Low-molecular-weight heparin for the treatment of acute ischemic stroke. *N Engl J Med.* 1995;333:1588–93.

Lewandowski C, Barsan W. Treatment of acute ischemic stroke. *Ann Emerg Med.* 2001; 37:202–16.

McCarthy ST, Turner J. Low-dose subcutaneous heparin in the prevention of deep-vein thrombosis and pulmonary emboli following acute stroke. *Age Ageing.* 1986;15:84–8.

Mayberg MR, et al. Guidelines for the management of aneurismal subarachnoid hemorrhage. A statement for healthcare professional from a special writing group of the stroke council, American Heart Association, *Circulation.* 1994;90:2592–605.

Multicentre Acute Stroke Trial – Italy (MAST-I) Group. Randomised controlled trial of streptokinase, aspirin, and combination of both in treatment of acute ischaemic stroke. *Lancet.* 1995;346:1509–14.

Publications Committee for the Trial of ORG 10172 in Acute Stroke Treatment (TOAST) Investigators. Low molecular weight heparinoid, ORG 10172 (Dsanaparoid), and outcome after acute ischemic stroke. *JAMA.* 1998;279:1265–72.

The Abciximab in Ischemic Stroke Investigators. Abciximab in acute ischemic stroke: a randomized, double-blind, placebo-controlled, dose-escalation study. *Stroke.* 2000;31:601–9.

The NINDS rt-PA Stroke Study Group. Tissue plasminogen activator for acute ischemic stroke. *N Engl J Med.* 1995;333:1581–7.

13 Movement Disorders

Sid M. Shah, Roger Albin, and Susan Baser

INTRODUCTION

Movement disorders (MD) encountered in the emergency department (ED) range from the familiar Parkinsonism and drug-induced dystonias to rare disabling hemiballism secondary to a stroke. A movement disorder is typically the sign of an underlying neurological or nonneurological disorder, rather than a diagnosis itself. Movement disorders, dystonia in particular, are often misdiagnosed as being hysterical or psychiatric in origin. In the ED, movement disorders are diagnosed on the basis of clinical evaluation, with relatively few contributions from laboratory and radiographic studies.

Movement disorders are classified as hypokinetic disorders, hyperkinetic disorders, tremor, and myoclonus. Characteristics of various movement disorders are described and drug-induced movement disorders, which commonly present to the ED, are reviewed in greater detail.

Evaluation

Vital signs and the adequacy of the airway are assessed on arrival in the emergency department. A seizure disorder is distinguished from a MD by obtaining a thorough history and by performing a focused physical examination. MD is usually diagnosed on the basis of clinical evaluation, with little additional information provided by laboratory and radiographic studies.

Important features of the history include the manner and temporal nature of symptom onset, the location of symptoms and body parts most affected, and mitigating and exacerbating factors. Inquire if the symptoms are present at rest, with sustained posture, with movement, or only during the execution of specific tasks. Possible association to environmental factors, toxins, or medication use is determined. Drug ingestion, substance abuse, and environmental toxins such as carbon monoxide are associated with different types of movement disorders. Family, social, and psychiatric history is reviewed. In a pediatric patient, evidence of premature birth, perinatal injury, or behavioral problems is sought. Use of psychotropic medications or antiemetics is questioned. A careful physical

Table 13.1. Classification of Movement Disorders

Hypokinetic Movement Disorders/Parkinsonism	Hyperkinetic/Choreic Movement Disorders
Parkinson's disease	Chorea
Drug-induced Parkinsonism	Athetosis
Parkinsonism syndromes	Ballism (hemiballism is more common)
	Dystonia
	Tics
Tremors	**Myoclonus**
Resting tremors	Generalized
Postural tremors	Segmental
Kinetic tremors	Focal
Task-related tremors	

examination can reveal signs of metabolic or endocrine derangements, or toxic exposures.

A careful neurological examination with accurate characterization of the abnormalities is the basis of evaluating movement disorders. The character of the involuntary movement(s) or movement problem is first assessed by observation of the patient's head, trunk, and limbs. Eye movements (saccadic and pursuit movements), tone, gait (casual, toe, heel, and tandem), and fine coordination (rapid finger tapping, alternating pronation and supination of the hands) are tested. The role of neuroimaging studies in the evaluation of movement disorders is limited. Some movement disorders occur acutely from focal structural lesions such as stroke. Typically, they are present in a localized body area or follow a "hemi-distribution," as in hemidystonia or hemiballism. Urgent brain imaging can be helpful following the acute onset of symptoms with a focal distribution of findings.

Classification of Movement Disorders

Movement disorders can be classified into four broad categories based on phenomenological features, clinical pharmacology, and neuropathology (Table 13.1):

1. Hypokinetic disorders, which are identical with the syndrome of *Parkinsonism*
2. Hyperkinetic/choreic movement disorders
3. Tremors
4. Myoclonus

Descriptive features of individual movement disorders are summarized in Table 13.2. Chorea, athetosis, and ballism are appropriately viewed as part of a spectrum of involuntary movements with a common pathophysiology.

Parkinsonism (Hypokinetic MD)

Characteristics. Parkinsonism is a syndrome associated with deficient dopamine innervation or dopamine effect within the striatum (caudate and putamen). The cardinal features are: (1) bradykinesia, slowness of movement with a paucity of

Table 13.2. Phenomenology of Movement Disorders

Movement Disorder	Features	Areas of Involvement	Anatomical Localization
Parkinsonism	Bradykinesia, rigidity, often resting tremor, often postural instability, stooped posture, masked facies, hypophonia	Often asymmetrical at onset but can be generalized	Basal ganglia – interruption of or interference with nigrostriatal dopaminergic neurotransmission
Dystonia	Sustained, spasmodic, repetitive contractions causing involuntary abnormal postures	Any voluntary muscle can be affected; usually head, neck, face, and limbs	Presumed to be basal ganglia – associated with putamen lesions in some cases
Tremor	Involuntary, rhythmic, and roughy sinusoidal movements; some are action-induced	Head, hands, limbs, and voice	In Parkinsonian resting tremor – basal ganglia Most other tremors may involve cerebellar dysfunction
Chorea	Involuntary, irregular, rapid, jerky movements without a rhythmic pattern; dancelike	Generally limbs, but any body part can be affected	Basal ganglia – striatum or subthalamic nucleus
Athetosis	Akin to chorea but distinct "writhing" movements	Limbs, but any body part can be involved	Identical with chorea
Myoclonus	Brief, rapid, shocklike jerks	Generally involves very small muscles	Can result from dysfunction at any level of the central nervous system
Tics	Intermittent, brief, sudden, repetitive, stereotyped movements or sounds	Any body part can be affected; phonation sounds	Presumed to be basal ganglia
Hemiballism	Uncontrollable, rapid, large-amplitude flinging movements of a limb	Generally a limb	Basal ganglia – subthalamic nucleus striatum

spontaneous movements such as arm swing when walking; (2) rigidity, a form of increased resistance to passive manipulation in which the increased tone has a "plastic quality or "cogwheel" rigidity (in which resistance has a ratchet-like characteristic); (3) tremor, typically a 4- to 6-Hz resting tremor of the hands/arms, legs, or chin that improves with use of the affected body part; and (4) impairment of postural reflexes, manifested by falls or near falls, and difficulty in maintaining a stable stance when displaced backward on examination. Symptoms and findings are often asymmetrical, with onset on one side of the body. Patients commonly complain of incoordination, notably with fine motor tasks. Loss of facial expression (hypomimia or masked facies) or loss of voice amplitude (hypophonia) is common. Historical features often useful include difficulty with initiating or halting movement, especially getting in or out of chairs, and a history of micrographia.

The primary differential diagnosis is idiopathic Parkinson's disease, drug-induced Parkinsonism, and rare neurodegenerative disorders involving the basal ganglia. Medication history seeking history of exposure to antipsychotics, antiemetics, and some antihypertensives that can interfere with dopaminergic neurotransmission are documented.

Management. Drug therapy with dopamine replacement and/or dopamine agonists provides excellent symptomatic relief for several years. Many patients develop marked fluctuations in response to therapy, with periods of complex involuntary movements (dyskinesias). These dyskinesias have features of both dystonia and chorea occurring in close temporal association with periods of severe bradykinesia and rigidity. Decreasing medication doses or lengthening the dosing interval can improve choreic dyskinesias.

Nausea is a common problem associated with use of carbidopa/L-dopa or dopamine agonists. Orthostatic hypotension, another common complication can lead to syncope and falls, with their attendant consequences. All medications used in the treatment of Parkinson's disease can cause altered mental status. Frequent falls are a cause of minor, sometimes unnoticed, head trauma.

Many patients with Parkinson's disease can manifest varied pain symptoms such as muscle spasms, cramps, and burning paresthesias. Severe localized limb pain, chest pain, or abdominal pain in the patient with Parkinson's disease can cause confusion in the evaluation of such a patient. Discontinuation of dopamine replacement therapy can cause the neuroleptic malignant syndrome, which is a medical emergency (see Chapter 37, "Neurotoxicology").

Hyperkinetic Movement Disorders

The hallmark of hyperkinetic movement disorders is the intrusion of involuntary movements into the normal flow of motor acts. Hyperkinetic movement disorders include dystonia, chorea, hemiballism, and tics. See Table 13.2. A specific hyperkinetic movement disorder may not be present at all times in its standard form, and overlap of some of these disorders is common.

Dystonia

Dystonia is characterized by sustained (tonic), spasmodic (rapid or clonic), patterned, or repetitive muscular contractions that frequently result in a wide range of involuntary twisting, repetitive movements, or abnormal postures (e.g., neck torsion, forced jaw opening, or inversion and dorsiflexion of the foot).

Dystonia is one of the most frequently misdiagnosed neurological conditions. It can be misinterpreted as a psychiatric or a hysterical condition because of (1) the patient's bizarre movements and postures, (2) the finding of "action-induced dystonia" (the exacerbation of symptoms with stress and improvement with relaxation), (3) diurnal fluctuations, and (4) frequent effectiveness of various sensory tricks. See Table 13.3.

Specific Dystonias

➤*Idiopathic torsion dystonia (dystonia musculorum deformans).* Most common among Ashkenazi Jews, this is usually an autosomal dominant trait with variable penetrance. This is the most common childhood-onset primary dystonia.

Table 13.3. Etiologies of Seleted Dystonias

Dystonia Due to Degenerative Disorders of CNS	Dystonia Due to Nondegenerative Disorders of CNS
Parkinson's disease	Traumatic brain injury
Huntington disease	History of perinatal anoxia
Progressive supranuclear palsy	Kernicterus
Other degenerative disorders of the basal ganglia and midbrain	Stroke (cerebral infarction)
Wilson's disease	Arteriovenous malformation
Storage diseases	Encephalitis
GTP cyclohydrolase deficiency	Toxins (e.g., manganese)
Lesch-Nyhan disease	Brain tumors
Mitochondrial disorders	Multiple sclerosis
Leigh's syndrome	Drugs
	Peripheral trauma

➤*Focal dystonia.* Focal dystonia refers to the involvement of a specific part of the body. A primary dystonia that begins in adulthood is usually focal (e.g., spasmodic torticollis). Torticollis can mimic a variety of orthopedic and neurological disorders that are important to recognize in the ED (Table 13.4).

➤*Blepharospasm and oromandibular dystonia.* Blepharospasm (blinking that progresses to clonic and then tonic closure of the eyelids) is the second most common focal dystonia, either isolated or associated with oromandibular dystonia. Blepharospasm-oromandibular dystonia syndrome is commonly referred to as Meige syndrome.

➤*Torticollis.* Torticollis refers to dystonia-producing abnormal neck postures. Specifically, torticollis is rotation of the neck with anterocollis (flexion), retrocollis

Table 13.4. Disorders Simulating Dystonic Torticollis (Cervical Dystonia)

Neurological disorders:
    Posterior fossa tumor
    Focal seizures
    Bobble-head syndrome (third ventricular cyst)
    Syringomyelia
    Congenital nystagmus
    Extraocular muscle palsies
    Arnold-Chiari malformation
Musculoskeletal/structural:
    Herniated cervical disc
    Rotational atlantoxial subluxation
    Congenital muscular or ligamentous absence, laxity, or injury
    Bony spinal abnormalities: degenerative neoplastic infectious
    Cervical soft tissue lesions: adenitis, pharyngitis
    Labyrinthine disease
    Abnormal posture in utero

Source: Adapted from Weiner W, Lang A. *Movement Disorders: A Comprehensive Survey.* Mount Kisco, NY: Futura Publishing Company; 1989.

(extension), or laterocollis (lateral flexion). See Table 13.4 for causes and differential diagnosis of torticollis.

➤ *Secondary dystonias.* Secondary dystonias are a consequence of underlying metabolic disorders, degenerative processes, or structural lesions. Sudden onset, presence of dystonia at rest, rapid progression, or an unusual distribution such as hemidystonia in an adult suggests secondary dystonia. Hemidystonia suggests a focal lesion such as a mass, infarction, or hemorrhage of the basal ganglia.

Management. Treatment of drug-induced acute dystonia are reviewed in a later section. The patient with torticollis due to orthopedic or neurosurgically treatable disorders is referred to the appropriate specialist. Anticholinergic medications are frequently successful in ameliorating dystonia. Botulinum toxin is an effective therapy for treating focal dystonias.

Chorea

Chorea, the Greek term for dance, consists of involuntary irregular, rapid, jerky movements without a rhythmic pattern, randomly distributed with a flowing "dancelike" quality that involves multiple body parts. Athetosis (writhing movement) and ballism are part of the spectrum of chorea and appear to share a common pathophysiology, usually involving the striatum or subthalamic nucleus. Unlike primary dystonia, chorea/athetosis/ballism are regarded as symptoms of an underlying neurological disorder.

Evaluation and Differential Diagnosis. Chorea can be a presenting symptom of a variety of neurological and nonneurological disorders. See Table 13.5. L-dopa-induced chorea in patients with Parkinsonism is the "chorea" most commonly encountered in the emergency department. Systemic lupus erythematosus (SLE) and primary antiphospholipid antibody syndromes can be associated with chorea. Case reports of transient chorea due to multiple sclerosis have been reported. Structural lesions from cerebral infarctions involving the basal ganglia and thalamus can produce chorea. Stroke is likely the most common cause of hemichorea-hemiballismus. See Table 13.5 for other possible causes of chorea. Chorea gravidarum refers to choreiform movements associated with pregnancy (see Chapter 36, "Pregnancy-Related Neurological Emergencies").

Sydenham's chorea is a form of autoimmune chorea preceded by group A streptococcus infection, typically rheumatic fever. Sydenham's chorea occurs several months after the onset of acute streptococcal infection and usually affects patients between 5 and 15 years of age, girls more frequently than boys. There appears to be a familial prevalence, suggesting hereditary susceptibility. It tends to occur abruptly, worsens over 2–4 weeks, and usually resolves spontaneously in 3–6 weeks. Measurement of antistreptolysin-O titers can help physicians to detect recent streptococcal infection. However, Sydenham's chorea can occur six months after the streptococcal infection, and measurements of antistreptolysin-O and antistreptokinase antibody concentrations obtained later may not be helpful.

Hereditary and Degenerative Causes of Chorea. Huntington's disease (HD) is a hereditary neurodegenerative disorder characterized by chorea, incoordination,

Table 13.5. Differential Diagnosis of Chorea

Hereditary choreas
  Huntington's disease (classic choreiform movement)
  Neuroacanthocytosis
  Wilson's disease
  Binign familial chorea
  Inborn errors of metabolism
  Porphyria
  Ataxia-telangiectasia
  Tuberous sclerosis
Metabolic choreas
  Hyper- and hypothyroidism
  Hyper- and hypoparathyroidism
  Hypocalcemia
  Hyper- and hyponatremia
  Hypomagnesemia
  Hepatic encephalopathy
  Renal encephalopathy
Infectious or immunological choreas
  Sydenham'a chorea (postrheumatic fever)
  Chorea gravidarum
  Systemic lupus erythematosus
  Polycythemia vera
  Multiple sclerosis
  Sarcoidosis
  Viral encephalitis
  Tuberous meningitis
Cerebrovascular choreas
  Basal ganglia infarction
  Arteriovenous malformation
  Venous angiomata
  Polycythemia
Structural choreas
  Posttraumatic
  Subdural and epidural hematoma
  Tumor (primary CNS or metastatic)
Drugs/medications
  Phenytoin, phenothiazines, lithium,
  Amphetamines, oral contraceptives, levodopa
Toxins
  Mercury, carbon monoxide
Infections
  Neurosyphilis
  Lyme disease
  Subacute sclerosing panencephalitis

dementia, and numerous psychiatric problems. HD is the most common cho-reiform neurodegenerative disorder.

Patients with HD are evaluated in the ED for complications for their dis-ease that can require immediate care. Swallowing dysfunction leads to poor nutrition and/or aspiration pneumonia, and sometimes asphyxia. Poor balance and coordination cause frequent falls. Because of cerebral atrophy, these patients are prone to subdural hematomas. Severe dysarthria, dysphagia, dementia, and loss of ambulation occur in the final stages of the disease. Psychiatric disorders are common and associated with a high rate of suicide (see Table 13.5). The dopamine receptor antagonist haloperidol is the medication most frequently used to control symptoms in HD. Dopamine-depleting agents such as reserpine or tetrabenazine can also be effective.

Hemiballism

Characteristics. Uncontrollable, rapid, large-amplitude proximal flinging movements of a limb characterize this movement disorder. Unilateral involvement is termed hemiballism, whereas rare bilateral involvement is called biballism. Typically, the face is not affected. Hemiballism is an extreme form of hemichorea and is part of a spectrum that includes chorea and athetosis. Hemiballism can occur from lesions in parts of the basal ganglia and the thalamus.

Evaluation and Management. The most common cause of hemiballism is stroke, generally a lacunar infarct in the subthalamic nucleus. Hemiballism occurs most frequently in individuals over 60 years of age with risk factors for stroke. Neuroleptic medication such as haloperidol is the most effective drug therapy.

Tics

Tics characterized by intermittent, sudden, repetitive, stereotyped movements (motor tics) or sounds (vocal tics) are the most common movement disorders. Tics can be abrupt and fast, or slow and sustained. Tics can result from contraction of only one group of muscles, causing simple tics, which are brief, jerklike movements or single, meaningless sounds. Complex tics result from a coordinated sequence of movements. Tics can be suppressed temporarily, and often wax and wane in type, frequency, and severity. Disorders associated with tics are listed in Table 13.6.

The most well-known tic disorder is *Gilles de la Tourette's syndrome*. Tourette's syndrome (TS) is a disorder characterized by childhood onset of motor and vocal tics. Obsessive-compulsive disorder (OCD) and attention deficit hyperactivity disorder (ADHD) are strongly associated with TS. Tics tend to worsen in adolescence and abate in adulthood. Haloperidol is used in doses ranging from 0.25 to 2.5 mg per day for control of symptoms. Higher doses can be used acutely. Clonidine, an alpha$_2$-adrenergic receptor agonist, is also used in treating TS. Selective serotonin reuptake inhibitors such as fluoxetine are widely used to treat OCD, which is frequently associated with TS.

Tremors

Characteristics. Tremors are defined as involuntary, rhythmic, and roughly sinusoidal movements. They are characterized as resting, postural, kinetic (goal-oriented activity), or task-related. *Intention tremor* is an imprecise term generally used to describe wide oscillations that occur when a limb approaches a precise destination.

Table 13.6. Etiological Classification of Tics

Primary tic disorders
Tourette's syndrome
Various chronic tic disorders

Secondary tic disorders

Inherited:	Huntington's disease
	Neuroacanthocytosis
	Torsion dystonia
	Chromosomal abnormalities
Acquired:	*Drugs* – neuroleptics, stimulants, anticonvulsants, levodopa
	Trauma
	Infections – encephalitis, Creutzfeldt-Jakob disease, Sydenham's chorea
	Developmental – mental retardation, static encephalopathy, autism, pervasive developmental disorder
	Stroke
	Degenerative – Parkinsonism, progressive supranuclear palsy
	Toxic – carbon monoxide poisoning

Source: Adapted with permission from Kurlan R, ed., *Treatment of Movement Disorders*, Philadelphia, Pa: JB Lippincott; 1995.

Physiological tremor, a normal phenomenon due to the viscoelastic properties of joints and limbs, can worsen because of anxiety, fatigue, or stress (Table 13.7). Hypoglycemia, hyperthyroidism, and pheochromocytoma can enhance physiological tremors (Tables 13.7 and 13.8).

Essential tremor (ET) is characterized by postural and kinetic tremor with no identifiable cause or neurological findings. ET is a slowly progressive disorder with variable clinical expression. Patients typically complain of difficulty with eating, writing, and drinking. A useful diagnostic maneuver is to have patients drink a cup of water. Affected individuals will have a marked exacerbation of tremor while holding the cup, which worsens as the cup approaches the mouth. Findings that support the diagnosis of ET include improvement with the use of alcohol, propranolol, or primidone.

➤ *Orthostatic tremor* is a rare but frequently misdiagnosed condition. It occurs more frequently in women, and the onset is typically in the sixth decade. It manifests as tremor of the legs triggered by standing.

Table 13.7. Conditions that Can Enhance Physiological Tremor

Mental state: anger, anxiety, stress, fatigue, excitement
Metabolic: fever, thyrotoxicosis, pheochromocytoma, hypoglycemia
Drugs and toxins: (see Table 13.8)
Miscellaneous: caffeinated beverages, monosodium glutamate, nicotine

Source: Adapted from Weiner W, Lang A. *Movement Disorders: A Comprehensive Survey*. Mount Kisco, NY: Futura; 1989.

Table 13.8. Well-Known Causes of Tremor

Physiological
Pathological
   Essential tremor
   Parkinson's disease
   Wilson's disease
   Midbrain tremor
   Peripheral neuropathy
   Multiple sclerosis
   Cerebellar infarction
   Cerebellar degenerative disorders
Drugs and toxins
   Neuroleptics
   Lithium
   Adrenocorticosteroids
   Beta-adrenergic receptor agonists
   Theophylline
   Ethanol
   Calcium channel blockers
   Valproic acid
   Thyroid hormone
   Caffeine
   Nicotine
   Tricyclic antidepressants
Psychogenic

➤*Cerebellar tremor* is a common consequence of injury to the cerebellum or its outflow pathways. This type of tremor can have resting, postural, and kinetic components associated with ataxia, dysmetria, and other signs of cerebellar dysfunction.

➤*Psychogenic tremor* is the typical hysterical movement disorder. Careful observation of the patient with psychogenic tremor reveals marked fluctuation of the tremor. See Table 13.9.

Myoclonus

Myoclonus is defined as brief, very rapid, sudden, and shocklike jerks that involve very small muscles or the entire body. These movements can be caused by active

Table 13.9. Features of Psychogenic Tremor

1. History of many undiagnosed conditions
2. History of multiple somatizations
3. Absence of significant finding on physical examination or imaging study
4. Presence of secondary gain (pending compensation or litigation)
5. Spontaneous remissions and exacerbations
6. Employment in the health care delivery field
7. History of psychiatric illness

muscle contractions (positive myoclonus) or lapses in posture or muscle contractions (negative myoclonus or asterixis). Hiccup (diaphragmatic myoclonus) is a good example of physiological myoclonus. Myoclonus is a descriptive term and not a diagnosis.

Classification and Clinical Features. The four broad categories of myoclonus are (1) physiological, (2) essential or idiopathic, (3) epileptic, and (4) symptomatic.

➤*Physiological myoclonus* occurs in normal people and includes sleep (hypnic) jerks, anxiety-induced myoclonus, exercise-induced myoclonus, and hiccup.
➤*Essential (idiopathic) myoclonus* is likely a hereditary disorder, which begins at a young age and generally has a benign course.
➤*Epileptic myoclonus*, as the term suggests, occurs in the setting of a seizure disorder and is a component of several different epileptic syndromes. Myoclonus can occur as a component of a seizure or as the sole manifestation of a seizure.
➤*Symptomatic myoclonus,* the most common cause of myoclonus, refers to syndromes associated with an identifiable underlying disorder. Symptomatic myoclonus resulting from metabolic derangements such as uremia, hepatic coma, hypercapnia, and hypoglycemia usually produce multifocal, arrhythmic myoclonic jerks predominantly affecting the face and proximal musculature. Changes in mental status are characteristic. The myoclonus resolves as the encephalopathy is corrected.

Posthypoxic myoclonus resulting from global cerebral hypoxia from any cause occurs in two forms. Transient rhythmic myoclonic jerks, signifying a very poor prognosis, can appear immediately following the hypoxic injury, while the patient is comatose. The second clinical form is delayed posthypoxic myoclonus, known as Lance-Adams syndrome, which is observed in patients during recovery from coma following cerebral hypoxic injury.

Asterixis, or negative myoclonus, was described originally in patients with hepatic encephalopathy but occurs in numerous other metabolic or toxic disorders. Asterixis can occur in the recovery phase of general anesthesia, with sedative or anticonvulsant drug administration, and in normal drowsy individuals.

Management. Although rare, intractable myoclonus (as in viral encephalitis) can cause hyperthermia, hyperkalemia, hyperuricemia, systemic hypotension, and renal failure secondary to rhabdomyolysis. In certain situations, valproic acid and clonazepam are effective in treating symptomatic myoclonus. Physiological myoclonus does not require specific treatment.

Movement Disorders Caused by Commonly Used Drugs

The cause-and-effect relationship between the drug and the movement disorder is poorly understood, but preexisting central nervous system (CNS) pathology likely predisposes to the development of movement disorders.

Commonly prescribed medications that result in movement disorders include (a) antiepileptics, (b) neuroleptic, (c) stimulants, (d) oral contraceptives, (e) antihistaminics and anticholinergics, and (f) antidepressants.

Antiepileptic Agents

Cerebellar signs including nystagmus, dysarthria, and ataxia are commonly associated with toxic levels of antiepileptics, most typically phenytoin and carbamazepine. Asterixis and spontaneous myoclonic jerks are common in the toxicity of phenytoin, phenobarbital, primidone, and carbamazepine. Chorea and dystonia can be observed with antiepileptic drug use. Chorea is generally associated with the chronic use of multiple antiepileptics. Postural tremor, similar to benign essential tremor or enhanced physiological tremor, is observed in approximately 20–25% of patients taking valproate.

Neuroleptic Agents

The literal meaning of neuroleptic is "that which grips the nerve." There are five major categories of movement disorders associated with the use of neuroleptic medications: (i) acute dystonic reaction (ADR); (ii) akathisia; (iii) drug-induced Parkinsonism; (iv) tardive disorders, and (v) neuroleptic malignant syndrome (NMS).

(i) ADR. Of episodes of ADR, 95% occur within 96 hours of initiation of therapy. ADR has a familial incidence and is more common in children, and young males, and in relatives of patients with idiopathic torsion dystonia (ITD). Females between the ages of 12 and 19 years are more prone to metoclopramide (Reglan)-induced ADR. A history of ADR with neuroleptic therapy is an indicator for future risk. Cocaine abuse increases the risk of neuroleptic-induced ADR. ADR typically involves cranial or truncal musculature. Children tend to have more generalized involvement, particularly the trunk and extremities. ADR is the most common cause of oculogyric crisis, which consists of forced conjugate eye deviation upward or laterally, often accompanied by extension or lateral movements of the neck, mouth opening, and tongue protrusion. ADR typically follows a varied course, with symptoms lasting from minutes to hours. ADR can be difficult to diagnose in the ED because abnormal movements can subside or fluctuate spontaneously.

The risk of developing ADR increases with the potency of the neuroleptic and occurs more frequently with parental neuroleptics than with oral medications. ADR resolves spontaneously when the offending drug is withheld. The duration of symptoms depends on the half-life of the drug. Symptoms of ADR can be controlled quickly by parenteral administration of anticholinergics such as benztropine (cogentin). This is given as initial dose of 2 mg intravenously, with a maintenance dose of 1–2 mg orally twice daily for 7–14 days. Benztropine is to prevent recurrence. Alternatively, diphenhydramine is given in a dose of 25–50 mg parenterally for rapid control of symptoms, and a maintenance dose of 25–50 mg orally 3–4 times daily for a few days.

(ii) Akathisia. Akathisia is a subjective sensation of restlessness commonly associated with the inability to remain seated. Abnormal limb sensation, inner restlessness, dysphoria, and anxiety are the commonly described symptoms associated with akathisia.

(iii) Drug-Induced Parkinsonism. Drug-induced Parkinsonism (DIP) can be caused by several different medications including neuroleptic medications, rarely

prescribed calcium channel blockers such as cinnarizine and flunarizine, anti-nausea medication (metoclopramide), and antihypertensive agents (reserpine). The features of DIP are generally indistinguishable from those of idiopathic Parkinsonism. A rhythmic, perioral, and perinasal tremor mimicking a rabbit chewing, termed rabbit syndrome, is typical of DIP.

(iv) Tardive Dyskinesia. Tardive dyskinesia (TD) occurs following prolonged use of neuroleptic medications in about 20% of patients treated with these drugs. TD is often precipitated or worsened when the dose of the neuroleptic is reduced or the drug is withdrawn. Increasing age increases the risk for developing tardive dyskinesia.

Involuntary stereotypical movements involving orofacial, neck, trunk, and axial muscles constitute the typical tardive dyskinesia.

(v) Neuroleptic Malignant Disorder. Neuroleptic malignant disorder is reviewed in Chapter 37, "Neurotoxicology."

Stimulants

Dextroamphetamine, methylphenidate (Ritalin), pemoline, and cocaine are all stimulant (dopaminomimetic) drugs with peripheral and central actions. Chorea, orofacial dyskinesia, stereotyped movements, dystonia, and tics are associated with these medications.

Oral Contraceptives

Chorea is the most frequently experienced movement disorder caused by the use of oral contraceptives in otherwise healthy young females. A unilateral distribution of chorea suggests the possibility of preexisting basal ganglia pathology. Symptoms generally abate within a few weeks following discontinuation of the contraceptive.

Antihistaminics and Anticholinergics

The use of chlorpheniramine, brompheniramine, phenindamine, and mebhydroline is associated with the development of orofacial dyskinesia, blepharospasm, ticlike movements, dystonia, and involuntary, semipurposeful movements of the hands. The H_2 receptor blockers cimetidine and ranitidine are associated with the development of postural and action tremor, dystonic reactions, Parkinsonism, confusion, and cerebellar dysfunction. The movement abnormalities induced by these agents are generally short-lived and resolve after the responsible medication is discontinued.

(F) Antidepressants

The use of monoamine oxidase (MAO) inhibitors is associated with tremors and less often with myoclonic jerks. Tricyclic antidepressants such as amitriptyline, imipramine, and nortriptyline cause choreiform movements infrequently, particularly orofacial dyskinesia.

PEARLS AND PITFALLS

- Movement disorders resulting from an acute event such as a stroke are rare but are commonly manifested in a localized body area or follow a "hemidistribution," as in hemidystonia or hemiballism.

- An emergency imaging study is most likely to yield positive results following the acute onset of focal, abnormal movements.

- Prescribed medications are the most common cause of mental status change in a patient with Parkinson's disease.

- Many patients with Parkinson's disease manifest varied pain symptoms such as painful muscle spasms, cramps, and burning paresthesias. Localized limb pain, chest pain, and abdominal pain can be difficult to diagnose. Falls due to impaired postural reflexes can result in significant trauma.

- Torticollis is a focal dystonia producing abnormal neck postures that can be due to orthopedic and other neurological conditions.

- Neuroleptic medications and phenothiazines are responsible for most of the acute dystonic reactions evaluated in the emergency department.

- Although chorea can be a manifestation of immunological, infectious, metabolic, degenerative, or drug- and toxin-induced disorders, the most common "chorea" evaluated in the emergency department is L-dopa-induced chorea in a patient with Parkinson's disease.

- Chorea can be associated with the chronic use of numerous antiepileptic drugs.

- Transient tic disorder is common in children, with an estimated prevalence of 5–24% in school-age children. Conditions such as chronic cough or behavioral disorders can mimic this disorder.

- Asterixis, or negative myoclonus, was described originally in patients with hepatic encephalopathy but occurs in toxic and metabolic derangements including those related to drugs.

- Many movement disorders commonly evaluated in clinical practice are due to medication use.

SELECTED BIBLIOGRAPHY

Bradley W, Daroff R, Fenichel A, Marsden CD, eds. *Neurology in Clinical Practice*. Boston, Mass: Butterworth-Heinemann; 1991.

Caviness J. Myclonus. *Mayo Clin Proc*. 1996;71:679–88.

Dewey RB, Jankovic J. Hemiballism–hemichorea. Clinical and pharmacologic findings in 21 patients. *Arch Neurol*. 1989;46:862.

Elbe RJ, Koller WC. *Tremor*. Baltimore, Md: Johns Hopkins University Press; 1990.

Fahn S. The varied clinical expressions of dystonia. *Neurol Clin*. 1984;2:541–54.

Jankovic J, Tolosa E, eds. *Parkinson's Disease and Other Movement Disorders*. Baltimore, Md: Urban and Schwarzenberg; 1987.

Johnson WG, Fahn S. Treatment of vascular hemiballism and hemichorea. *Neurology*. 1977;27:634.

Koller WC. Sensory symptoms in Parkinson's disease. *Neurology*. 1984;34:957.

Kurlan R, ed. *Treatment of Movement Disorders*. Philadelphia, Pa: JB Lippincott; 1995.

Kurlan R, Lichter D, Hewitt D. Sensory tics in Tourette's syndrome. *Neurology*. 1989;39:731.

Marsden CD, Fahn S, eds. *Movement Disorders*. London: Butterworth; 1982.

Pranzatelli MR, Snodgrass SR. The pharmacology of myoclonus. *Clin Neuropharmacol*. 1985;8:99–130.

Shoulson I. On Chorea. *Clin Neuropharmacol*. 1986;9:585.

Weiner WJ, Lang AE. *Movement Disorders: A Comprehensive Survey*. Mount Kisco, NY: Futura; 1989.

Young RR, Shahani BT. Asterixis: one type of negative myoclonus. *Adv Neurol*. 1986;43:137.

14 Peripheral Nervous System and Neuromuscular Disorders

John J. Wald and James W. Albers

INTRODUCTION

The hallmarks of peripheral nervous system (PNS) disorders and neuromuscular diseases are weakness, numbness, or pain. These patients present to the emergency department (ED) when (1) there is rapid progression of disease, (2) the disease process is associated with pain, and (3) speech, swallowing, or breathing are involved. Identifying abnormal eye movements, facial movements, and phonation is important since these are affected by nerve, muscle, or neuromuscular junction disease. Extraocular eye movements are commonly abnormal early in myasthenia gravis. Understanding the underlying disease mechanisms and the typical course of these disorders directs testing, diagnosis, treatment, and disposition.

Selective characterization and associated disorders of the PNS include:

1. *Nerve roots* (dorsal or sensory, ventral or motor) exit the brainstem or spinal cord. Disorders of nerve roots give rise to radiculopathies.
2. *Mixed nerves* are formed by the dorsal and ventral nerve roots and exit from the skull or the spinal column. Examples of a collection of mixed nerves are the brachial plexus and lumbosacral plexus (in the subclavicular and retroperitoneal areas, respectively). Disorders involving a plexus is called a plexopathy.
3. *Peripheral nerves* travel from the plexus to end organs, including afferent (sensory), efferent (motor), and autonomic nerve fibers. Disorders affecting peripheral nerves are the various polyneuropathies (such as Guillain-Barré syndrome) and mononeuropathies.
4. *Neuromuscular junction* transduces motor-nerve depolarization to muscle contraction. Examples of disorders of defective neuromuscular transmission are myasthenia gravis and botulism.
5. *Muscle* is the end organ producing contraction and movement. Disorders involving the muscle are the various myopathies and certain systemic disorders.
6. *Motor neuron* disorders that primarily involve the PNS also affect the central nervous system (CNS). A disorder specifically involving motor neurons is amyotrophic lateral sclerosis (ALS).

Evaluation

Acute exacerbation of a neuromuscular disorder can have a rapid transition from unlabored breathing to decompensation and hypoventilation because of muscular fatigue (e.g., myasthenia gravis), or with aspiration of oral secretions in patients with marginal ventilatory function (e.g., ALS). As decompensation can occur abruptly, respiratory rate can provides false reassurance. It is important to ask patients if they are tiring and to note increasing anxiety. The forced vital capacity (FVC) and maximal negative inspiratory force (NIF) are useful quantitative measures of ventilatory muscle function. An FVC of less than 15 ml/kg or NIF of less than 15 mm Hg indicates the need for elective intubation. Aspiration can occur in the patient with dysphagia even with adequate ventilatory function and requires tracheal intubation (with placement of nasogastric feeding tube) to protect the airway.

Other factors requiring emergent attention include cardiac arrhythmias and volatile blood pressure changes that can result from autonomic nervous system involvement in peripheral nerve disorders. Rhabdomyolysis occurs after muscle injury due to trauma, overexertion, prolonged excessive external pressure (e.g., unconscious or obtunded patient), internal pressure (e.g., compartment syndrome), alcohol, drug (prescribed or illicit) and toxin exposure, and infections. Unprovoked rhabdomyolysis occurs with metabolic and mitochondrial muscle disorders. Treatment consists of hydration, which may begin in the field, and forced diuresis with alkalinization.

Information regarding underlying neuromuscular illness, whether controlled or quiescent, is important. Patients with neuromuscular junction, peripheral nerve, or muscle disorders are prone to unexpected "toxicities" after administration of certain agents and prescribed medications. For example, questions often arise when choosing antibiotics for patients with myasthenia gravis, anticonvulsants for patients with porphyria, or cholesterol-lowering agents for patients with myopathies.

Focused Examination of PNS

Strength Testing. Strength testing is performed by assessing the power of several proximal and distal muscle groups and by noting patterns of weakness and asymmetry. A screening examination includes shoulder abduction, elbow flexion/extension, wrist flexion/extension, hip flexion/extension, knee flexion/extension, and ankle plantar flexion/dorsiflexion. Symmetrical weakness that is diffuse and greatest proximally suggests myopathy. Weakness that is greatest distally suggests neuropathy. Asymmetrical weakness in the distribution of one or several nerve root(s) or specific nerve(s) is consistent with localized disease such as a herniated disk causing radiculopathy, or local compression causing mononeuropathy (Table 14.1). Weakness that is made worse by repeated testing suggests abnormal fatigability as seen in neuromuscular junction disorders.

Sensory Testing. Numbness indicates the need for sensory testing to determine the patient's ability to perceive sensory stimuli. Pain is tested by gently touching the patient with a pin or other sharp object, inquiring whether the sensation produced is similar with side-to-side and proximal-to-distal comparisons. Sensation carried by the large nerve fibers is tested using a vibrating 128-Hz tuning fork.

Table 14.1. Nerve Root Distribution Suggested by Pattern of Weakness and Reflex Change

Nerve Root	Weakness	Reflex Diminished or Absent
Upper extremity		
C5,6	Shoulder abduction, elbow flexion	Biceps, brachioradialis
C7	Elbow, wrist extension	Triceps
C8	Wrist, finger flexion	Triceps
T1	Finger, thumb abduction, adduction, opposition	
Lower extremity		
L2,3,4	Hip flexion, knee extension	Patellar
L5	Ankle dorsiflexion, inversion, eversion	Internal hamstring
S1	Ankle plantar flexion	Achilles

Sensory loss that is diffuse, symmetrical, and greatest distally suggests a peripheral polyneuropathy. Sensory loss that is asymmetrical or "focal" in the distribution of one or several nerve root(s) or specific nerve(s) is more consistent with localized disease and requires more refined sensory testing to determine which dermatome (Figure 14.1) or cutaneous nerve distribution (Figure 14.2) is affected. Detailed sensory testing fatigues the patient and examiner, and except for observable responses (e.g., grimacing), the results of clinical sensory testing are subjective.

Reflexes. Upper motor neuron involvement (e.g., ALS, stroke) is suggested when the reflex is unexpectedly brisk; nerve root, plexus, or nerve involvement is suggested by a diminished reflex. Reflex loss or diminution that is diffuse, symmetrical, and greatest distally suggests polyneuropathy. Deep tendon reflex (DTR) loss that is asymmetrical or "focal" in the distribution of one or several nerve root(s) or specific nerve(s) suggests localized disease (Table 14.1). Several cutaneous reflexes are tested. The Babinski response is tested by scratching the sole of the foot; great toe extension indicates an upper motor neuron abnormality.

The findings of the neurological examination are integrated into a neuroanatomical localization and differential diagnosis. Weakness in the distribution of a given nerve root that is accompanied by the appropriate sensory and DTR abnormalities is consistent with radiculopathy. Proximal weakness with normal sensation and normal DTRs is most likely due to myopathy (Figure 14.3).

Differential Diagnosis and Management

Specific anatomical and physiological changes, as well as diagnostic and management considerations, are grouped by disease entity, beginning with the nerve roots and proceeding peripherally.

[A] Disorders Involving Nerve Roots

Radiculopathy
Acute pain radiating into the dermatomal distribution of a given nerve root, with associated weakness, sensory loss, and diminished DTRs (when available for the

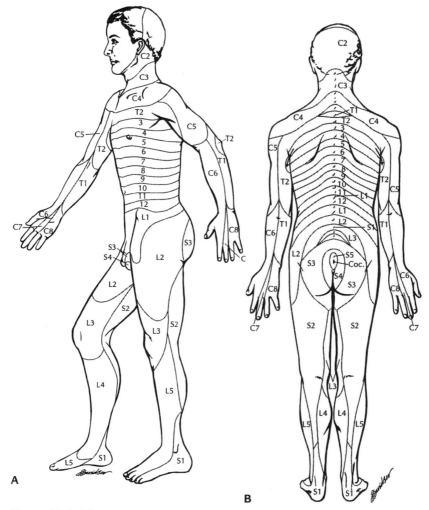

Figure 14.1. Diagram of dermatomes, anterior (A) and posterior (B) views.

root in question), is the hallmark of compressive radiculopathy due to disk herniation or bony degenerative disease. The nerve roots can be involved in several
other neuromuscular disorders (Table 14.2). Pain is variable. Bowel and bladder
functions are evaluated. Diffuse or progressive symptoms and signs require neurological consultation or hospital admission for documentation of progression,
pain control, and further neurological evaluation.

[B] Disorders of Mixed Nerves

Plexopathy
The brachial plexus and lumbosacral plexus are the regions distal to the nerve
roots where the roots intermix to form specific nerves. Plexopathy is considered when muscle weakness or sensory loss is in a distribution greater than
a single nerve root or peripheral nerve. Definitive diagnosis typically requires

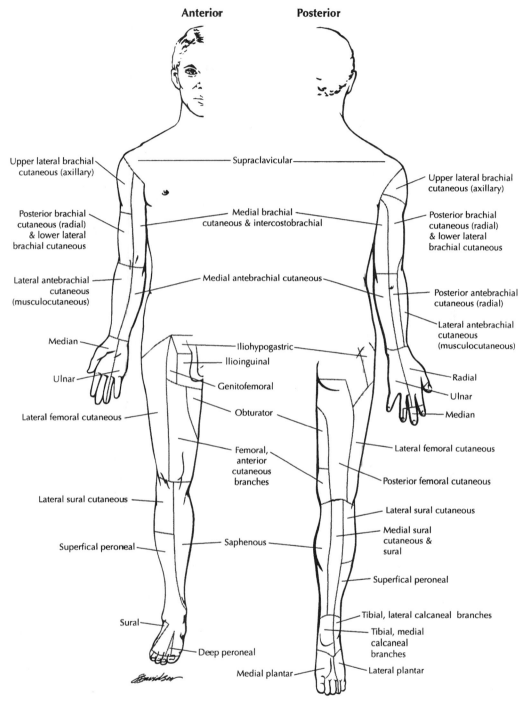

Figure 14.2. Diagram of peripheral nerve sensory distribution, anterior and posterior views.

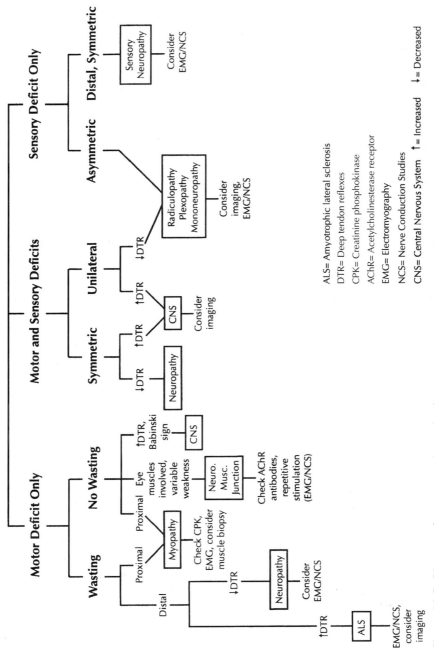

Figure 14.3. Diagram of neuromuscular evaluation.

ALS= Amyotrophic lateral sclerosis

DTR= Deep tendon reflexes

CPK= Creatinine phosphokinase

AChR= Acetylcholinesterase receptor

EMG= Electromyography

NCS= Nerve Conduction Studies

CNS= Central Nervous System   ↑= Increased   ↓= Decreased

Table 14.2. Etiologies of Radiculopathy

Etiology	Signs/Symptoms	Diagnostic Aids	Treatment
Trauma, spinal degenerative disease	Pain, weakness, numbness, diminished DTRs	Imaging, EMG	Bed rest, physical therapy, analgesia, surgery
Infectious (herpes zoster, CMV, HIV, Lyme)	Pain, weakness, numbness, diminished DTRs	Spinal fluid, skin change, evidence of systemic disease	Treat underlying infection
Inflammatory (GBS, CIDP)	Weakness, numbness, diminished DTRs, +/2pain	EMG/NCS, spinal fluid	See text
Metabolic (diabetes mellitus)	Anterior thigh pain, thoracic pain, +/2evidence of polyneuropathy	EMG/NCS, spinal fluid, evidence of diabetes	Analgesia, improved glucose control
Malignant invasion	Pain, weakness, numbness, diminished DTRs	EMG/NCS, spinal fluid, evidence of systemic malignancy	Analgesia, treatment of malignancy

electromyograph (EMG) evaluation. Multiple radiculopathies or mononeuropathies can mimic a plexopathy, often requiring extensive evaluation and imaging for precise localization. Historical features such as trauma, limb positioning, recent immunization, underlying medical conditions (malignancy, collagen vascular disease), and exposure to radiotherapy are helpful in arriving at a diagnosis. The pattern of weakness can suggest the region of the plexus involved (Table 14.3).

Brachial Plexus. The most common etiologies of brachial plexopathy are traumatic or radiation-induced injury, idiopathic (presumed to be inflammatory, occasionally preceded by immunization), and infiltration or compression by malignancies. Trauma is a common cause of brachial plexus injury. Forces causing downward shoulder movement (such as a forceful blow) injure the upper trunk, causing weakness of shoulder and proximal arm muscles and proximal sensory loss. Upward shoulder displacement (reaching for a handhold when falling) injures the lower trunk causing hand muscle weakness and sensory loss along the ulnar (medial) side of the hand. Shoulder and neck trauma, as in contact sports, can cause transient burning or stinging of the shoulder, arms, or hands ("burners" or "stingers"), which are likely milder, transient forms of plexus injury.

Table 14.3. Distribution of Weakness in Brachial Plexopathy

Trunk	Clinical Findings
Upper	Weakness of arm abduction, elbow flexion; diminished biceps reflex
Middle	Weakness of elbow, wrist, and finger extension; diminished triceps reflex
Lower	Weakness of intrinsic hand muscles

Idiopathic Brachial Plexopathy. Idiopathic brachial plexopathy, also called Parsonage-Turner syndrome or idiopathic brachial plexus neuritis, usually begins acutely with severe unilateral neck and shoulder pain. Weakness develops within days, most prominent proximally, with only mild sensory impairment. Weeks later, atrophy becomes noticeable. Many patients have had an antecedent surgery, immunization, infection, or trauma, suggesting an autoimmune etiology similar to that in Guillain-Barré syndrome (GBS). Most patients have good recovery of function; pain subsides in several weeks, and strength returns slowly, usually within 12 months, consistent with the rate of reinnervation.

Lumbosacral Plexus. Lower extremity symptoms/signs involving the distribution of several nerves (e.g., sciatic and femoral) suggest lumbosacral plexus localization, although polyradiculopathy is also considered. Etiologies of lumbosacral plexopathy are similar to those of brachial plexopathy but also include retroperitoneal hemorrhage in patients receiving anticoagulant therapy and "diabetic amyotrophy" in diabetic patients. Traumatic lesions of the lumbosacral plexus are commonly associated with major pelvic trauma. The most common nontraumatic lumbosacral plexopathy is diabetic amyotrophy, presenting with proximal leg pain followed by weakness beginning days later.

[C] Disorders of Peripheral Nerves

Polyneuropathy

The hallmarks of polyneuropathy are distal weakness and numbness. Examination findings are weakness, distal sensory loss, and hyporeflexia or areflexia. The most common acute presentations are the acute or chronic inflammatory demyelinating polyneuropathies. The patients with the acute form of inflammatory polyneuropathy (GBS) typically develop respiratory failure, requiring ventilatory support, and clinically significant dysautonomia. See Chapter 15, "Guillain-Barré Syndrome."

Chronic Inflammatory Demyelinating Polyneuropathy. Chronic inflammatory demyelinating polyneuropathy (CIDP) is a progressive or relapsing polyneuropathy that resembles GBS.

Mononeuropathy

Mononeuropathies produce abnormal motor or sensory function, usually both, in the distribution of a peripheral nerve. Etiologies are diverse, including acute trauma, repetitive minor trauma, and injury related to metabolic (diabetes) or vascular disease. Compressive or traumatic mononeuropathy can produce pain and nerve tenderness at the site of injury. Compressive injury commonly occurs during sleep or decreased consciousness. Features of several common mononeuropathies are described in Table 14.4. When several mononeuropathies are present, mononeuritis multiplex, or "multiple mononeuropathies," is considered. *Mononeuritis multiplex* refers to involvement of several isolated nerves, which can be widely separated, such as right median and left femoral nerve. Motor and sensory abnormalities are confined to the area innervated by the individual nerve. This syndrome is associated with diabetes, malignancy, and collagen vascular disorders. Disseminated vasculitis is believed to be the underlying pathology.

Table 14.4. Selected Examples of Mononeuropathy

Nerve Involved	Common Sites of Compression, Entrapment	Distribution of Weakness	Distribution of Sensory Loss	Frequent Cause	Clinically Useful Muscle(s)
Facial	Stylomastoid foramen	Face	None	Idiopathic	Face
Median	Wrist	Thumb abduction, opposition	Digits 1 and 2	Wrist flexion/extension, compression at ventral wrist, diabetes	Abductor pollicus brevis
Ulnar	Wrist, elbow	Hand, intrinsic muscles	Digits 4 and 5	Elbow trauma, compression from limb positioning	First dorsal interossei (abduct index finger)
Radial	Spiral groove (lower humerus)	Extensors of wrist and fingers	Dorsal arm and hand	Arm draped over back of chair, bed partner's head on outstretched arm, lead intoxication	Weak brachioradialis, wrist extensors normal triceps (innervated above spiral groove)
Femoral	Inguinal ligament, retroperitoneal space	Knee extension, hip flexion	Anterior thigh	Hip abduction, external rotation, direct compression, hemorrhage into the iliacus, retroperitoneal tumors, or diabetes mellitus (diabetic amyotrophy)	Quadriceps
Sciatic		Leg flexor (hamstring), all muscles below the knee	Lower leg and foot	Fracture, dislocation, surgery (at hip), compression in unconscious patient, IM injections, aneurysm, hematoma	
Peroneal	Fibular head (knee)	Foot dorsiflexion, eversion	Lateral leg, dorsum of foot	Prolonged squatting, bed rest, crossed legs	Ankle dorsiflexors

Facial. Facial nerve mononeuropathy *(Bell's palsy)*, a relatively common mono-neuropathy produces acute or subacute facial weakness. The etiology and patho-physiology of Bell's palsy remain unknown, although compression or swelling of the nerve within the facial canal may play a role. There can be associated pain behind the ear, hyperacusis, and altered taste sensation, depending on which area of the facial nerve is involved. Hyperacusis results from weakness of the stapedius muscle which is no longer able to contract adequately to tighten the ossicular chain and protect the inner ear from loud noises.

Facial weakness due to facial nerve involvement (i.e., not due to CNS disease) involves the entire face, including muscles that furrow the brow. Involvement of other cranial nerves (true facial numbness, diplopia, speech/swallowing abnor-malities) or more diffuse weakness suggests alternate diagnoses and requires more extensive evaluation.

Supranuclear facial palsy (central facial palsy) refers to a lesion in the supranu-clear corticobulbar lesions producing contralateral paresis of the lower portion of the face with sparing of the upper facial muscles. The upper part of the face is spared because its supranuclear control has both ipsilateral and contralateral representation, whereas the lower face has mainly contralateral supranuclear con-nections. Supranuclear facial palsy is essentially a "central" event and evaluation proceeds in that direction.

Treatment of Bell's palsy is controversial. Many advocate prednisone in doses of approximately 1 mg/kg followed by a rapid taper. Others suggest that the good prognosis without treatment (>80% with complete recovery) militates against steroid therapy. Acyclovir has been used in conjunction with steroid therapy. However, its effectiveness has not been fully established. All patients with facial weakness require corneal protection until eye closure returns. This is accom-plished with moisturizing drops (artificial tears) and ointment, or patching at night.

[D] Disorders of Neuromuscular Transmission

Neuromuscular junctions transduce a nerve action potential into muscle mem-brane depolarization and subsequent muscle contraction. Defective function in this region leads to weakness without numbness or pain. When a patient with weakness is evaluated, neuromuscular junction disorders such as myasthenia gravis (MG), anticholinesterase toxicity, Lambert-Eaton myasthenic syndrome (LEMS), and botulism are considered.

Myasthenia gravis is one of the best understood autoimmune disorders. It is characterized by a rapid fatigability and weakness of voluntary muscles. These symptoms of MG are related to the binding of antibodies to acetylcholine recep-tors (AChRs). See Chapter 16, "Myasthenia Gravis."

Lambert-Eaton Myasthenic Syndrome. LEMS is another disease characterized by defective neuromuscular junction transmission, although this defect is associated with impaired release of acetylcholine (ACh). LEMS is characterized by progressive weakness and autonomic features including dry mouth and impotence. Patients with LEMS can resemble those with MG, although bulbar muscles are usually spared in the former.

Treatment of patients with LEMS includes anticholinesterase medications (although they are less effective in patients with LEMS compared to the positive response in patients with MG), immunosuppression protocols similar to those used in MG, and 3,4-diaminopyridine (which improves presynaptic ACh release). Any identified underlying disorder (such as a small cell carcinoma) is addressed, and treatment of these conditions can lead to significant improvement or resolution of the LEMS symptoms.

Botulism. Botulinum toxin can produce acute, diffuse weakness associated with presynaptic neuromuscular junction dysfunction. Although rare, botulism is considered in the differential diagnosis of MG and GBS. Exposure (in adults) usually occurs from improper home canning. Clinically, extraocular and pupillary muscle involvement is important in differentiating botulism intoxication from other causes of acute weakness. Antibiotic and antitoxin therapies can be instituted following diagnosis.

[E] Disorders Involving Muscle and Muscle Function

Myopathy

Myopathies cause weakness and, at times, muscle discomfort (myalgia). Important factors in determining etiology include time course, recent trauma, medication or toxin exposure, underlying medical conditions, and recent infection. Patients typically have proximal muscle weakness. Ventilation or swallowing is affected infrequently. Myopathies range from those present at birth that remain relatively static to acquired inflammatory myositis associated with other medical conditions.

Inflammatory Myopathy. Inflammatory myopathy denotes three diseases: dermatomyositis (DM), polymyositis (PM), and inclusion body myositis (IBM). In these diseases, primarily (but not exclusively) skeletal muscle invasion by inflammatory cells occurs. DM is a humoral autoimmune attack directed primarily against muscle blood vessels. PM is a cell-mediated disease directed against muscle fibers. IBM is a distinct form of inflammatory myopathy with "inclusions" apparent on muscle biopsy, although the role of autoimmunity is unknown. Proximal muscle weakness is present in most patients with myopathy. Serum creatinine phosphokinase (CPK) and other cellular enzymes, such as, lactate dehydrogenase (LDH), are elevated in up to 90% of patients. A high erythrocyte sedimentation rate (ESR) or the presence of autoantibodies suggests the presence of an associated collagen vascular disorder. Corticosteroids, cytotoxic agents (azathioprine, cyclophosphamide, and methotrexate), and intravenous immunoglobulin (IVIG) are commonly used treatments.

Necrotizing Myopathy. Necrotizing myopathy, an acute or subacute onset of painful weakness with necrosis of muscle fibers, is commonly caused by myotoxins. A broad range of medications has been implicated in causing necrotizing myopathy. Lipid-lowering agents, including HMG-CoA-reductase inhibitors (particularly when given concurrently with cyclosporin or other immunosuppressants), nicotinic acid, and clofibrate have been associated with necrotizing myopathy. Other commonly encountered toxins producing necrotizing myopathy include substances of abuse such as cocaine, heroin, amphetamines, and alcohol.

Metabolic Myopathy. Metabolic myopathy implies muscle disease due to abnormal glycogen, lipid, or purine metabolism. There are many potential enzymatic defects, most of which are rare. Patients with metabolic myopathy can present with exercise-induced muscle pain, exercise intolerance, or progressive weakness.

Mitochondrial myopathy is a specific form of metabolic myopathy. Mitochondria are the site of the electron transport chain, generating adenosine triphosphate (ATP) through oxidative phosphorylation. Mitochondrial disorders can be inherited or acquired. Exacerbation of symptoms such as worsening weakness, pain, or altered consciousness leads to evaluation in the ED. Rapid determination of the blood glucose, lactic acid, pyruvate, and ammonia levels can lead to diagnosis and possibly direct further treatment (e.g., discovering hypoglycemia, a potential exacerbating factor, or lactic acidosis). Furthermore, obtaining a urine organic acid screen and a serum acyl-carnitine screen (which may be normal between attacks) can be helpful in diagnosis (however, these screens cannot assist with immediate diagnosis or treatment).

Dystrophy. Muscular dystrophies are inherited disorders causing progressive muscle weakness. Other organ systems are often involved. The best-understood dystrophy is Duchenne muscular dystrophy (DMD), an X-linked disorder of young males causing progressive weakness. As in most myopathies, DMD is characterized by elevated CPK and proximal muscle weakness. Diagnosis is made by analysis for muscle dystrophin, a cytoskeletal protein that is absent in DMD. Joint contractures, scoliosis, intellectual impairment, and electrocardiogram (EKG) abnormalities are common. Becker muscular dystrophy presents with less rapidly progressive weakness and is due to decreased or abnormal dystrophin.

Myotonic muscular dystrophy is the most common adult muscular dystrophy. It is a multisystem disorder characterized by limb weakness, facial muscle wasting, and weakness and frontal balding, producing a "hatchet face."

Periodic Paralysis. Acute, severe weakness with a history of similar previous attacks following exercise or carbohydrate meals is the hallmark of periodic paralysis. Commonly, there is a family history of similar attacks. Several conditions associated with altered potassium levels or metabolism are likely to produce these attacks, and these periodic paralyses are commonly classified according to the potassium abnormality present with the acute weakness (hypo-, normo-, and hyperkalemic periodic paralysis). Thyrotoxicosis, common in Asians, is related to a similar syndrome. There is considerable overlap between the hyperkalemic forms of periodic paralysis and rare myotonic conditions.

Respiratory muscle involvement is uncommon during attacks; cardiac arrhythmias are more common. During an episode of weakness, it is critical to obtain serial electrolyte measurements. In hypokalemic periodic paralysis, the potassium level is often less than 3.0 mEq/l, but can be "normal." Relative changes in the potassium concentration correlated with changes in the neurological examination are more significant than the actual potassium level. Treatment consists of normalizing the potassium level, either acutely during an attack of weakness or chronically to prevent attacks.

Systemic Conditions. Many underlying systemic conditions and their medical treatment can lead to myopathy. Hypo- or hyperthyroidism, hypo- or hyperkalemia, hypo- or hyperparathyroidism, hypo- or hypercalcemia, hypophosphatemia, hypomagnesemia, excess or insufficient adrenal function, and chronic renal insufficiency can be associated with underlying symptoms referable to muscle, including weakness. Medications, corticosteroids in particular, can cause myopathic weakness.

[F] Motor Neuron Disease

Motor neuron diseases involve diffuse, painless degeneration of the motor neurons without sensory involvement. Motor neuron disease is rarely diagnosed in the ED, but respiratory distress or aspiration of gastric contents requires evaluation in the ED. The most common motor neuron disease is ALS, also known as Lou Gehrig's disease.

Weakness is the hallmark of ALS. ALS involves degeneration of the upper motor neurons (causing hyperreflexia, spasticity, pseudobulbar affect) and lower motor neurons (causing weakness, wasting, and fasciculations). The pattern of hyperreflexia in weak, wasted limbs is fairly specific for ALS, although diagnosis requires exclusion of conditions such as lymphoma, viral infection, and spinal degenerative disease (e.g., cervical spondylosis), which can mimic this disorder.

When disease onset is bulbar, dysarthria and dysphagia are early symptoms. Upper motor neuron disorder presents with spasticity and hyperreflexia, but there is no muscle wasting, sensory change, or pain. The findings of hyperreflexia, muscle wasting, and fasciculations are most important in diagnosing this condition. EMG and nerve conduction studies (NCS) are helpful in excluding other conditions (myasthenia gravis, polyneuropathy) and in documenting the distribution and severity of disease. Thyroid and parathyroid function, serum calcium, serum protein electrophoresis, and measurement of anti-G_{M1} antibodies can exclude "mimicking" disorders. Magnetic resonance imaging (MRI) helps to exclude local pathology as an etiology of the upper and lower motor neuron degeneration. Treatment is primarily symptomatic and supportive. Riluzole, a benzothiazole, is currently available for treatment of ALS. Excessive emotional lability related to upper motor neuron and frontal lobe and involvement can be treated with tricyclic antidepressants. Excessive oral secretions are treated with anticholinergic medications. Cramps can be treated with quinine or phenytoin. Patients who have progressive bulbar dysfunction with aspiration and inadequate nutrition require a feeding gastrostomy tube.

PEARLS AND PITFALLS

Nerve Disease
- Patients with normal Achilles reflexes rarely have a clinically significant polyneuropathy.
- It can take up to 7 days for NCS changes to become evident after nerve injury, unless the nerve can be stimulated proximal to the injury.
- It can take up to 21 days for needle EMG abnormalities (fibrillation potentials, positive waves) to develop after nerve injury.
- Diabetes is the most common cause of polyneuropathy in the developed countries.
- GBS is considered in patients with newly recognized ascending numbness, weakness, or reflex loss.

Neuromuscular Junction Disease
- Rapid transition can occur from unlabored breathing to hypoventilation because of muscular fatigue (e.g., MG), or with aspiration of oral secretions. Normal blood gas measurements provide false reassurance.
- Consider potential neuromuscular blocking effects when prescribing any medication for a patient with MG.
- Any cause for elevated body temperature (infection, increased ambient temperature) worsens symptoms of MG.

Muscle Disease
- Proximal, painless, symmetrical, weakness suggests myopathy.
- Exertional muscle pain suggests metabolic myopathy; serum CPK, lactate, glucose, ammonia, and urine myoglobin should be measured.
- Consider potassium-sensitive paralysis in patients with acute severe weakness and a history of similar attacks.

Motor Neuron Disease
- Motor neuron disease is considered in any patient with painless, progressive asymmetrical weakness.

SELECTED BIBLIOGRAPHY

Aranason BGW, Soliven B. Acute inflammatory demyelinating polyradiculopathy. In: Dyck PJ, Thomas PK, Griffin JW, Low PA, Podulso JF, eds. *Peripheral Neuropathy*, 3rd ed. Philadelphia, Pa: WB Saunders; 1993;1437–97.

Asbury AK, Arnason BGW, Karp HR, McFarlin DE. Criteria for diagnosis of Guillain-Barré syndrome. *Ann Neurol*. 1978;3:565–6.

Dalakas MC. Current treatment of the inflammatory myopathies. *Curr Opin Rheumatol*. 1994;6:595–601.

DiMauro S, Moraes CT. Mitochondrial encephalomyopathies. *Arch Neurol*. 1993; 50:1197–208.

Drachman DB. Myasthenia gravis. *N Engl J Med*. 1994;330:1797–810.

Katusic SK, Beard M, Wiederholt WC, Bergstralh EJ, Kurland LT. Incidence, clinical features, and prognosis in Bell's palsy, Rochester, Minnesota, 1968–1982. *Ann Neurol*. 1986;20:622–7.

McEvoy KM. Diagnosis and treatment of Lambert-Eaton myasthenic syndrome. *Neurol Clin*. 1994;12:387–99.

Mendell J. Neuromuscular junction disorders: a guide to diagnosis and treatment. *Adv Neuroimmunol*. 1994;1:9–16.

Riggs JE. The periodic paralyses. *Neurol Clin*. 1988;6:485–98.

Ropper AH. The Guillain-Barré syndrome. *N Engl J Med*. 1992;326:1130–6.

Tsairis P, Dyck PJ, Mulder DW. Natural history of brachial plexus neuropathy. Report on 99 patients. *Arch Neurol*. 1972;27:109–17.

Wilbourn AJ. The diabetic neuropathies. In: Brown WF, Bolton CF, eds. *Clinical Electromyography*. Boston, Mass: Butterworth; 1987:329–64.

15 Guillain-Barré Syndrome

Sandeep Rana and Sid M. Shah

INTRODUCTION

Guillain-Barré syndrome (GBS) is a form of acute inflammatory (demyelinating) polyneuropathy. An acquired neuromuscular disorder, GBS is the most common disorder causing rapidly ascending numbness and weakness. GBS can affect any level of the peripheral nervous system, including the cranial nerves, nerve roots, peripheral nerves, and the autonomic nervous system. Acute, early presentation of GBS can be "atypical" with no pathognomonic features, confounding its diagnosis in an emergency setting. Failure to recognize a neurological illness is a common error in the early phase. Hence, GBS should be considered seriously in the differential diagnosis of new onset weakness in an otherwise healthy individual. The most important emergency concern in GBS is potential respiratory compromise due to muscular and diaphragmatic weakness.

Viral upper respiratory infection, gastroenteritis, and other antecedent events occur in more than 75% of the cases of GBS in the month prior to the onset of symptoms. *Campylobacter* enteritis has been linked to a fulminant form of GBS. Human immunodeficiency virus (HIV), systemic lupus erythematosus (SLE), Hodgkin's disease, sarcoidosis, and vaccinations may also trigger GBS (Table 15.1).

Emergency Presentation

The illness typically begins with diffuse paresthesias in the toes or fingertips, muscle pain, and cramps ("charley horse"), often in association with back pain. This is followed by weakness that makes walking or climbing stairs difficult. Most cases have distal to proximal ascending paralysis; however, variants are frequent. Pain is common, particularly in large muscles of the legs, arms, and back. Cranial

Table 15.1. Selected Clinical Entities Associated with GBS

Infection	Collagen Vascular Diseases	Vaccination Related	Others
Nonspecific viral illness	Systemic lupus erythematosus	Influenza vaccination	Hodgkin's lymphoma
Cytomegalovirus	Wegener's granulomatosis	Oral polio vaccination	Surgery, epidural anesthesia
Epstein-Barr virus	Sarcoidosis	Tetanus toxoid	Medication and drugs: Captopril, thrombolytic agents, heroin
HIV	Hashimoto's disease	Botulinum toxin therapy	Head trauma
Varicella			Henoch-Schönlein purpura
Hemophilus influ. type B			
Mycoplasma			
Hepatitis A, B, C			
Campylobacter			
Helicobacter jejuni			

nerves are commonly involved, producing facial weakness, difficulty chewing, and dysphagia. On rare ocassions extraocular muscles and pupillary muscles are involved. Deep tendon reflexes are absent or hypoactive. Sensory impairment is variable but generally there is minimal loss of sensation despite extensive paresthesias. The autonomic nervous system is involved in two-thirds of patients manifested as labile blood pressure (BP), cardiac arrhythmias, and bowel or bladder dysfunction (Table 15.2).

Weakness rarely progresses beyond 4 weeks with maximal weakness usually occurring by 7 to 14 days. Almost a third of patients develop respiratory insufficiency and require mechanical ventilation.

Table 15.2. Common Clinical Features of Typical GBS

Paresthesias	Initially "toes and fingers" then extremities "Charley horse" particularly in legs
Pain	Large muscle groups of arms and legs; muscle pain "crampy" Back pain may simulate sciatica
Weakness	Distal to proximal; variable Variable arm, facial, oropharyngeal Vital capacity – compromised
Autonomic symptoms	Bowel or bladder dysfunction Labile blood pressure, arrhythmias
Sensation	Variable; generally minimal loss

Table 15.3. Variants of GBS

Miller-Fisher syndrome	Ophthalmoplegia, ataxia, areflexia, little weakness

Weakness without paresthesias or sensory loss
Isolated weakness of arm, leg, or oropharynx
Bilateral facial weakness with distal paresthesias
Severe ataxia and sensory loss

Emergency Evaluation and Differential Diagnosis

In the early phase, a high index of suspicion for GBS is essential in the presence of ascending numbness and weakness because ancillary tests may not help. A normal cerebrospinal fluid (CSF) protein level in the early phase or a finding of numerous lymphocytes does not exclude the diagnosis of GBS. By end of first week of illness, CSF analysis usually reveals normal CSF pressure and elevated protein without leukocytosis termed albuminocytological dissociation. The extent of protein elevation varies; however, values greater than 2.5 g per liter raise suspicion of spinal cord compression. Pleocytosis can signify Lyme disease, neoplasia, HIV infection, sarcoid meningitis, and other diseases.

Blood count, chemistry profile, and other laboratory tests do not enhance the diagnosis of GBS but may be indicated for other associated conditions (Table 15.3). Computerized tomography (CT) imaging of the brain is not routinely recommended. Nerve conduction studies and electromyography (required to confirm the diagnosis) reveal prolonged distal latencies, slowing of conduction velocities, and conduction blocks with abnormal temporal dispersion (Tables 15.4 and 15.5).

Management

Despite advances in the treatment of GBS, good supportive care is still the most important determinant of favorable outcome. Cardiac monitoring is routine for patients with severe findings. Respiratory status is assessed with periodic vital capacities. Elective endotracheal intubation for ventilatory support is considered when the vital capacity is below 15 ml/kg. Manifestations of autonomic instability (i.e., labile BP and cardiac arrhythmias) are treated aggressively. Patients with severe weakness receive prophylaxis for deep vein thrombosis.

Two forms of immunomodulation, intravenous immunoglobulins and plasmapheresis, are efficacious in shortening the disease course. Patients presenting within 2 weeks of illness are treated with either one. It may be reasonable to treat beyond 2 weeks particularly when weakness progresses. The role of corticosteroids in the treatment of GBS has always been controversial and is generally not recommended.

Causes of death in patients with GBS include unrecognized respiratory failure, complications of artificial ventilation, pulmonary infection (usually nosocomial), cardiac arrhythmias, and pulmonary embolism.

Table 15.4. Diagnostic Criteria for Typical GBS

Features required for diagnosis
　　Progressive weakness in both arms and legs
　　Areflexia

Features strongly supporting the diagnosis
　　Paresthesias in legs and arms
　　Muscle pain, back pain
　　Progression of symptoms over days to 4 weeks
　　Relative symmetry of symptoms
　　Absent or mild sensory findings
　　Cranial nerve involvement, especially bilateral weakness of facial muscles
　　Autonomic dysfunction
　　Absence of fever at the onset
　　Elevated CSF protein level with < 50 cells per cubic mm
　　Typical electronmyograph and nerve conduction studies

Features making the diagnosis doubtful
　　Distinct sensory level
　　Persistent asymmetry of clinical findings
　　Severe bladder and bowel dysfunction
　　More than 50 cells per cubic mm in CSF

Table 15.5. Differential Diagnosis of GBS

Spinal cord lesions	Early involvement of sphincters
	Definite sensory level
	Babinski sign
Botulism (usually foodborne)	Symmetric weakness
	Extraocular eye muscle
	Weakness
	Pupillary (vision) changes
	Dysarthria
	Descending weakness (variable)
	Normal CSF and creatine phosphokinase (CPK)
	More fulminant course others affected
Acute necrotizing myopathy	Markedly elevated CPK
	Normal CSF
Periodic paralysis	Symmetric weakness (reverses quickly)
	Normal CSF and CPK
	No respiratory compromise
Myasthenia gravis	Fluctuating weakness
	Absence of sensory involvement
Chronic inflammatory demyelinating polyneuropathy (CIDP)	Stepwise course, progresses beyond 4 weeks
	Indistinguishable from GBS in the early phase

PEARLS AND PITFALLS

- In patients with GBS, deep tendon reflexes are absent or hypoactive. If reflexes are brisk, the diagnosis should be questioned.

- Weakness usually progresses over a few days. In some severe cases, rapid weakness may occur over a period of hours.

- Good supportive care is still the key to favorable prognosis.

- Most patients with GBS recover gradually over a period of months. Mortality rate is estimated to be about 5%. Usual cases of death are respiratory failure, sepsis, and cardiac arrhymias.

- Monitor respiratory status by serial measurement of vital capacities. Decisions regarding intubation should not be based on blood gas abnormalities as these often are late to occur.

SELECTED BIBLIOGRAPHY

Dyck PJ, Thomas PK, eds. *Peripheral Neuropathy,* 3rd ed. Philadelphia, Pa: WB Saunders; 1993.

Hughes R. *Guillain-Barré Syndrome.* London: Springer-Verlag; 1990.

Victor M, Ropper A, eds. *Adams and Victor's Principles of Neurology*, 7th ed. New York, NY: McGraw Hill; 2001.

16 Myasthenia Gravis

George A. Small and Mara Aloi

INTRODUCTION

Myasthenia gravis is the prototypic neuromuscular junction disorder and the most well-studied autoimmune disease. It causes varying diplopia, speech and swallowing difficulty, and commonly, respiratory failure. When properly recognized, the disease can be controlled, minimizing mortality and morbidity. When not, unexpected deaths and prolonged hospitalizations do occur. Myasthenia gravis is caused by antibodies that bind to postsynaptic acetylcholine receptors of the neuromuscular junction of skeletal muscle. These antibodies are detected in less than 50% of patients with ocular myasthenia and in 75% of patients with limb weakness. Because serologic testing for these antibodies takes days to be reported and may not be conclusive, emergency department (ED) evaluation is based on the recognition of the symptoms and signs of myasthenia gravis.

The prevalence of myasthenia gravis is 8 per 100,000 persons. It occurs most commonly in young women but also in older men, resulting in a bimodal incidence distribution. *Neonatal* myasthenia gravis is caused by the passive transfer of acetylcholine receptor (AChR) antibodies in utero from myasthenic mothers to the fetus. A weak cry or difficulty swallowing typically develops in the first 3 days of life and lasts for less than 5 weeks but can be severe. *Congenital* myasthenia gravis is a nonautoimmune disorder of infants born to mothers without myasthenia gravis and presents with cranial neuropathies and, at times, respiratory failure. The hallmark of this disease is fatigability. It is typically less severe than the neonatal form but is refractory to therapy.

The role of the thymus in the pathogenesis of the disease has not been fully elucidated. It has been hypothesized that the thymus is the site of autoantibody formation, but this remains unproven. Some degree of thymus abnormality is seen in up to 65% of patients with myasthenia gravis. Following the diagnosis of myasthenia gravis, patients should be evaluated for thymic pathology.

Classification

Group I – ocular involvement alone

Group IIA – mild generalized weakness

Group IIB – moderately severe generalized myasthenia gravis (Patients present with ocular myasthenia followed by gradual involvement of pharyngeal and limb muscles.)

Group III – patients with acute generalized myasthenia gravis with development of pharyngeal weakness, arm and leg weakness, and respiratory weakness

Group IV – patients with group III disease who progress despite the best medical therapy

Evaluation

The majority of patients with myasthenia gravis present to the ED with an exacerbation of the disease or complications of their medications. On rare occasions, a patient presents with undiagnosed disease. Although a myriad of symptoms and signs are possible, most have bulbar weakness and decreased exercise tolerance that improves with rest. Ptosis and painless intermittent diplopia suggest myasthenia gravis. Loss of visual acuity, pain, and any pupillary changes suggest alternative diagnoses. Approximately 30% of patients present with progressive proximal upper and/or lower extremity weakness manifested as difficulty arising from a seated position or combing one's hair. Ten percent of patients with ocular symptoms only for two years or more rarely go on to develop respiratory failure or limb weakness. General complaints of fatigue frequently accompany physical findings.

The most ominous presentation of myasthenia gravis is subtle, progressive respiratory failure due to diaphragmatic and intercostal muscle weakness. Agitation, diaphoresis, and increased respiratory rate frequently occur prior to shortness of breath. This is a classic presentation of restrictive lung disease. Abnormal arterial blood gases do not reliably predict the need for mechanical ventilation. Patients frequently delay medical attention until respiratory failure is inevitable. Drooling will occur when pharyngeal muscle weakness prevents normal reflex swallowing mechanisms.

Differential Diagnosis

Brainstem stroke can present with altered mental status, ptosis, diplopia, and pupillary abnormalities. MRI with diffusion-weighted imaging can reliably distinguish acute brainstem stroke from myasthenia gravis.

Subacute meningitis with multiple cranial neuropathies can mimic myasthenia gravis; however, bacterial meningitis usually has distinguishing symptoms and signs. More subtle forms of chronic meningitis associated with carcinoma, sarcoidosis, or Lyme disease may be difficult to distinguish from myasthenia gravis. Spinal fluid analysis in myasthenia gravis is normal and is frequently diagnostic in other conditions.

The Miller-Fisher variant of the Guillain-Barré syndrome is a form of postinfectious inflammatory polyneuropathy that can present with abnormalities of ocular movement that may or may not fluctuate. Although pupillary dysfunction can occur, it may be absent, mimicking myasthenia gravis. Lack of tendon reflexes, ataxia, and high cerebrospinal fluid (CSF) protein levels associated with normal cellularity distinguish this condition from myasthenia gravis.

Botulism is the prototypic presynaptic neuromuscular junction disorder caused by the toxin elaborated by the anaerobic bacterium *Clostridium botulinum*, which decreases the release of acetylcholine at the neuromuscular junction. Botulism typically presents with painless eye movement abnormalities and ptosis but frequently will also affect the muscarinic receptors of the ciliary muscle, thereby preventing pupillary constriction. These patients appear to have pupillary dilatation unreactive to light, helping one distinguish myasthenia gravis from this disease. Electrophysiologic testing can also help distinguish prejunctional neuromuscular junction disorders such as botulism from postjunctional neuromuscular junction disorders such as myasthenia gravis, especially since botulism can cause the same limb weakness and respiratory failure that myasthenia gravis causes. Unfortunately, spinal fluid analysis and clinical examination at times cannot distinguish the two diseases. A careful medical history regarding ingestion of poorly canned foods may be the only way to reliably distinguish the two entities when pupillary function is normal. However, lack of any eye movement for days is exceedingly rare in myasthenia gravis and may be a clinical clue to aid in diagnosis.

Primary muscle diseases such as inherited *ocular myopathies, oculopharyngeal muscular dystrophy*, and the most common form of muscular dystrophy in adults, *myotonic muscular dystrophy*, can present with ptosis and eye movement abnormalities, but these diseases progress over the years without fluctuation. Electromyography (EMG)/nerve conduction velocity testing will reliably distinguish muscle disease from neuromuscular junction disease. Other disease entities that may present with symptoms similar to myasthenia gravis include *amyotrophic lateral sclerosis, hypokalemia*, and *myxedema*.

Diagnostic Testing

One reliable diagnostic tool for myasthenia gravis is the edrophonium (Tensilon) test, which may help to differentiate a cholinergic crisis (i.e., overmedication of cholinesterase inhibitors) from a myasthenic crisis and guide subsequent therapy. An acetylcholinesterase inhibitor, edrophonium quickly prevents enzymatic degradation of acetylcholine at the neuromuscular junction, prolonging its interaction with muscle cell receptors thus allowing improved muscle contraction. The drug is given intravenously. Approximately 2–3 mg is injected, and an effect should be seen within 1–2 minutes. In the myasthenic patient, bulbar weakness is observed to change suddenly, such that eyelid drooping will dramatically improve and double vision may resolve as well. This effect is transient and may last only 15 minutes. If no improvement is observed, further medication is given to a maximum of 10 mg. Lack of response to the maximum dosage of edrophonium indicates that the patient's weakness is not due to myasthenia gravis. Increased weakness or the development of excessive muscarinic symptoms after edrophonium administration identifies a patient in cholinergic crisis.

Side effects due to the muscarinic effects of edrophonium can occur, including bradycardia, abdominal cramps, and the sensation of the need to defecate or urinate. Wheezing may occur, especially in those prone to bronchospasm. Respiratory failure can develop, especially in those already in cholinergic crisis. It is mandatory to have 1–2 mg of atropine available in the event that overwhelming muscarinic side effects develop. Cardiac monitoring is important throughout the entire test because of possible bradycardia. Occasionally, a patient will present with sudden respiratory failure or limb weakness; a longer acting acetylcholinesterase inhibitor such as neostigmine can be administered intramuscularly. A starting dose of 2 mg is frequently used. After 1 hour, weakness should be assessed for improvement. Pre- and posttreatment pulmonary function testing may also be performed to identify any improvement.

Another diagnostic tool that is readily available in any ED is the *ice pack test*. The utility of this modality is based upon the fact that neuromuscular transmission can be improved by cooling. In a patient presenting with ocular signs of presumed myasthenia gravis, placement of an ice pack over one eyelid should result in improvement of ptosis. This may be seen in up to 80% of affected patients, but false-positive results may occur in those with other conditions.

Confirmatory electrophysiologic testing of involved muscles is helpful in diagnosis, but is not practical in the ED setting. The patient's forced vital capacity and negative inspiratory force are the best indicators of the restrictive lung disease in myasthenia gravis. Although these are not useful in the diagnosis, they may guide further therapy and identify those patients in need of airway management. Measurement of AChR antibody titers is not practical in the ED. There is no clear correlation between titers and clinical severity of disease.

Management

Supportive Measures

Careful attention to airway support is of primary importance in the myasthenic patient. Whether it results from a cholinergic or a myasthenic crisis, the potential for respiratory depression and aspiration is great. Beta-agonist bronchodilators (albuterol) and inhaled anticholinergic medications (ipratropium) may improve respirations and bronchospasm due to excessive cholinergic effects. Suctioning is performed in the presence of copious oropharyngeal secretions. Any evidence of poor respiratory effort or inadequate ventilation mandates intubation and mechanical ventilation. Useful gauges include pulse oximetry, peak expiratory flow measurements, and p_{CO_2} level measurements. Medications for rapid sequence intubation should be altered. Due to the relative lack of functioning AChRs, succinylcholine, a depolarizing paralytic agent, may have less predictable results in the myasthenic patient. Moreover, paralysis may be prolonged. Rapid-onset nondepolarizing agents such as rocuronium are the agents of choice to induce paralysis in these patients.

Fever should be aggressively controlled as high temperatures worsen muscle strength by impairing neuromuscular transmission. The presence of fever indicates that an infectious process may be responsible for the myasthenic exacerbation. Pulmonary infection is most common, and a chest radiograph should be obtained, even in the absence of any pulmonary symptoms because it may detect a thymoma, seen as an anterior mediastinal mass. It is crucial to remember that antibiotics such as flouroquinolones and aminoglycosides can worsen neuromuscular transmission and should be avoided in patients with myasthenia gravis. Once the patient has been stabilized, emergent consultation with a neurologist should be sought.

Potential Therapeutics

The Tensilon test is carried out as outlined previously. A careful neurological exam both before and after administration of the drug is critical for gauging effects as results may be subtle. Those patients that manifest improvement after administration of edrophonium will require further cholinesterase-inhibiting medication. Long-term symptomatic treatment may be attained with the use of pyridostigmine (Mestinon), an anticholinesterase medication. The initial dose is 60 mg orally every 3–6 hours. Higher doses may be given but may be limited by weakness. Increased motor strength should be seen within 1 hour.

Immunosuppressive agents are useful for long-term suppression of the disease. Low-dose prednisone should be initiated at a dose of 10–20 mg daily and gradually increased to 1–2 mg/kg daily. Effects may not be observed for 3–4 weeks. Inpatients unable to tolerate oral intake should be given methylprednisolone, usually at a starting dose of 60 mg q8 intravenously. Other agents such as azathioprine and cyclosporine have been used to control exacerbations of the disease but are rarely initiated in the ED.

Adjunctive therapy includes plasmapheresis, which is thought to remove autoantibodies from the circulation, thereby resulting in control of acute myasthenia exacerbations. Intravenous immunoglobulin has also been used to diminish activity of the disease. The dosing regimen is variable, and administration of this drug should be done in conjunction with neurology consultation. Thymectomy results in some degree of clinical improvement in the majority of patients and may even induce remission of the disease in up to 60% of cases. It should be considered in patients with thymoma and in patients past puberty without thymoma but who have generalized mysathenia.

Disposition

Most patients with exacerbations of myasthenia gravis require admission to the hospital because of the variable course of the disease. All patients with airway compromise require intensive case unit (ICU) admission. Those patients with infectious processes, especially pneumonia, should be considered for admission. The immunosuppressive agents used by these patients increases their risk for a more complicated course. However, with good supportive care and the medical regimen outlined here, myasthenia patients have a near-normal life span.

PEARLS AND PITFALLS

- Rapid transition can occur from unlabored breathing to hypoventilation because of muscular fatigue or with aspiration of oral secretions. Normal blood gas measurements can provide false reassurance.
- When applicable, distinguish between a cholinergic crisis and a myasthenic crisis.
- Consider potential neuromuscular blocking effects when prescribing any medication for a patient with MG.
- Any cause for elevated body temperature worsens symptoms of MG.

SELECTED BIBLIOGRAPHY

Daroff RB. The office Tensilon test for ocular myasthenia gravis. *Arch Neurol*. 1986; 43:843–4.

Drachman DB. Myasthenia gravis. *N Engl J Med*. 1994;330:1797–810.

Kelly JJ Jr, Daube JR, Lennon VA, Howard FMJ, Younge BR. The laboratory diagnosis of mild myasthenia gravis. *Ann Neurol*. 1982;12:238–42.

Lewis RA, Selwa JF, Lisak RP. Myasthenia gravis: immunological mechanisms and immunotherapy. *Ann Neurol*. 1995;37:S51–S62.

Lindstrom JM. Pathophysiology of myasthenia gravis: the mechanisms behind the disease. *Adv Neuroimmunol*. 1994;1:3–8.

Vincent A, Newsom-Davis J. Acetylcholine receptor antibody as a diagnostic test for myasthenia gravis: results in 153 validated cases and 2967 diagnostic assays. *J Neurol Neurosurg Psychiatry*. 1985;48:1246–52.

17 Musculoskeletal and Neurogenic Pain

Robert G. Kaniecki and L. R. Searls

INTRODUCTION

Acute pain is often accompanied by anxiety and sympathetic hyperactivity. Chronic pain is often associated with affective and vegetative symptoms of depression. *Nociceptive* (somatic) pain involves activation of the peripheral receptors often secondary to tissue damage. *Neuropathic* pain arises from aberrant somatosensory processing in the peripheral or central nervous system. A definitive diagnosis of musculoskeletal or neuropathic pain syndrome in the emergency department is difficult. However, this does not preclude successful management of the pain.

Facial Pain

See Table 17.1.

Nociceptive Syndromes

Odontalgia is the most common cause of orofacial pain in adults. Simple cases are treated with analgesics, antibiotics, and dental referral. Intravenous antibiotics are used for cases with fever and facial swelling along with abscess incision and drainage when appropriate followed by urgent dental referral.

Acute sinusitis is diagnosed by localized pain and tenderness, nasal congestion, purulent rhinorrhea, and fever. Leukocytosis is variable. Blood tests and radiographs are not needed in immunocompetent patients who appear healthy. Treatment is with decongestants and oral antibiotics. Frontal or sphenoidal acute sinusitis is an emergent condition with a potential for intracranial spread.

Temporo-mandibular joint dysfunction is frequently diagnosed, but a controversial source of facial pain due to the nebulous nature of the clinical findings. However, the pain is generally localized at the joint and is associated with abnormal radiographic findings and two of the following four criteria: pain with joint movement, tenderness on joint palpation, decreased range of motion, and/or crepitus on joint movement. Treatment is providing supportive measures.

Table 17.1. Common Causes of Facial Pain	
Nociceptive	**Neuropathic**
Odontalgia	Trigeminal neuralgia
Sinusitis	Herpetic neuralgia
TMJ syndrome	Glossopharyngeal neuralgia
Disorders of the neck, salivary glands	Geniculate neuralgia
Eyes and ears	

Disorders of the neck, salivary glands, eyes, and ears can also be sources of facial pain.

Neuropathic Syndromes

Trigeminal neuralgia is characterized by sudden paroxysms of lancinating pain lasting seconds to minutes, often recurring many times a day. Pain can occur spontaneously or be provoked by sensory stimulation of facial trigger points. The antiepileptic drug (AED) carbamazepine is the initial drug of choice, although other AEDs are also effective. Analgesics are helpful adjuncts. Intravenous fluids may need to be considered for those at risk for dehydration due to inability to take fluids orally.

Acute herpetic neuralgia most often involves the first division of the trigeminal nerve. Supportive treatment includes the use of local heat or cold, soothing emollients, nonsteroidal or opioid analgesics, and antiviral drugs. Neuropathic pain, which persists beyond one month of the initial episode of herpetic infection, is called postherpetic neuralgia. The elderly are particularly prone to this. Tricyclic antidepressant drugs provide the most benefit.

Neck and Upper Extremity Pain

Although the most common sources of pain in the neck and upper extremities are musculoskeletal or neurogenic, referred pain from ischemic processes of visceral organs is often confounding. See Table 17.2.

Nociceptive Syndromes

The most common cause of neck pain is cervical strain, characterized by transient cervical pain, stiffness, and posterior cervical muscle spasm. Local application of heat and anti-inflammatory analgesics are generally effective.

Cervical osteoarthritis is the most common cause of neck pain in individuals over 40 years of age. Pain from the apophyseal joints typically is isolated to the neck and shoulders; further radiation into the upper extremities suggests nerve root irritation. Compression fractures from osteoarthritis or osteoporosis rarely cause symptoms other than acute pain. Chronic pain is best managed with nonsteroidal anti-inflammatory drugs (NSAID); acute exacerbation of pain often requires narcotics analgesics.

Table 17.2. Common Causes of Neck and Upper Extremity Pain

Nociceptive	Neuropathic
Disorders of cervical spine	Cervical radiculopathy
Cervical strain	Brachial plexus disorders
Cervical osteoarthritis	Erb-Duchenne (upper plexus) palsy
Rheumatoid arthritis	Dejerine-Klumpke (lower plexus) palsy
Ankylosing spondylitis	Radiation plexitis
Disorders of upper extremities	Idiopathic brachial plexitis
(a) Inflammatory causes	Thoracic outlet syndome
Septic arthritis	Reflex sympathetic dystrophy
Noninfectious arthritides	Suprascapular nerve palsy
Tendonitis	Radial nerve neuropathies
Bursitis	Ulnar nerve neuropathies
Tenosynovitis	Median nerve neuropathies
(b) Ischemic (vascular) causes	
Acute arterial dissection	
Subclavian steal syndrome	
(c) Traumatic causes	

Rheumatoid arthritis (RA) (see also Chapter 26, "Nontraumatic Spinal Cord Emergencies") is an erosive, systemic polyarthritis primarily involving small joints. The cervical spine is the second most common area of involvement; small joints of the hand being the first. Bony and ligamentous disruption from spinal involvement in RA result in several distinct syndromes, which are reviewed in Chapter 26.

Ankylosing spondylitis (AS) (see also Chapter 26, "Nontraumatic Spinal Cord Emergencies") is a spondyloarthropathy classified along with Reiter's syndrome, psoriatic arthritis, and the arthritis of inflammatory bowel disease. These disorders share the characteristics of spondylitis, sacroiliitis, tendon insertion inflammation, asymmetrical oligoarthritis, and often extraarticular manifestations such as uveitis, urethritis, and mucocutaneous lesions. Although cervical involvement may occur, dysfunction of the lower thoracic and lumbar sacral regions is much more common. Pain and limited range of motion are frequent findings; spinal cord compression due to ossification or epidural hemorrhage is uncommon. Typical "bamboo spine" appearance on plain radiographs is a classic finding in AS. NSAIDs, most commonly indomethacin, and physical therapy remain the cornerstones of effective management.

Nociceptive pain in the upper extremity can also arise either from inflammatory or ischemic disorders. Local infection and disruption of arterial or venous circulation in the upper extremity typically exhibit obvious findings. Acute arterial dissection, subclavian steal syndrome, and Raynaud disease are examples of such vascular disorders.

Nonbacterial septic arthritis (rubella, Epstein-Barr virus, hepatitis) involving the joints of an extremity is associated with systemic findings. The inflammatory arthritides are generally self-limited and respond to immobilization and NSAIDs. The bacterial septic arthritides are commonly divided into gonococcal and nongonococcal (staphylococcal or streptococcal species) groups, with both requiring joint fluid analysis. Surgical drainage is often necessary.

Extremity sites prone to develop nonspecific or "overuse" inflammatory conditions include the shoulder (supraspinatus or bicipital head), elbow

Table 17.3. Localization of Cervical Nerve Root Pathology

Disc Involved	Nerve Root Involved	Area of Pain	Area of Sensory Change	Motor	DTR
C3–4	C4	Shoulder	Variable	± Deltoid	None
C4–5	C5	Shoulder, lateral upper arm	Shoulder	Deltoid ± biceps	Biceps
C5–6	C6	Shoulder, upper arm, lateral forearm, thumb, and index finger	Lateral forearm, thumb	Biceps, triceps wrist extensors	Brachio-radialis and biceps
C6–7	C7	Postero-lateral upper arm, shoulder, neck	Index and middle fingers	Wrist flexors, finger extensors, triceps	Triceps
C7–T1	C8	Ulnar forearm and hand	Medial forearm, small finger	Hand intrinsics, finger flexors, wrist extensors	None

(epicondylitis, or "tennis elbow"), and thumb (de Quervain disease). Flares of systemic rheumatoid or osteoarthritic disease can cause local limb pain. Acute shoulder tendonitis can present with a dramatic onset of severe incapacitating pain over the anterolateral shoulder and aching in the deltoid and lateral arm. Motion of the shoulder, especially arm abduction, is exquisitely painful, and tenderness is noted at the insertion points of the biceps or supraspinatus tendons. The illness is self-limited but requires NSAIDs and possible immobilization of the shoulder in the sling for up to 2 weeks. Subsequent physical therapy or corticosteroid injections may be necessary.

Neuropathic Syndromes

Lesions of the cervical spinal cord generally result in deep segmental pain that is poorly localized and infrequently influenced by positional changes or Valsalva maneuvers. Segmental weakness, sensory loss, and hyporeflexia are generally present in the upper extremities. The lower extremities may exhibit spasticity, weakness, sensory loss, hyperreflexia, and a positive Babinski sign. Urinary or fecal incontinence occur relatively late in the course. Extramedullary or intramedullary tumors, arteriovenous malformations, syringomyelia, central disc herniations, or severe cervical spondylosis and spinal stenosis are visualized by magnetic resonance imaging (MRI) or computerized tomography (CT) myelography.

Cervical radiculopathy is most often caused by cervical spondylosis and cervical disc disease. Cervical herniated nucleus pulposus (HNP) can occur either from trauma or from disc degeneration. Upper limb radiation of the pain in a segmental fashion and neck pain are reported in most cases. Clinical findings include segmental sensory loss, motor weakness, and reflex changes (Table 17.3). The lower cervical roots of C6–8 require the most attention because C6–7 HNP accounts for 70% of all cases and C5–6 HNP accounts for 20% of cases. Physical exam includes the "chin-chest" maneuver, which involves provocation of pain with neck flexion. The "head-tilt" maneuver generates discomfort upon lateral flexion toward the side of the radiculopathy. Head compression (Spurling's maneuver) worsens pain; manual cervical traction may alleviate pain by altering the diameter of the foraminal spaces. Significant sensory loss (seen in 25% of patients), weakness (seen in 75%), or intractable pain requires cervical MRI or CT myelography followed by neurosurgical evaluation.

Thoracic outlet syndrome is an uncommon condition observed most often in thin adult women with drooping shoulders. Compression of the lower trunk of the brachial plexus and subclavian artery is observed in varying combinations, usually from impingement due to cervical or abnormal first thoracic rib, clavicle, fascia, or abnormal scalene muscle. Pain in the shoulder and arm, paresthesias in the median or ulnar nerve distributions, and weakness, atrophy, and vascular changes in the distal forearm and hand are common. Diagnostic maneuvers include the Wright or "hold up" maneuver (abduct and externally rotate the arm 90 degrees with the elbow flexed 90 degrees) and the Adson maneuver (extension and rotation of the head to the effected side while holding an inspiration) while palpating for a weakened pulse. Plain radiographs of the cervicothoracic area may demonstrate a cervical rib. Treatment includes analgesics, flexibility exercises, and postural and ergonomic changes. Surgery is necessary occasionally.

Reflux sympathetic dystrophy (RSD) also known as shoulder-hand syndrome (Sudek's atrophy) causes neurologically mediated shoulder and arm pain characterized by vasomotor and dermal changes and premature osteoporosis. RSD is defined as an otherwise unexplained syndrome of ongoing pain that is not limited to a single nerve distribution, disproportionate to an initial noxious event, and associated with abnormal vascular or pseudomotor (sweat gland) activity.

Causalgia, identical to Sudek's atrophy, arises as a result of direct nerve injury. Clinical findings include burning pain with hyperesthesia, dysesthesia, and edema with trophic changes in the hair, skin, and nails, and eventually muscle atrophy with joint motion. Urgent treatment involves exercise, supplemented by nonsteroidal or opioid analgesics.

Entrapment syndromes in the upper extremity involve several nerves causing shoulder and upper extremity pain (see also Chapter 14, "Peripheral Nervous System and Neuromuscular Disorders"). The suprascapular nerve is compressed resulting in pain at the glenohumeral or acromioclavicular joints and weakness in abduction and external rotation at the shoulder. Radial nerve palsy occurs at the level of the spiral groove of the humerus (Saturday night palsy), the radial tunnel (posterior interosseous syndrome), or the wrist (cheiralgia paresthetica). Ulnar neuropathy may be reflected as pain at the elbow when compressed in the cubital tunnel, or pain at the wrist when impingement occurs in Guyon's canal. Median nerve compression can become symptomatic as the pronator teres syndrome, which results in proximal arm pain on pronation and both weakness and sensory loss in the hand, or the anterior intraosseous syndrome, which results in similar weakness without sensation as it is generally painless. Carpal tunnel syndrome is the most common nerve entrapment in the upper extremity and is reviewed in Chapter 14.

Table 17.4. Thoracic and Truncal Pain

Nociceptive	Neuropathic
Tumors of the spine	Tumors of the spine (spinal cord compression)
Diffuse idiopathic skeletal	Thoracic disc disease (HNP)
hyperosteosis (DISH)	Herpetic neuralgia
	Epidural abscess
	Transverse myelitis
	Spinal cord infarction

Thoracic and Truncal Pain

Nociceptive Syndromes

Tumors of the axial skeleton are commonly metastatic in origin. Occasionally benign tumors cause pain. Presentation includes slowly progressive back pain, which is often worse when the patient is supine, localized tenderness to percussion, and, in patients with malignancy, weight loss, malaise, and fevers or night sweats. Plain radiographs are unremarkable. Urgent MRI or myelography is indicated when neurological deficits are identified. Disorders of the heart and pericardium, lungs and pleura, esophagus, gallbladder, and rib cage can also present as thoracic pain (Table 17.4).

Neuropathic Syndromes

The thoracic region is the most common spinal location for metastatic disease; 70% of spinal cord compression cases arise from thoracic cord involvement. (See Chapter 26, "Nontraumatic Spinal Cord Emergencies.")

Thoracic disc disease or HNP is uncommon in the thoracic spine. Vague back pain with or without radiation along one or more of the intercostal nerves is the typical presentation. Tenderness and local sensory deficit may be present, and respiratory excursion may worsen the pain. MRI is the test of choice for imaging this area.

The thoracic region is also a common location of acute herpetic or postherpetic neuralgias. The discomfort follows dermatomal patterns and occasionally precedes the rash. Other clinical features and treatment recommendations were discussed previously.

Epidural abscess is more common at the thoracic level and causes thoracic or upper abdominal pain (see Chapter 26, "Nontraumatic Spinal Cord Emergencies").

Spinal cord infarction is a rare event, presenting as acute partial (anterior) myelopathy (sparing vibratory and proprioceptive sensation) with chest, abdominal, or back pain (see Chapter 26, "Nontraumatic Spinal Cord Emergencies"). It is commonly accompanied by limb ischemia or diminution of peripheral pulses, with aortic dissection as the underlying cause of spinal cord infarction. Atheroembolic disease, fibrocartilaginous emboli from disc herniation, vasculitis, sepsis, and complication of vascular catheterizations or epidural anesthesia are the other etiologies.

Table 17.5. Common Causes of Low Back and Lower Extremity Pain

Nociceptive	Neuropathic
Disorders of the lumbar spine	Disorders of the lumbar spine
Lumbosacral strain	Conus medullaris syndrome
Trauma	Cauda equina syndrome
Discogenic disease	Spinal stenosis
Systemic arthritides (RA, AS)	Lumbar HNP
Congenital spinal diseases	Disorders of the lower extremities
Degenerative spinal disorders	Lateral femoral cutaneous
Spinal stenosis	neuropathy
Vertebral osteomyelitis	Peroneal neuropathy
Sacroiliitis	Joplin's neuroma
Tumors	Morton's neuroma
Abdominal aortic aneurysm	
Peptic ulcer disease	
Disorders of the kidneys	
Disorders of female reproductive tract	
Prostatitis	
Diverticulitis	
Hemoglobinopathies	
Psychogenic	
Disorders of the lower extremities	
Vascular (ischemic): acute arterial	
occlusion	
Deep venous thrombosis	
Systemic and septic arthritides	
Acute gout	
Tendinitis, bursitis, and tenosynovitis	

Low Back and Lower Extremity Pain

Nociceptive Syndromes

Lumbar strain or sprain is the most common source of "benign" backache. The pain is either acute or subacute with a pattern of recurrent attacks superimposed on chronic discomfort. The pain radiates to lower extremity, but rarely below the knee, thus distinguishing it from radiculopathy of discogenic pain. Physical examination reveals reproducible tenderness and spasm in the paraspinal muscles with restricted range of motion. Plain radiograph of the lumbosacral region are typically unremarkable, and their routine use is discouraged. Bed rest, application of cold and heat, and liberal use of NSAIDs and analgesics provide supportive care. Children and adolescents are most likely to have congenital malformations, postural abnormalities, or other conditions such as osteochondritis. Young adults are prone to lumbosacral strains or direct trauma, discogenic disease, or systemic disorders such as rheumatoid arthritis, ankylosing spondylitis, and Reiter's syndrome. Older adults are most likely to experience osteoarthritis with spondylitic changes, spinal stenosis, and vertebral metastases (Tables 17.5 and 17.6).

Vertebral osteomyelitis presents as a subacute pain progressing over weeks to months, worsening with activity, and not disappearing with rest. Comorbid conditions include diabetes, intravenous drug use, and, commonly, recent infection of the skin, urinary tract, or lungs. The likely pathogens include

> **Table 17.6.** Indications for Plain Radiographs in Back Pain
>
> Unable to assess the patient clinically
> History of significant trauma
> Suspected pathological lesions (carcinoma)
> Age >50 (a relative indication)
> History of cancer with suspected metastasis to bone
> Suspected infection
> Immunocompromised patients
> Patients on dialysis
> Patients with recent spine surgery
> Intravenous drug users
> Children (age <15) (a relative indication)
> Neurological deficit
> Suspected ankylosing spondylitis (sclerosis of sacroiliac joints)

Staphylococcus and *Pseudomonas* species (see Chapter 26, "Nontraumatic Spinal Cord Emergencies").

Sacroiliitis presents as back, buttock, or leg pain. In young adults this may reflect the onset of ankylosing spondylitis; in older adults it generally arises from nonspecific inflammation. Local tenderness and stress on the joint when the patient is prone or supine are helpful diagnostic points. Treatment programs generally use NSAIDs and physical therapy.

Lumbar pain has additional causes such as abdominal aortic aneurysm, peptic ulcer disease, pancreatitis, disorders of the kidneys or female reproductive tract, prostatitis, or diverticulitis. Hemoglobinopathy, such as sickle cell disease and thalassemias can also present as back pain. Psychogenic pain is a diagnosis of exclusion.

Nociceptive pain in the lower limb most often has vascular or inflammatory origins. Acute arterial occlusion is more common in the leg than arm, as is deep venous thrombosis. Septic arthritis was discussed previously, as were the systemic arthritides.

Tendinitis, tenosynovitis, and *bursitis* can involve the hip, knee, ankle joints, as well as the foot. Trochanteric bursitis at the hip, prepatellar bursitis at the knee, and calcaneal bursitis at the heel are the most common sites of involvement. Joint rest and NSAIDs are essential. A local injection of 10–40 mg of Triamcinolone plus 1 ml of 1% lidocaine often provides immediate relief.

Acute gouty arthritis typically presents as an attack of excruciating pain in the foot or ankle. A history of gout may be present, and attacks can be precipitated by stress, excess food or alcohol intake, surgery, or dehydration. Diagnosis is based on clinical findings and elevated serum uric acid level. Initiation of high-dose, rapid-acting NSAIDs may abort the attack within hours. Indomethacin is considered a drug of choice, and colchicine is also useful early in the course of the disease. Allopurinol should not be given during an acute attack.

Neuropathic Syndromes

Because the spinal cord ends at the L1–2 level, myelopathies are rarely seen in the disorders of the lumbosacral spine.

Merskey H, Bogduk N. *Classification of Chronic Pain. Descriptions of Chronic Pain Syndromes and Definitions of Pain Terms*. Seattle, Wash: IASP Press; 1994.

Solomon S, Lipton RB. Facial pain. *Neurol Clin*. 1990;8:913–28.

Wall PD, Melzack R, eds. *Textbook of Pain*, 3rd ed. New York, NY: Churchill; 1994.

Wiens DA. Acute low back pain: differential diagnosis, targeted assessment, and theraupeutic controversies. *Emerg Med Reports*. 1995;16(14):129–40.

18 Neuro-Ophthalmological Emergencies

Dennis Hanlon and Eric R. Eggenberger

INTRODUCTION

Diplopia, visual loss, and pupillary asymmetry are important presentations of neuro-ophthalmologic emergencies. Monocular diplopia usually results from an ophthalmologic cause while binocular diplopia results from ocular misalignment. This misalignment is produced either by lesions of cranial nerves III, IV, or VI or dysfunction of the extraocular muscles, the neuromuscular junction, or internuclear connections. Neuro-ophthalmologic visual loss refers to visual loss not related to an obvious abnormality on physical examination of the eye. This visual loss can be divided anatomically into lesions of the prechiasmal, chiasmal, or postchiasmal area. Pupillary abnormalities are commonly observed in the emergency department. These abnormalities are evaluated, in the context of the patient's overall clinical condition with particular attention to any systematic illnesses.

Neuro-ophthalmologic disorders can be divided into eye movement disorders (efferent diseases), visual loss (afferent diseases), and pupillary dysfunction. The ED evaluation defines the extent of the dysfunction, rapidity of onset, and any associated findings.

Emergency Evaluation

History

The medical history and the list of medications are essential aspects of evaluation and serve to highlight predisposing conditions for neuro-ophthalmic diseases. Family history can provide critical information for patients with hereditary or genetic diseases. Aspects of the patient's social history such as alcohol, tobacco, and caffeine use provide clues to specific diagnoses.

Visual Acuity

The measurement of visual acuity is one of the most important aspects of the emergency eye examination. Visual acuity is tested in each eye separately with the patient's corrective lens by using a Snellen chart or a near card. When optimal correction is not available, pinhole testing is used. Patients with vision less than 20/400 are quantified according to their ability to count fingers, detect hand movements (specify distance and quadrant), or perceive light.

Pupils

When evaluating pupillary dysfunction, the size of the pupil under conditions of light and dark, and reactivity in response to light and near stimuli are considered. When the pupil fails to respond normally to light, a near target is used to assess reactivity. Near-light dissociation (NLD) exists when the pupil reacts to a near target, but not to light. The differential diagnosis for NLD is discussed in the later section on pupils. The swinging flashlight test is used to check for apparent "paradoxical" pupillary dilation in response to light (relative afferent pupillary defect, or RAPD, also referred to as the *Marcus-Gunn pupil*). This test is the only objective confirmation of monocular anterior visual dysfunction. This test is performed in a dark room by shining a bright light in one of the patient's eyes for 1–2 seconds, then swinging the light to stimulate the other eye. A normal response is initial constriction with light stimulation in each eye. Pupil dilation that occurs when the light is presented indicates an afferent (sensory) visual lesion (most commonly an optic neuropathy).

Visual Fields

Monocular confrontational testing of visual fields is one of the most important aspects of the neurological examination for localizing abnormalities. Prechiasmal lesions cause monocular visual field defects. A lesion at the optic chiasm causes bitemporal hemianopsia. Postchiasmal lesions of the optic tract, optic radiation, or occipital cortex produce homonymous hemianopsia. Associated symptoms and signs, and neuroimaging help distinguish the various locations of abnormality. Formal visual field testing with either Goldmann or Humphrey perimetry may be required to detect or quantify visual field defects accurately.

Motility

Neuro-ophthalmological examination of the patient with binocular diplopia emphasizes ocular alignment and movement of the eyes through the nine cardinal positions of gaze. Ductions refer to the excursion of each eye separately; versions refer to conjugate eye movements (e.g., leftward or upward). Occasionally, especially in patients with complete nerve lesions, the eye is unable to move in a characteristic direction (Figure 18.1). Other patients with diplopia have only subtle misalignment in a particular position of gaze, and general assessment in the positions of gaze is unrewarding. In such patients, formal measurements of ductions and ocular alignment are valuable.

Ductions can be measured according to the extent of movement limitation, either as a percent of normal, or in millimeters of "scleral show" remaining at the end of the ocular movement. Ocular alignment refers to the angle of deviation of one eye in relationship to the other eye. Exotropia (XT) indicates an outward deviation of the eye ("wall-eyed"); esotropia (ET) is the inward turning of the

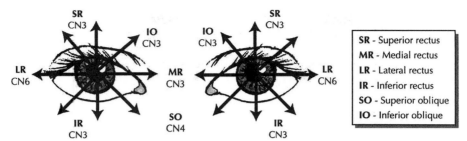

Figure 18.1. Depiction of extraocular muscle innervation by cranial nerves III, IV, VI, and the direction of eye movements that result with contraction of the different extraocular muscles.

eye ("cross-eyed"). Hypertropia refers to one eye that is higher than the other eye. Techniques to dissociate the eyes, such as alternate cover or red Maddox rod testing, are required to quantify the amount of ocular misalignment.

Lids and External Eye Examination

Ptosis can result from disorders of the nerve (cranial nerve III or sympathetic nerve dysfunction as in Horner's syndrome), neuromuscular junction (e.g., myasthenia gravis), or muscle (e.g., dehiscence of the levator palpebrae muscle from its tendon, mitochondrial myopathy or muscular dystrophies). Lid retraction is typically a symptom of thyroid eye disease; however, certain medications or hydrocephalus (as part of Parinaud's syndrome) can also produce this sign. Proptosis can result from either traumatic (orbital hemorrhage, bony displacement, or carotid-cavernous fistula) or nontraumatic mechanisms (infection, tumor, carotid-cavernous fistula, thyroid eye disease, or other myopathy).

Fundus

The optic disc is examined for distinctness of margins, and color. Papilledema refers to disc edema due to increased intracranial pressure (ICP) and is a neurological emergency. In the early stages of disc edema, the margins of the nerve head appear indistinct due to disc elevation (the direct ophthalmoscope resolves in only two dimensions and therefore cannot provide elevation details). In advanced cases of disc edema, the retinal vessels are obscured as they pass over the disc margin, and splinter hemorrhages can be observed.

Evaluation and Differential Diagnosis of Diplopia

When evaluating a patient with diplopia, the most important initial step is to determine whether the diplopia is monocular or binocular. Binocular diplopia resolves when either eye is covered. Monocular diplopia usually results from ophthalmologic causes or refractive errors (Table 18.1). The evaluation of monocular diplopia is relatively straightforward (Figure 18.2).

Binocular diplopia results from ocular misalignment. There are many causes of misalignment. Lesions of cranial nerves III, IV, VI, and their internuclear connections or dysfunction of the extraocular muscles or the neuromuscular junction can produce this misalignment (Table 18.2). The associated neurological findings

Table 18.1. Monocular Diplopia:
Differential Diagnosis

Cataract
Subluxed/dislocated lens
Keratoconus
Iridodialysis
Macular disease
Hysteria (diagnosis of exclusion)

are the most important factors in determining etiology. The evaluation of binocular diplopia demands a focused history and examination (Figure 18.3).

Diplopia is most pronounced when looking in the direction of the limited extraocular movement regardless of cause. The false image is projected peripherally to the true image and appears less sharp. These images may be separated vertically, obliquely, or horizontally.

Cranial Neuropathies

Cranial nerve palsies are the most common cause of binocular diplopia. A thorough knowledge of extraocular muscle innervation and movements is essential (Figure 18.1).

Oculomotor Nerve: Cranial Nerve III

Other associated neurological findings are the single important factors in determining etiology of cranial nerve (CN) III dysfunction. The presentation of third nerve palsy varies depending on the location and degree of involvement, producing a combination of ptosis, mydriasis, and diplopia. This diplopia may be vertical, horizontal, or oblique. Third nerve fibers are vulnerable to lesions

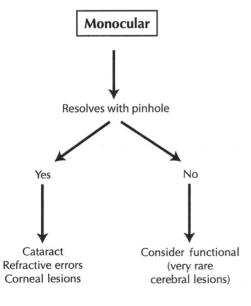

Figure 18.2. Evaluation of monocular diplopia.

> **Table 18.2.** Binocular Diplopia: Differential Diagnosis
>
> Cranial Nerve Palsy III, IV, or VI
> Internuclear ophthalmoplegia
> Posttraumatic mechanical defects
> Orbital cellulitis
> Orbital pseudotumor
> Tolosa-Hunt syndrome
> Cavernous sinus thrombosis
> Dysthyroid eye disease
> Myasthenia gravis
> Miller–Fisher syndrome
> Botulism
> Wernicke's encephalopathy
> Ophthalmoplegic migraine
> Skew deviation
> Vertebrobasilar artery insufficiency
> Miscellaneous CNS lesions

anywhere along their course, and associated symptoms and signs help distinguish among midbrain, subarachnoid space, cavernous sinus, or orbital lesions.

CN III can be referred to as the vasculopathic cranial nerve due to its vulnerability to compression by an aneurysm and the ischemic third nerve palsies commonly seen in diabetics. Since the pupillomotor fibers travel on the outside of the third nerve fascicle, the pupil is involved in most compressive third cranial nerve lesions. Any patient with a pupil-involved third nerve palsy is considered to have a posterior communicating artery aneurysm until angiography proves otherwise. With a "vasculopathic" or ischemic CN III palsy, microvascular disease affects the interior of the nerve; thus, the pupil is spared. If ocular motility is completely affected, and the pupil is not involved, then the cause is microvascular disease and not "compressive lesion." Ischemic third nerve palsies generally resolves within three months without sequelae. If ocular motility is only partially affected, the patient must be followed very closely for any evidence of pupillary involvement.

Trochlear Nerve: Cranial Nerve IV

Trauma is the most common cause of fourth cranial nerve palsy. Microvascular disease associated with diabetes and hypertension may also cause this palsy. Isolated fourth cranial nerve palsy is easily missed as no obvious impairment of ductions is noted with the nine cardinal positions of gaze. Vertical diplopia is noted while reading or going down stairs. On physical exam, the affected eye may appear elevated, and the head may be tilted to the opposite side as compensation. Evaluation and management depends on the underlying etiology (Table 18.3).

Abducens Nerve: Cranial Nerve VI

Sixth nerve palsies produce binocular horizontal diplopia that becomes worse with gaze toward the side of the lesion. Increased ICP from any cause can

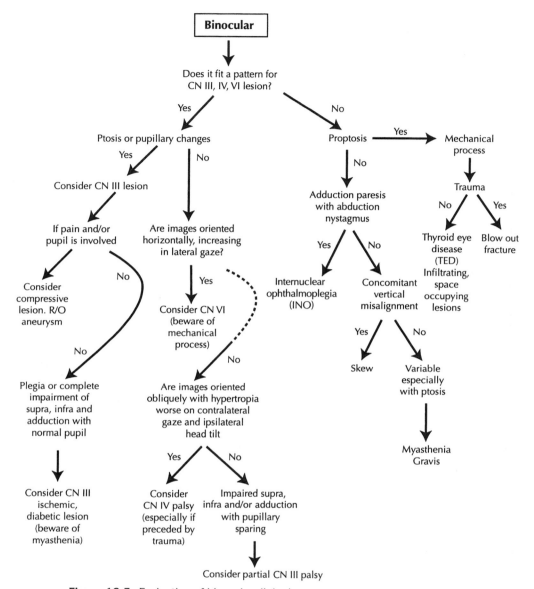

Figure 18.3. Evaluation of binocular diplopia.

produce a "false localizing" sixth nerve palsy. This cranial nerve is referred to as the "tumor" nerve since it can be affected by direct compression or secondary to increased ICP. Ischemia and Wernicke encephalopathy are also considered (Table 18.3).

Internuclear Ophthalmoplegia

Medial longitudinal fasciculus (MLF) dysfunction produces an internuclear ophthalmoplegia (INO). INO is a pattern of ocular misalignment causing impaired ipsilateral adduction and contralateral abducting nystagmus. In younger patients,

Table 18.3. Binocular Diplopia

Lesion	Resting Position Of Eye	Weakness	Pupillary Involvement	Other Findings	Causes
CN III	"Down & Out"	Adduction Supraduction Infraduction	Compressive (yes) Microvascular (no)	Ptosis Aberrant regeneration (compressive)	Aneurysm Ischemia (diabetic) Neuritis Tumor Trauma
CN IV	Hypertropia (relatively elevated)	Depress & intort	No	Head tilt to opposite side Difficulty in downward gaze	Trauma Ischemia Hydrocephalus Aneurysm (rare)
CN VI	Esotropia	Abduction	No	Compensatory turning of head toward paretic side	↑ ICP ("False localizing") Trauma Tumors Vascular Wernicke's Postviral (pediatrics)
MLF	Generally normal	Impaired adduction lateral gaze	No	Nystagmus of abducting eye in lateral gaze	MS (age <40) Ischemia (age >60) Children (glioma)

multiple sclerosis is the most common etiology, while ischemia is the most frequent cause in older adults. In pediatric patients, gliomas must be considered (Table 18.3).

Diplopia from Other Causes

Dysfunction of the extraocular muscles, the neuromuscular junction, and orbital pathology also cause diplopia. Myasthenia gravis can cause a painless, pupil-sparing, binocular diplopia of virtually any pattern. Some authorities recommended that all patients with unexplained diplopia or ptosis have a Tensilon test. The Miller-Fisher syndrome (MFS) is a variant of Guillain-Barré syndrome (GBS) characterized by ophthalmoplegia, ataxia, and areflexia without extremity weakness. The most common early neurological complaints of botulism are diplopia and weakness. Orbital pathology from trauma, infection, or thyroid disease may also cause diplopia.

Neuro-Ophthalmologic Visual Loss

The thrust of initial evaluation is to determine whether the symptoms are due to an ocular or neurological cause (Table 18.4). Neuro-ophthalmologic

Table 18.4. Neuro-ophthalmologic Visual Loss

Prechiasmal Disease
➤ AION (see Table 18.5)
    Nonarteritic
    Arteritic
➤ Optic Neuritis
➤ Compressive optic neuropathy
➤ Traumatic optic neuropathy
➤ Toxic optic neuropathy
Chiasmal Disease
➤ Tumor
➤ Pituitary apoplexy
Postchiasmal Disease
➤ Infarction
    Cortical blindness (bilateral)
➤ Tumor
➤ AVM
➤ Migraine Disorders

visual loss is defined as visual loss not explained by ocular pathology. This visual loss is divided into prechiasmal, chiasmal, or postchiasmal etiologies. Monocular visual loss indicates a lesion anterior to the chiasm; lesions posterior to the chiasm result in binocular visual field loss without diminution of visual acuity.

Prechiasmal Visual Loss

Anterior Ischemic Optic Neuropathy

Ischemia is a common cause of optic nerve dysfunction that almost exclusively affects the optic nerve head or anterior portion of the nerve. While the nonarteritic form is the most common cause of sudden visual loss in the elderly, the

Table 18.5. Anterior Ischemic Optic Neuropathy

	Nonarteritic	Arteritic
Systemic symptoms	No	Yes
Pain	No	Yes (but may be poorly localized)
RAPD	Yes	Yes
Visual acuity	Decreased	Decreased to markedly decreased
Visual field defects	Often altitudinal	Often altitudinal
Funduscopic exam	Edema of optic nerve Small optic cups are predisposed	Edema of optic nerve
Bilateral	10–15% Sequential	One-third Sequential over hours to days
Labs	Normal ESR	Marked ↑ ESR (20% normal)
Treatment	Aspirin	High dose IV steroids

arteritic form, associated with giant cell arteritis (GCA) is a medical emergency (Table 18.5). See Chapter 6, "Headache."

Optic Neuritis

Optic neuritis is a common cause of visual dysfunction, especially among patients between 18 and 45 years of age. The classic presentation is progressive visual loss over several hours to days with painful extraocular movements. Visual acuity reaches nadir in 1 week and improves to 20/40 or better in 85% of patients. The degree of visual loss may range from minimal decrease to profound loss. Ocular exam reveals decreased vision, RAPD, and a normal appearing disc in two-thirds of the cases. One-third of the patients will have a swollen disc. Optic neuritis may be idiopathic; 35% of patients with optic neuritis will develop multiple sclerosis (MS).

Compressive Optic Neuropathies

Compressive optic neuropathies (e.g., meningiomas, pituitary adenomas, aneurysms) produce gradually declining monocular vision. These compressive neuropathies tend to involve multiple cranial nerves. Unlike most compressive optic neuropathies, pituitary apoplexy causes sudden visual loss in addition to headache, diplopia, and decreased level of consciousness. Immediate neuroimaging, neurosurgical consultation, and attention to endocrine status (cortisol levels) are needed.

Chiasmal Visual Loss

Visual acuity is unaffected, but some type of bitemporal visual field defect is the hallmark of chiasmal compression. The classic visual field defect is bitemporal hemianopsia. The patient may be unaware of bitemporal hemianoptic defects due to overlapping visual fields. The most common cause of such compression is tumor with pituitary tumors accounting for 50% of these cases.

Postchiasmal Visual Loss

Postchiasmal lesions produce a homonymous hemianopsia. Common causes include infarction, tumor, arteriovenous malformation, and migraine disorders. Cortical blindness is visual loss from bilateral occipital infarction. Since pupillary reflexes remain intact and the funduscopic examination is normal, this entity may be misdiagnosed as functional visual loss. *Anton syndrome* is cortical blindness with denial of the blindness (Table 18.6).

Anisocoria

Pupils are evaluated for reactivity and size in light and dark environments. Anisocoria is defined as unequal pupil size. Anisocoria of 0.5 mm or less, consistent in both light and dark, can be physiologic if the pupils react normally and there are no associated symptoms or signs. It is important to determine which pupil is the abnormal one. If the anisocoria increases in bright light, then the larger pupil is abnormal. If the anisocoria is more pronounced in a dark environment, then the

Table 18.6. Sudden Loss of Vision

Central retinal artery occlusion
Central retinal venous occlusion
Retinal detachment
Vitreous hemorrhage
Macular hemorrhage
Anterior ischemic optic neuropathy
Optic neuritis
Optic neuropathies
Acute closed-angle glaucoma
Cytomegalovirus retinitis
Iritis
Endophthalmitis
Chiasmal lesions (visual field loss)
Postchiasmal lesions (visual field loss)
Cortical blindness
Functional visual loss (diagnosis of exclusion)

smaller pupil is abnormal. The flow diagram in Figure 18.4 can help determine the cause of anisocoria.

Sympathetic System and Horner's Syndrome

The sympathetic nervous system control of pupillary function involves three neurons and a very circumferential course, beginning in the posterolateral hypothalamus, and traversing the ipsilateral brainstem to synapse on second-order neurons within the ciliospinal center of Budge-Waller (C8–T2). Fibers ascend via the sympathetic chain to synapse on the third-order neuron in the superior

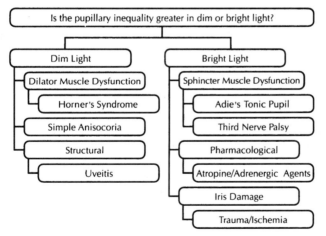

Figure 18.4. Anisocoria: The first step in evaluation of anisocoria is the pupillary measurement in light and dark illumination. The muscles of dilation are innervated by the sympathetic nervous system, and dysfunction of these nerves results in a Horner's syndrome. The pupillary sphincter muscles are innervated by the parasympathetic nerves; third nerve palsies and Adie's pupil are common manifestations of parasympathetic dynsfunction.

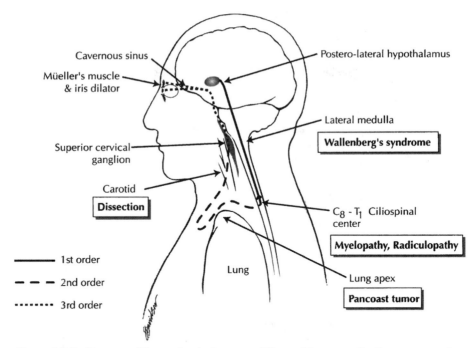

Figure 18.5. Diagram of the anatomical course of fibers of the sympathetic nervous system involved in the control of pupillary function. Different pathological conditions are indicated that can alter the normal function of the sympathetic fibers at various sites along their course from the hypothalamus to the pupil.

cervical ganglion. The third-order sympathetic fibers ascend with the carotid artery to enter the cavernous sinus. The fibers enter the orbit via the superior orbital fissure to innervate dilators of the iris and Müller's muscle (partial lid elevator) (Figure 18.5).

Horner's syndrome consists of miosis, minimal ptosis (1–2 mm), and anhidrosis. Dilation lag is a classic finding with anisocoria greater at 5 seconds than after 15–30 seconds in a dark environment. The extensive course of the sympathetic fibers suggests that a lesion at several locations can produce a Horner's syndrome. Associated symptoms and signs and pharmacological testing of the pupils are required for accurate localization to the first-, second-, or third order segments of the nerve.

Third-order Horner's syndrome can result from carotid dissection, cavernous sinus, or orbital diseases. Second-order Horner's syndrome can result from carotid dissection, C8–T1 radiculopathy, brachial plexus lesions, or apical lung mass. First-order Horner's syndrome can result from lateral medullary infarction (Wallenberg's syndrome) or other lesions within the brain.

Parasympathetic System

The oculomotor nerve (cranial nerve III) innervates the pupillary constrictors via fibers emanating from the Edinger-Westphal nucleus. Pupillary involvement is a point of special importance when evaluating the patient with a third nerve palsy;

however, isolated pupillary dysfunction is rarely indicative of a third nerve palsy. The dilated pupil due to third nerve dysfunction is typically MID position (not maximally dilated), poorly reactive, and accompanied by other symptoms and signs of oculomotor palsy. *Adie's tonic pupil* is a more common cause of an isolated light-fixed pupil. Adie's pupil results from postganglionic parasympathetic denervation and produces mydriasis with poor light reactivity but retained pupillary reactivity to a near target (convergence, accommodation, and miosis). An isolated unilateral tonic pupil is typically a benign condition. Adie's syndrome refers to Adie's pupil plus generalized areflexia. Bilateral Adie's pupils or Adie's syndrome can result from viral or syphilitic infection or can be associated with more widespread autonomic dysfunction. Adie's pupil can be confirmed with instillation of dilute pilocarpine solution. Adie's pupil is one of several syndromes resulting in NLD (greater reaction to near than to light stimuli). The differential diagnosis for NLD includes Parinaud syndrome, tonic pupils (e.g., Adie's), Argyll Robertson pupils (syphilis), diabetic or other peripheral neuropathies, anterior visual pathway injury, or aberrant regeneration of the oculomotor nerve.

Pharmacological Causes of Anisocoria. Inadvertent or deliberate instillation of several drugs can produce a widely dilated and unreactive pupil. Atropine-like agents such as scopolamine (used for motion sickness) are a common cause of pharmacologically dilated pupils. The pharmacologically dilated pupil is maximally dilated; other aspects of the examination, including motility and eyelid function, are normal (with the exception of diminished near vision in the affected eye). Proof of pharmacological instillation may be obtained through the use of 1% pilocarpine. This agent constricts most other causes of a widely dilated pupil, with the exception of pharmacological blockade or mechanical iris damage (e.g., iris scar or trauma).

Structural Anisocoria. Iris trauma or scar can produce a poorly reactive pupil. Typically, this pupil dilates and constricts incompletely, and interruption or thinning of sections of the iris can be visible under slit lamp microscopy. Previous iritis can also result in synechiae that inhibit pupillary reaction.

Physiological Anisocoria. A significant percent (approximately 20%) of the population has minimal anisocoria without pathology, termed physiological or simple anisocoria. This is generally less than or equal to 0.5 mm, and the amount of anisocoria remains essentially the same in light and dark (or is slightly greater in dark). The side of the larger eye can change over time in some patients. Old photographs such as a driver's license viewed with a magnifying glass can be helpful in establishing the date of onset of the anisocoria. The remainder of the examination is normal in patients with physiological anisocoria. Only physiological anisocoria or Horner's syndrome produce anisocoria with normally reactive pupils; the associated ptosis and lack of response to cocaine ophthalmic drops in the latter is helpful diagnostically.

PEARLS AND PITFALLS

- Binocular diplopia can result from nerve, muscle, neuromuscular junction, or internuclear or supranuclear (skew) dysfunction.
- Important historical features of diplopia include monocular or binocular characteristics and vertical, horizontal, or oblique separation of images.
- Visual acuity is the most important test in patients with blurred vision.
- Transient visual loss due to ischemia (amaurosis fugax) rarely lasts more than seconds to minutes.
- Visual field examination has important localization value.
- Isolated pupillary dysfunction rarely is caused by a third nerve palsy.
- Third nerve palsy with pupillary involvement is due to an aneurysm until proven otherwise.

SELECTED BIBLIOGRAPHY

Brunette DD, Ghezzi K, Renner GS. Ophthalmologic disorders. In: Rosen P, Miller NR, Newman NJ, eds. *Walsh and Hoyt's Clinical Neuro-Ophthalmology*, 5th ed. Baltimore, Md: Williams & Wilkins; 1998.

Catalano RA. Neuro-ophthalmologic and nontraumatic retinal emergencies. In: Catalano RA, ed., *Ocular Emergencies*, Philadelphia, Pa: WB Saunders; 1992:335–89.

Leigh RJ, Zee DS. *The Neurology of Eye Movements*, 2nd ed. Philadelphia, Pa: FA Davis; 1991.

Richardson LD, Joyce DM. Diplopia in the emergency department. *Emerg Med Clin North Am*. 1997;15:507–26.

Thompson HS, Kardon RH. Clinical importance of pupillary inequality. *American Academy of Ophthalmology: Focal Points*. 1992;10:1–10.

19 Multiple Sclerosis

Thomas F. Scott

INTRODUCTION

Multiple sclerosis (MS) is a common disorder, characterized by inflammatory lesions of the central nervous system (CNS) (brain and spinal cord), affecting approximately 0.1% of the population in the United States. The disease has a peak incidence in the second and third decades of life, typically presenting in this age group as relapsing-remitting disease (RRMS). Patients with RRMS present to the emergency department with acute exacerbations of their illness. Good recovery from attacks is typically seen following the initial attacks. Attack frequency decreases with time, but many patients begin to accumulate permanent disability. In patients over 50 years of age, the disease most commonly presents as a slow chronic progressive illness (CPMS). Approximately 10–15% of patients have CPMS. Patients with chronic progressive MS present to the emergency department with commonly occurring problems associated with their illness and with worsening neurological symptoms caused by infection and other illnesses.

MS is diagnosed primarily from clinical data. The criteria developed by the Schumacher panel in 1965 are the most widely used clinical guidelines for the diagnosis of MS. According to these guidelines, a patient must exhibit neurological abnormalities attributable to the CNS involving two or more areas (primarily white matter), and two or more episodes of associated dysfunction must occur, each lasting more than 24 hours. Alternatively, a stepwise progression of neurological disability over a 6-month period or more can qualify a patient for the diagnosis. Several diagnostic tests are used to help establish the diagnosis of MS. These include cerebrospinal fluid testing, evoked potential studies, and magnetic resonance imaging (MRI). In 1983, there were elaborated a new set of diagnostic criteria that included the use of these tests and characterized patients as having either probable or definite MS.

Pathophysiology

The primary pathological event in MS lesion development is an immune-mediated destruction of the neuronal myelin sheath. Some scattered remyelination takes place, but this is probably of minor importance following MS attacks. Axonal transection occurs frequently within inflammatory perivenular lesions composed mainly of T lymphocytes. Wallerian degeration of many injured neurons ultimately leads to cerebral and spinal cord atrophy. Lesions of MS may be present throughout the white matter of the CNS, but they have a predilection for the optic nerve, periventricular white matter, spinal cord, and brainstem. Based on pathological or immunological criteria, it is difficult to differentiate between lesions of MS and other demyelinating diseases such as Devic's disease (neuromyelitis optica), acute transverse myelitis (ATM), and encephalomyelitis. Differentiation between MS and these rarer entities is achieved primarily on a clinical, not a histopathological, basis.

Evaluation and Management

The inflammatory lesions of MS can affect any part of the CNS and optic nerves, resulting in a wide variety of presenting symptoms. The first symptoms of MS are commonly weakness, paresthesias, visual loss, incoordination, vertigo, and sphincter impairment. Onset of symptoms occurs most typically over days, but strokelike onset may evolve over minutes to hours. Symptoms referable to MS involving the spinal cord commonly present in an asymmetrical fashion (i.e., partial transverse myelitis). Lhermitte's sign (electric-like sensations radiating up and down the spine, often exacerbated by neck flexion) is commonly observed. A "sensory-level" or hemi-spinal cord (Brown-Séquard) syndrome may also be observed. Other presenting symptoms include speech disturbance, a wide variety of pain syndromes (including radicular pain), and transient acute nonpositional vertigo. Psychiatric manifestations of MS include depressive illness, manic-depression (observed much less frequently), and psychosis (observed rarely).

Neurological Examination

The neurological examination of patients with MS may be normal, minimally abnormal, or markedly abnormal. Focused testing of cranial nerve function, strength, coordination, gait, and sensation, and an evaluation for pathological reflexes are important. It is best to record corrected visual acuity with a Snellen chart and to determine whether optic nerve head pallor exists. Assessment for red desaturation is carried out by asking the patient to view a red object with each eye in an alternating fashion and indicate any subjective change in depth of color. A decrease in perceived redness in one eye suggests impairment of vision in that eye. The typical visual field loss in optic neuritis is a central scotoma. Occasionally, a junctional defect (a small temporal area of field loss opposite a more severe and generalized field loss) may be observed. Rarely, altitudinal defects, arcuate defects, or peripheral visual loss are noted. Disc swelling is present in about 10–50% of patients with MS, and sometimes optic disc pallor from an old asymptomatic injury is observed. Hemorrhages are rare and typically linear. An afferent pupillary defect (Marcus-Gunn pupil) is often found. Internuclear ophthalmoplegia (INO) is a classic finding in patients with MS.

Table 19.1. Differential Diagnosis for New-Onset MS Categorized by Neuroanatomical Presentation

Hemispheric or brainstem focal lesion
  Mass lesion
  Cerebrovascular event
    Ischemic stroke
    Intracerebral hemorrhage
Hemispheric or brainstem multiple lesions
  Neoplastic (multifocal primary or metastatic)
  Infectious (abscess)
  Cerebrovascular
    Cardioembolic (consider infectious endocarditis and atrial
      lesions)
    Coagulopathies (often resulting in cardiac emboli)
    Vasculitis/connective tissue diseases
    Moya-moya disease
Spinal cord lesion
  Acute transverse myelitis (acute transverse myelopathy)
  Ischemic injury/vascular malformation
  Mass lesion
  Connective tissue disease/sarcoidosis/vasculitis
Ocular onset
  Amaurosis fugax/vascular
  Papilledema
  Viral papillitis
Spinal cord and ocular combined
  Devic's disease (neuromyelitis optica)
  Vasculitis/sarcoidosis/connective tissue disease
  Metastatic disease
Spinal cord and brain
  Encephalomyelitis
  Vasculitis/sarcoidosis/connective tissue disease
  Metastatic disease

Common Presentations and Differential Diagnosis

Optic Neuritis

The onset of MS is heralded by a bout of optic neuritis in about 20% of patients with MS, and more than 50% of patients with optic neuritis eventually develop the disease. MRI can usually identify those at increased risk. Typically, optic neuritis is associated with pain either preceding, during, or following the onset of visual loss. The pain is often accentuated with eye movement, and the eye may be tender. The onset of visual loss can be sudden but is more often gradual over one or more days, especially when progressing to blindness. Visual problems are described initially as blurred vision or a sensation of looking into a fog. The differential diagnosis for optic neuritis primarily includes anterior ischemic optic neuropathy (see Chapter 18, "Neuro-Ophthalmological Emergencies"), viral papillitis, and central retinal artery occlusion (see Table 19.1). Anterior ischemic optic neuropathy is unlikely to occur in young patients and is associated with risk factors for arterial disease. Central retinal artery occlusion is generally a disorder of the elderly and is associated with a pale retina and a cherry-red spot in the macula.

Strokelike Syndromes

The most important and difficult diagnostic decisions made in the emergency department involve distinguishing the acute onset of RRMS from symptoms due to CNS ischemia. Although several episodic or multifocal CNS disease processes can resemble MS, stroke is the most common cause of acute focal or multifocal neurological dysfunction in young people, approaching the incidence of MS. An apoplectic onset of MS is rare, and this is the most important historical feature distinguishing the two processes. Clinical features suggesting a single lesion in the CNS favor a diagnosis of stroke in the acute setting. The presence of risk factors associated with stroke is sought, as is a complete review of systems to assess for features of connective tissue disease or coagulopathy. A history of migraine or "complicated" migraine is sought in patients with acute or rapidly evolving deficits because complicated migraine can mimic a transient ischemic attack (TIA) or acute MS symptoms. However, a prominent headache component is unusual in MS and is more commonly associated with complicated migraine or stroke.

Chronic Progressive Multiple Sclerosis

CPMS presents a different set of differential diagnoses than RRMS. It occurs primarily in patients over 40 years of age and is the most common form of MS observed in patients over 55 years of age. Patients are affected primarily in the lower extremities with weakness and spasticity, and occasionally signs of cerebellar dysfunction are also observed. These patients are typically evaluated in an outpatient setting and rarely present to the emergency department for their initial evaluation. Spinocerebellar degenerative syndromes are the most difficult to distinguish from this form of MS. Insidious spinal cord compression due to cervical stenosis is also an important condition to consider in the differential diagnosis.

Myelopathy

An urgent evaluation for spinal cord compression by a mass lesion is necessary when signs of acute or subacute spinal cord dysfunction are present. If a compressive lesion is not found by MRI or myelography, ATM and MS are considered as possible causes of myelopathy. These conditions are often identified by the increased signal observed in the spinal cord on T2-weighted MRI. MS presenting as a spinal cord lesion is much more likely to be associated with asymmetrical motor and sensory signs. In ATM, a sensory level is almost always present, motor findings are symmetrical, and sphincter dysfunction is also usually present. Urinary retention requiring bladder catheterization is commonly present.

Fatigue Syndromes

Fatigue is a very common symptom in patients with MS. Symptoms associated with fatigue are often mistaken for depression in patients with MS. Because many patients who have MS also have anxiety, an initial misdiagnosis of a hysterical condition or depression is common. When evaluating patients with fatigue, consideration is given to thyroid function, electrolyte imbalance, hematological abnormalities, and connective tissue disease.

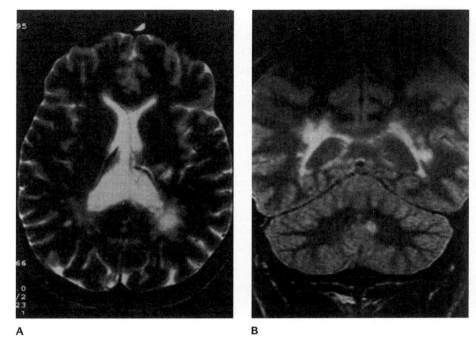

A   **B**

Figure 19.1. T2-weighted MRI scan showing (A) typical globular periventricular white matter lesions primarily in the posterior white matter, axial view. (B) Coronal view using proton density imaging showing periventricular white matter lesions and a lesion in the cerebellar white matter.

Other Conditions

In the emergency department, new-onset MS is most often suspected in young patients (second and third decades of life) with acute or subacute neurological dysfunction. The differential diagnosis includes causes of stroke in young patients, which include cardiac emboli, coagulopathies (e.g., antiphospholipid antibody syndrome), and connective tissue diseases (e.g., vasculitis and other vasculopathies associated with systemic lupus erythematosus, periarteritis nodosa, etc.). Encephalomyelitis is a monophasic, often postinfectious disorder resembling MS in its histopathology and MRI findings and is considered in the differential diagnosis of MS (see Table 19.1). Lyme disease is also rarely a consideration in the differential diagnosis of MS. Lyme disease mimicking MS but lacking other features suggestive of Lyme disease is exceedingly uncommon. Sarcoidosis involving the CNS can be exceedingly difficult to distinguish from MS when systemic signs are absent; however, the prevalence of CNS sarcoidosis is very low.

Ancillary Tests

MRI or computerized tomography (CT) of the brain (without and with contrast), when available, provides the most comprehensive assessment in the emergency department. Neuroimaging assists in differentiating MS from mass lesions, infections, or strokes. MRI is a sensitive test for demonstrating lesions due to MS and is fairly specific for diagnosing MS in young patients (see Figure 19.1). MRI is more sensitive in detecting MS than is CT scanning, cerebrospinal fluid (CSF) analysis, and evoked potential studies. A concise battery of rheumatological screening tests including antinuclear antibody testing, erythrocyte sedimentation rate, Lyme titers, angiotensin-converting enzyme level (sarcoidosis), and SS-A and SS-B autoantibody titers (Sjögren's disease) is considered when the patient's history suggests the possibility of a rheumatological or a collagen vascular condition. A complete blood count including platelets and a coagulation profile are important in assessing possible hematological or coagulation defects. Lumbar puncture is considered but is rarely required in the emergency setting for suspected MS. CSF findings in acute phases of MS include a slightly increased protein level, a mild lymphocytosis, and a normal glucose level. Test results for oligoclonal bands and other abnormalities of CSF immunoglobulins are not immediately available in the emergency department. Oligoclonal IgG bands are present in the CSF but not in the plasma in up to 95% of patients with MS. The finding of oligoclonal bands is nonspecific and present in many inflammatory conditions of the CNS.

Management

Patients with RRMS who experience an acute exacerbation of their illness present with either recurrence or worsening of old symptoms, or entirely new neuro-logical symptoms (Figure 19.2). Although the role of intravenous or oral corti-costeroids is controversial in the treatment of acute relapses, many patients are "steroid-responsive," and the use of corticosteroids should be strongly considered in this group of patients. The role of corticosteroids in the treatment of chronic MS remains even more controversial. However, corticosteroids are widely used and given either intravenously at high doses over a period of several days or orally in moderate doses over variable periods of time. Decisions about the use and dosage of corticosteroids therapy is made in conjunction with a neurologist. Immuno-suppressive therapy with cyclophosphamide, azathioprine, or methotrexate in special situations is also considered, although the efficacy of these agents remains inconclusive. The first medication clearly shown to reduce the attack frequency in RRMS was interferon beta-1b. More recently approved, interferon beta-1a and Copolymer-1 also appear to decrease the frequency of exacerbations of MS.

Disposition

Patients with new neurological symptoms or signs referable to one or more areas of the CNS by history and examination are considered for admission to the hospital for a comprehensive diagnostic evaluation. Inpatient evalu-ation is based on the severity of symptoms and the overall clinical condi-tion. Patients with mild symptoms such as paresthesias and numbness can be considered for outpatient evaluation. Many patients with an established diagnosis of MS require hospital admission due to acute loss of ambulation, deterioration of swallowing function, or other disabling effects of an acute exacerbation. Many patients require initiation or adjustment of medications for management of specific symptoms such as spasticity, bladder dysfunc-tion, or psychiatric disturbance. Acute severe flexor spasms of the lower ex-tremities occur occasionally and may be managed effectively with benzodi-azepines or baclofen. Urinary tract infections are common in patients with

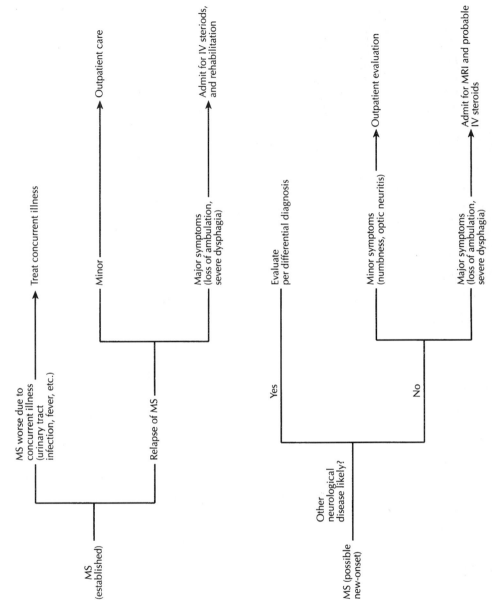

Figure 19.2. Multiple sclerosis management flowchart.

moderately advanced MS and may be associated with lethargy and exacerbation of weakness or spasticity. Bladder catheterization for urinary retention is commonly required. An urgent psychiatric consultation is prudent in cases of suicidal depression or psychosis. A search for coexisting diseases is undertaken, especially in patients with a recurrence of previous neurological symptoms; underlying infections often are responsible for this condition even in the absence of new CNS inflammation due to MS.

PEARLS AND PITFALLS

- Patients must have two bouts of neurological dysfunction referable to the CNS to be considered for the diagnosis of RRMS.

- Patients should have experienced at least six months of progressive or stepwise neurological dysfunction to be considered for the diagnosis of CPMS.

- Emergency physicians should attempt to review briefly the neurological history of patients presenting with established MS before treating new or acute problems. Causes of neurological dysfunction other than MS must be considered.

- In patients with poorly documented history, minimal neurological findings, or other equivocal factors in their past diagnosis of MS, documentation of an MRI scan consistent with the diagnosis of MS is the single most helpful factor.

SELECTED BIBLIOGRAPHY

Matthews WB, ed. *McAlpine's Multiple Sclerosis.* New York, NY: Churchill Livingstone; 1991:43–71.

Poser C, Presthus J, Horstal O. Clinical characteristics of autopsy-proved multiple sclerosis. *Neurology.* 1966;16:791.

Poser CM, Paty DW, Scheinberg L, et al. New diagnostic criteria for multiple sclerosis. Guidelines for research protocols. *Ann Neurol.* 1983;13:227–31.

Schumacher GA, Beebe G, Kibler RF, et al. Problems with experimental therapy in multiple sclerosis: report by the panel on evaluation of experimental trials of therapy in multiple sclerosis. *Ann NY Acad Sci.* 1965;122:552–68.

20 Dementia

Judith L. Heidebrink and Norman L. Foster

INTRODUCTION

Dementia is a common problem in the emergency department (ED) and must be distinguished from other cognitive disorders. Approximately 6% of individuals over age 65 and nearly 30% of all adults over age 85 have at least mild dementia. Unless there is a superimposed acute illness, the majority of patients with dementia can be managed as outpatients. In some cases of extreme agitation, treatment of behavioral symptoms is needed urgently.

Evaluation and Differential Diagnosis

Physical restraint is achieved in some cases of extreme behavioral problems upon the patient's arrival in the ED. Once vital signs have been noted and stable clinical condition is affirmed, haloperidol can be given safely as an intramuscular injection in progressively higher doses beginning at 1 mg. This will rapidly control acute agitation. This major tranquilizer is preferred over a benzodiazepine because it is less likely to cause significant sedation or worsen disorientation and does not risk respiratory compromise. It is safer to use "chemical restraints," through the use of tranquilizers like haloperidol (if there is no contraindication to its use) than to physically restrain an elderly patient for prolonged time.

Importance of Recognizing Dementia

Subtle dementia is often not easily recognized. Medical care suffers when a patient has dementia that is not recognized. An inaccurate history can confound the diagnosis. Medications may be prescribed without consideration of potential cognitive side effects. Therefore, it is important to look for dementia, and mental status is assessed routinely in those at greatest risk: the elderly, patients who require assistance for their care, and everyone with a history of delirium.

Definition of Dementia

Dementia is a decline in intellectual ability from a previous level of performance that causes an altered pattern of activity in a patient with unimpaired consciousness. There are several key points in this definition. First, dementia represents a decline in ability. Previous occupation and education can help in determining whether a decline has occurred, and information from family is critical. Second, the decline must be sufficient to alter daily activities such as employment, independence, or socialization. It is important to document the consequences of this intellectual decline. Third, dementia is impairment in overall "intellectual ability," and thus simultaneously involves multiple areas that contribute to intellect such as memory, judgment, language, and visuospatial skills. Finally, dementia can be identified only when consciousness is unimpaired. An altered level of consciousness suggests *delirium* rather than dementia (see differential diagnosis in this chapter and also in Chapter 5, "Altered Mental Status"). Dementia cannot be assessed until a patient is fully awake and stable.

Despite its complicated definition, dementia is a syndrome, not a specific diagnosis. There are more than 70 recognized disorders that cause dementia and the ultimate responsibility of determining the precise cause of dementia lies with a multidisciplinary team or dementia clinic.

Guidelines for Cognitive Testing

A routine history and general physical examination may elicit clear evidence of dementia. Mild dementia, however, is often missed unless mental status is formally assessed. Patients with dementia often do not complain of memory loss.

Determining the level of orientation is not sufficient. Significant memory impairments often occur before orientation is affected. Memory must be tested specifically. Ask the patient to recall personal information and general information, such as current events, geography, and historical dates. In addition, assess short-term memory by asking the patient to repeat 3 items and then recall them 5 minutes later. Any difficulty with these tasks suggests the need for further investigation, including questioning the patient and family members about symptoms of cognitive decline that support a diagnosis of dementia.

It is important also to assess several other areas of cognition. See Chapter 1, "Neurological Examination." This is best accomplished with a careful mental status examination; however, some find it easier to use a standard battery of screening questions (e.g., the Mini-Mental Status Examination, MMSE). This 30-point scale assesses orientation, memory, calculations, language, and visuospatial ability. In most cases, scores less than 26 reflect impairment in cognition, whether due to dementia or other causes. This battery, like others, is not perfect. Nevertheless, the score on the MMSE reflects severity of impairment and is an effective way to describe the patient's performance to other physicians.

Differential Diagnosis in Patients with a Cognitive Complaint

Dementia is only one possible explanation for cognitive deficits. Other disorders that cause impaired cognition include (a) transient global amnesia, (b) delirium, (c) acute psychosis, (d) aphasia, and (e) depression. Several of these

Table 20.1. Clinical Features Helpful in Distinguishing Dementia from Delirium and Acute Psychosis

Characteristic	Delirium	Dementia	Acute Psychosis
Onset	Acute	*Usually* insidious	Acute
Course over 24 hours	Marked fluctuations	Stable	Stable
Consciousness	Reduced	Normal	Normal
Attention	Usually impaired	Normal, unless dementia severe	May be disturbed
Cognition	Impaired	Impaired	Unimpaired if cooperative
Hallucinations	Visual, ±auditory	Often absent	Predominantly auditory
Psychomotor	Activity increased or reduced, shifts unpredictably	Often normal	Increased or reduced, but not rapidly shifting
Speech	Incoherent, slow or rapid	Word finding, normal pace	Normal, slow, or rapid

conditions also can occur as a complication of dementia. As a result, considerable clinical judgment is required to assess the presence or interaction of each.

Transient Global Amnesia. Transient global amnesia (TGA) is a rare, but dramatic entity with a benign prognosis. Recognition avoids expensive and unnecessary testing. TGA is characterized by abrupt, temporary inability to form new memories (anterograde amnesia) and variable impairment of recent and remote memory (retrograde amnesia). The entire episode persists for 1–8 hours, rarely lasting more than 12 hours. TGA typically affects individuals in their fifth to seventh decades of life. In contrast with dementia, TGA spares nonmemory functions, such as language and visuospatial skills. Level of consciousness and personal identity are maintained. Epileptic features are notably absent. Any focal neurologic signs exclude a diagnosis of TGA and warrant evaluation for ischemia. The etiology of TGA is controversial, yet patients with strictly defined episodes of TGA do not have an increased risk of vascular events or dementia. However, patients with recurrent, brief (less than 1 hour) episodes may develop epilepsy.

ED evaluation of patients with suspected TGA hinges on confirmation of the diagnosis by careful history and examination. No other diagnostic testing (e.g., head CT scan) is needed for typical cases of TGA. Patients whose memory deficits persist following ED assessment require short-term admission or extended observation, with consideration of a head CT and/or electroencephalogram (EEG) if symptoms have not substantially improved within 24 hours after onset.

Delirium. Delirium is an acute, fluctuating disorder of attention that causes an altered level of consciousness, disturbance of perception, altered psychomotor activity, disorientation, and memory impairment. Like dementia, it is common among the elderly and has many etiologies. It is crucial that the cognitive impairment from delirium not be attributed to dementia, as failure to evaluate delirium would neglect many potentially life-threatening conditions. Key features that distinguish delirium from dementia are summarized in Table 20.1.

Acute Psychosis. Patients with dementia may have severe behavioral disturbances, giving the impression that they suffer from acute psychosis rather than dementia. Distinguishing features are listed in Table 20.1. Cognition itself is preserved in an acute psychosis that is not superimposed on dementia. Auditory hallucinations are common in acute psychosis but are rare in mild dementia. Whereas dementia is common in the elderly, the onset of schizophrenia in late life is unusual and controversial.

Aphasia. Aphasia is an acquired disturbance of language due to a cerebral insult. In contrast to dementia, aphasia refers to impairment of a single element of cognition, with sparing of other aspects. The presence of aphasia necessitates use of nonverbal communication in assessing a patient's thinking abilities.

Depression. Depression is considered in any evaluation of memory loss. In the absence of a major depressive disorder, however, depression is seldom the sole cause of cognitive decline. Loss of interest rather than an actual loss of abilities suggests depression. Disorientation is rare in depression, but patients may exhibit a sense of hopelessness, quickly answering, "I don't know," when cognition is assessed. As always, vegetative symptoms and depressed mood are helpful in identifying depression.

Management and Disposition

Special Considerations

When dementia is suspected, the reliability of the patient's history must be assessed. Information about prior level of functioning and any recent changes in medications, environment, and health status is obtained from a collateral informant such as family or caregivers. Emergency personnel should provide simple explanations for procedures and supervision to prevent wandering. Avoid medications that may worsen cognition, particularly anticholinergic drugs. When extreme agitation requires pharmacologic treatment, haloperidol or another neuroleptic is preferable.

Unknown Etiology

Implications of Dementia of Unknown Cause. The ED physician routinely sees patients whose charts document "dementia" without a specific etiologic diagnosis. Further evaluation is needed to permit appropriate management of cognitive and behavioral disturbances. Treatment can reverse or prevent progression of some dementias.

Neurologic Consultation in the ED. The diagnostic evaluation of dementia is best done in the outpatient setting. Nonetheless, neurologic consultation in the ED sometimes is warranted, and head computerized tomography (CT) and lumbar puncture may be appropriate (Table 20.2). In addition, behavioral disturbances occasionally are so severe that inpatient psychiatric care is required. The combination of dementia and new seizures necessitates a head CT looking for neoplasm,

Table 20.2. Indications for ED Neurologic Consultation and Procedures in Patients with Dementia

Feature	Head CT[a]	Lumbar Puncture[a]
New onset seizure	+	±
Focal neurologic deficit	+	−
Gait disturbance	±	±
Subacute onset (less than 3 month duration)	+	+

[a] +: recommended procedure, ±: often recommended depending on clinical circumstances, −: not recommended. (See text for additional details.)

hematoma, or stroke. If negative, lumbar puncture is performed to assess for meningitis or encephalitis. Dementia and gait disturbance coexist in several disorders, and a specific diagnosis is often suggested by the pattern of gait disturbance. A neurologic consultation in the ED is advisable for consideration of additional testing or treatment.

Rapidly Progressive Dementia. This raises several etiologic possibilities requiring prompt attention (Table 20.3). Unless an inaccurate history or delirium is found to account for the rapid course, most patients need admission for further evaluation. In the ED, such patients receive a head CT scan followed by a lumbar puncture, unless a mass lesion is identified. Cerebrospinal fluid testing analysis to include cytology, cryptococcal antigen, and bacterial, fungal, and TB cultures is done. Polymerase chain reaction (PCR) testing for viral antigens such as herpes simplex is also considered. Special precautions are needed for lumbar puncture, since Creutzfeldt-Jakob disease (CJD) is a potential etiology (Table 20.4). This rare, but transmissible disease causes a rapidly progressive dementia with ataxia; visual disturbances, rigidity, and a myoclonic startle response to sudden noises. CJD is not transmitted by casual contact or routine nursing care.

Initiation of Outpatient Evaluation and Referral. Patients are referred for evaluation and management to a multidisciplinary dementia clinic. Diagnostic evaluation includes a series of laboratory studies focusing on medical causes of dementia and an imaging study of the brain to look for structural abnormalities.

Table 20.3. Differential Diagnosis of Rapidly Progressive Dementia

Creutzfeldt-Jakob disease
Meningitis/encephalitis (including TB, herpes, fungal, cryptococcal, carcinomatous, paraneoplastic)
Vasculitis
Primary or metastatic tumors, including CNS lymphoma
Subdural hematoma
Normal pressure hydrocephalus
Multi-infarct dementia (occasionally)
Alzheimer's disease (rarely)

Table 20.4. Laboratory Evaluation for Dementia

Serum chemistries: electrolytes, glucose, renal, and liver function
  tests
Complete blood count
Urinalysis
Thyroid stimulating hormone
Treponemal antibody test (nontreponemal tests are less sensitive
  for neurosyphilis)
Erythrocyte sedimentation rate
Vitamin B_{12} and folate levels
HIV testing (if indicated)

Known Etiology

Expected Clinical Course. When a specific etiology for a patient's dementia is known, it helps confirm that the patient's current presentation is consistent with the expected clinical course. Each disorder causing dementia has a unique course, and deviation from this course suggests either a misdiagnosis or a superimposed condition.

Alzheimer's disease is characterized by insidiously progressive cognitive decline. Short-term memory loss, mild naming difficulties, and visuospatial deficits arise early in the course, at a time when the patient is still independent in activities of daily living. Over time, impairments in language, orientation, and judgment necessitate patient supervision. As a guide, scores on the MMSE fall by roughly three points per year, unless modified by treatment. Alterations in personality and behavior become more prominent and range from agitation and hallucinations to passivity and social withdrawal. By 8 years after onset, more than 60% of patients with Alzheimer's disease reside in a nursing home.

Unexpected clinical changes in Alzheimer's disease require additional evaluation. Such changes include incontinence or gait disturbance occurring when cognitive deficits are mild, or focal weakness at any time. Seizures may indicate a superimposed illness, although they frequently occur in patients with Down's syndrome who develop Alzheimer's disease and can occur in others late in the course of the disease.

Multi-infarct dementia (MID) has an abrupt onset with stepwise decline, often after a known series of clinical strokes. Focal symptoms and signs are present, and both seizures and incontinence can occur early in the course. Cognitive impairment may remain remarkably stable in the absence of further ischemia. New, focal symptoms reflect a failure of therapy to prevent further strokes and may require additional evaluation or treatment modification.

Medical Complications and Exacerbation of Cognitive Deficits. Complications of dementia include falls, malnutrition, and infections. Common complications, such as pneumonia and urinary tract infection, are considered in demented patients with a precipitous decline in cognition. Medications with central nervous system actions are another frequent reason for decline. Agitation or worsening cognition also occurs acutely due to changes in environment.

Table 20.5. Pharmacologic Treatment of Alzheimer's Disease

Class/Name	Indication	Adverse Effects
Cholinesterase inhibitors	Cognitive impairment	
Tacrine (Cognex)		Hepatoxicity, nausea, diarrhea
Donepezil (Aricept)		Rare nausea, diarrhea
Rivastigmine (Exelon)		Nausea, diarrhea
Galanthamine (Reminyl)		Nausea, diarrhea
Dopaminergic agents	Extrapyramidal symptoms	
Levodopa (Sinemet)		Nausea, hallucinations, orthostasis
Neuroleptics	Hallucinations, paranoia	
Haloperidol (Haldol)		Extrapyramidal symptoms, sedation
Risperidone (Risperdal)		Extrapyramidal symptoms
Quetiapine (Seroquel)		Orthostasis, rare extrapyramidal symptoms
Anxiolytics	Anxiety, agitation	
Buspirone (Buspar)		Sedation
Anticonvulsants	Agitation, aggression	
Valproic acid (Depakote)		Nausea, thrombocytopenia
Carbamazepine (Tegretol)		Sedation, neutropenia
Antidepressants (serotonergic)	Agitation, depression	
Trazodone (Desyrel)		Sedation, orthostasis
SSRI's (Prozac, Zoloft)		Anxiety, insomnia

Diagnosis-Specific Treatments and Potential Complications. Some dementia-specific treatments are available. Alzheimer's disease is treated with cholinesterase inhibitors to increase cerebral acetylcholine levels. Tacrine (Cognex), donepezil (Aricept), rivastigmine (Exelon), and galanthamine (Reminyl) are presently available. Principal side effects include nausea, anorexia, and diarrhea. Tacrine also requires regular laboratory monitoring for hepatotoxicity. Cognitive benefits of these agents are modest, and none prevents disease progression. Table 20.5 summarizes indications and adverse effects of commonly used medications in Alzheimer's disease.

Treatment of MID is identical to that appropriate for stroke under other circumstances. Extrapyramidal symptoms seen in Parkinson's disease or Alzheimer's disease can be treated with dopaminergic agents such as levodopa (see Chapter 13, "Movement Disorders"). AIDS dementia is treated with combination antiretroviral therapy.

Management of Behavioral Disturbances. Behavioral disturbances usually do not require hospitalization. In some cases, environmental or activity modifications suffice. When pharmacologic intervention is necessary, agents with little or no anticholinergic activity are preferred. Neuroleptic agents have traditionally been the mainstay of treatment for agitation or hallucinations. However, the high-potency neuroleptic agents (which have the least anticholinergic activity) may exacerbate or precipitate extrapyramidal symptoms. Alternatives to neuroleptic agents include anxiolytics (buspirone), anticonvulsants (carbamazepine or valproic acid), and antidepressants (trazodone, fluoxetine). If the patient can no longer be safely managed on an outpatient basis due to severe agitation or aggression, hospitalization is pursued.

Disposition and Medical-Legal Issues

Consultation and Placement from the ED. Unless consultation and/or hospitalization are indicated (earlier), referral for outpatient management is appropriate. All patients with dementia and their caregivers are referred to community-based support services such as the Alzheimer's Association and the Area Agency on Aging.

Medical-Legal Issues. Before discharging a patient with dementia from the ED, driving restrictions, elder abuse, and patient competency must be addressed. Patients are informed not to drive until driving safety has been assessed in the context of a comprehensive dementia evaluation. Any suspicion of physical abuse by caregivers is reported to adult protective services. A durable power of attorney for financial and medical decision making should be recommended as soon as dementia is recognized. If the patient is no longer competent to make decisions himself, guardianship is necessary.

PEARLS AND PITFALLS

- Memory is specifically tested in patients at risk for dementia.
- Identifying the specific cause of dementia is necessary to guide appropriate management.
- Treating patients with dementia can enhance cognition, improve associated medical and psychiatric conditions, and reduce caregiver burden.
- Infectious precautions are required when evaluating patients with rapidly progressive dementia.
- Abrupt changes in cognition may signify a superimposed medical complication, not a worsening of the underlying dementia.
- Neuroleptics are preferable to benzodiazepines for acute management of severe agitation in patients with dementia.
- Dementia may go undetected on casual observation.
- Not all patients with dementia complain of memory loss.
- Many patients with dementia *do* complain of memory loss.
- Age-related changes in cognition do not significantly impair everyday activities.
- Level of orientation does not adequately test cognition.
- Impaired, fluctuating consciousness is an indicator of delirium, not dementia.
- Not all patients with dementia have Alzheimer's disease.
- Alzheimer's disease is *not* a diagnosis of exclusion; specific diagnostic criteria exist.
- Nonspecific terms such as *senility* and *organic brain syndrome* are inaccurate and useless.

Brain Tumors and Other Neuro-Oncological Emergencies

Herbert B. Newton

INTRODUCTION

Neuro-oncologic (N-ONC) emergencies are a diverse group of disorders that occur frequently in patients with brain tumors and other types of cancer. They are most often caused by direct effects of tumor on the nervous system but can also develop as a result of treatment, infection, metabolic disturbances, medication side effects, and other mechanisms. Alterations of mental status are the most common type of neuro-oncologic emergency, typically caused by toxicity from various medications, as well as other etiologies.

The most commonly encountered neuro-oncologic emergencies are divided into five categories:

1. Those causing alteration of mental status
2. Those associated with seizures and status epilepticus
3. Those associated with cerebrovascular events
4. Those associated with focal neurological deficits
5. Those associated with back pain and spinal cord compression

N-ONC Disorders Causing Alteration of Mental Status

Alterations of mental status are common in patients with brain tumors and other types of cancer. Mental status changes can be caused by structural abnormalities within the nervous system (e.g., tumor), de novo or treatment-related infections, seizures, metabolic or treatment-related encephalopathies, and other diagnostic considerations (see Table 21.1). The changes in mental status can range from slight lethargy or confusion in mild cases to encephalopathy or coma.

Evaluation and Differential Diagnosis

The differential diagnosis is extensive and includes structural changes within the parenchyma of the brain, infections, toxic encephalopathies, metabolic

Table 21.1. Disorders Associated with Alterations of Mental Status in Cancer Patients

Structural disease	*Toxic encephalopathy*
Primary/metastatic brain tumors	Sedative hypnotics
Elevated intracranial pressure	Narcotics
Hydrocephalus	Antidepressants
Intratumoral or parenchymal hemorrhage	Anticonvulsants
Leptomeningeal metastases	Neuroleptics
Cerebrovascular disorders	Antiemetics
Abscess	Steroids
Metabolic encephalopathy	*Infection*
Fluid/electrolyte disturbances	Neutropenic sepsis
Hypoxia	Meningitis
Renal failure/uremia	Encephalitis
Liver failure/hyperammonemia	Aspiration pneumonia
Endocrine disorders	
Wernicke's encephalopathy	
Treatment-Related Encephalopathy	*Seizure Disorder*
Radiation therapy	Postictal state
Chemotherapeutic agents	Subclinical status epilepticus

encephalopathies, treatment-related encephalopathies, and seizure activity (see Table 21.1). Many of these disorders can elevate intracranial pressure (ICP), which further contributes to alterations of mental status. The most common structural alterations that cause mental status changes are the presence of primary or metastatic brain tumors (see Table 21.2). If caused by tumor growth and associated edema formation, these changes are usually gradual, but they can be rapid if due to hemorrhage or hydrocephalus. Hydrocephalus can also be caused by other neuro-oncologic considerations such as leptomeningeal tumor, infection, and hemorrhage.

Table 21.2. Common Primary and Metastatic Brain Tumors

Primary Tumors	Metastatic Tumors
Adults	
Glioblastoma multiforme (35–40%)	Lung (64%)
Astrocytoma grades I–III (18–20%)	Breast (14%)
Meningioma (18%)	Unknown primary (8%)
Pituitary adenoma (9%)	Melanoma (4%)
Oligodendroglioma (5%)	Colorectal (3%)
Schwannoma (3–5%)	Hypernephroma (2%)
Ependymoma (2%)	
Children	
Astrocytoma, low-grade (15–30%)	Wilm's tumor (18.6%)
Astrocytoma, high-grade (8–15%)	Rhabdomyosarcoma (18.6%)
Medulloblastoma (18–25%)	Osteogenic sarcoma (16.3%)
Brainstem glioma (6–15%)	Germ cell tumors (16.3%)
Ependymoma (6–13%)	Ewing's sarcoma (9.3%)
Craniopharyngioma (6–9%)	Neuroblastoma (4.6%)
Pineal region (2–5%)	Hepatocellular carcinoma (4.6%)

Other infectious etiologies that cause alterations of mental status in cancer patients include sepsis, meningitis, viral encephalitis, and systemic infections (e.g., pneumonia). Aspiration pneumonia resulting from dysphagia can be clinically silent.

Encephalopathic states can result from various therapeutic interventions, medications, or metabolic disturbances (see Table 21.1). Radiation therapy can cause an acute encephalopathy, especially in the setting of a brain tumor with edema and mass effect, by further exacerbating ICP. Several chemotherapeutic agents are known to cause encephalopathy, including 5-fluorouracil, ifosfamide, methotrexate, cytosine arabinoside, α-interferon, and interleukin-2. Metabolic encephalopathy most often occurs in patients with electrolyte disturbances but can also be seen with uremia, hyperammonemia, and Wernicke's encephalopathy.

Evidence of systemic disease such as fever, meningismus, bilateral asterixis, or movement disorder (such as myoclonus) is sought. Focal findings help differentiate structural from metabolic alterations of mental status. Patients with focal, structural brain disease often have localizing signs (e.g., hemiparesis, facial weakness, sensory loss, or visual field defect).

Management

Laboratory tests include complete blood counts, electrolytes, renal and liver panels (including ammonia), blood cultures, blood gases, glucose, thyroid screen, lactate, coagulation profile (see later), vitamin B_{12}, folate, thiamine, and appropriate medication levels (e.g., anticonvulsants, digoxin). An enhanced computerized tomography (CT) or magnetic resonance imaging (MRI) scan can evaluate for enlargement or progression of primary or metastatic brain tumors. In cancer patients without nervous system disease, neuroimaging will screen for structural lesions and infection. Lumbar puncture is necessary for cerebrospinal fluid analysis in suspected cases of leptomeningeal metastases (cytology, tumor markers) and central nervous system (CNS) infection (gram stain, cultures, immunological tests).

Patients with elevated ICP require rapid stabilization to prevent brain herniation (see Chapter 23, "Increased Intracranial Pressure and Herniation Syndromes").

Metabolic causes of mental status changes (see Table 21.1) are corrected. Seizure activity is controlled as outlined in the next section. Antibiotics are administered after appropriate cultures have been drawn. Neutropenic patients receive hematologic support with granulocyte colony-stimulating growth factor (Neupogen; 5 μg/kg/per day by subcutaneous injection). Patients with toxic encephalopathy (see Table 21.1) need reduction in dosage or discontinuation of the causative medication.

N-ONC Disorders Associated with Seizures and Status Epilepticus

Seizures are common in patients with primary and metastatic brain tumors and occur as symptoms at presentation in 54% and 15–20% of patients, respectively. The frequency of seizure activity often increases with tumor growth, due to irritation of surrounding neural tissues. The seizures are classified most often as focal in origin and usually have localizing value related to tumor location (e.g., face, arm). Less often, purely generalized or partial complex seizures occur. Oncology patients without brain tumors may also be at risk for seizures due to disease-related metabolic disturbances, infections, and effects of treatment.

Evaluation and Differential Diagnosis

In patients with a diagnosed brain tumor, the most common cause for seizure activity is nontherapeutic or inadequate anticonvulsant levels. Less often, the seizure occurs as the first symptom de novo in a patient with brain tumor. Preictal symptoms such as fever, headache, nuchal rigidity, somnolence, or confusion are explored. The presence of new focal findings could represent Todd's postictal paralysis, tumor progression, or seizure-related ischemia. Metabolic conditions that can precipitate seizures include uremia, hyponatremia, hypoglycemia, hypoxia, hypocalcemia, and hypomagnesemia. Cerebral hemorrhage, infarction, infection, or leptomeningeal metastasis can also induce seizures. Treatment-related causes include brain radiation, chemotherapy (e.g., methotrexate, cisplatin), and analgesics (e.g., meperidine).

Management

Anticonvulsant levels, complete blood count (CBC), platelets, BUN and creatinine, electrolytes (including calcium and magnesium), and glucose are checked. Brain tumor patients with alterations of their baseline neurologic status need a screening CT or MRI scan to evaluate for tumor progression, hemorrhage, or hydrocephalus. All metabolic causes of seizure activity require correction of the underlying disorder. In patients with a history of cancer, a first seizure requires a screening CT or MRI scan and cerebrospinal fluid assessment if the metabolic screening tests are negative.

N-ONC Disorders Associated with Cerebrovascular Events

Cerebrovascular disorders are common in cancer patients and often occur in patients with brain tumors. Autopsy studies reveal cerebrovascular lesions in approximately 15% of all cancer patients. The most important predisposing factors for cerebrovascular disease in cancer patients are direct effects of tumors on blood vessels, tumor-induced coagulation disorders (hemorrhagic and thrombotic), and treatment-related injury to blood vessels. Cerebrovascular emergencies can have a variable presentation, appearing in most patients as a typical transient ischemic attack (TIA) or stroke and in others as a confusional state or encephalopathy.

Evaluation and Differential Diagnosis

The differential diagnosis includes tumor-related disorders, coagulation disorders, and treatment-related disorders (see Table 21.3). Tumor-related disorders can occur with primary brain tumors or metastatic disease producing a TIA or stroke-like presentation due to intra-tumoral hemorrhage or ischemia. Coagulation disorders can lead to intracranial thrombosis, ischemia, or hemorrhage. *Nonbacterial thrombotic endocarditis (NBTE)* is characterized by sterile fibrin vegetations on one

Table 21.3. Cerebrovascular Disorders with Associated Tumor Types and Symptoms

Cerebrovascular Disease	Tumor Types	Symptoms
Tumor-related		
Intratumoral parenchymal hemorrhage	CPP, Pit. Ad., oligo., mal. astro., melanoma, chorio., renal, germ	HA, obtundation, Sz, focal signs
Superior sagittal sinus occlusion	Neuroblastoma, CA, lymph.	HA, focal signs, Sz, confusion
Subdural hemorrhage	Carcinoma, leukemia, lymph.	Confusion, lethargy, focal signs
Ruptured neoplastic aneurysm	Chorio, lung CA, cardiac myx.	HA, obtundation, Sz, focal signs, meningismus
Coagulation disorders		
DIC, thrombocytopenia	Leukemia	Confusion, disorientation, focal signs, ?HA, ?Sz
NBTE	Mucin-producing CA	Focal signs, encephalopathy, Sz
Cerebral intravascular coagulation	Lymph, breast CA, leukemia	Encephalopathy, focal signs
Superior sagittal sinus occlusion	CA, leukemia, lymph	Sz, encephalopathy, focal signs
Treatment-related		
L-Asparaginase (infarction or hemorrhage)	Leukemia	Focal signs, ?HA, obtundation
RT-induced carotid occlusion	Head and neck tumors, lymph	Focal signs
Carotid rupture	Head and neck tumors, RT	Focal signs, obtundation
Mitomycin (hemolytic uremic syndrome)	Solid tumors	HA, focal signs, obtundation

Note: Abbreviations: DIC – disseminated intravascular coagulation; NBTE – nonbacterial thrombotic endocarditis; RT – radiation therapy; CPP – choroid plexus papilloma; Pit. Ad. – pituitary adenoma; oligo. – oligodendroglioma; mal. astro. – malignant astrocytoma; chorio. – choriocarcinoma; HA – headache; Sz – seizure; germ – germ cell tumor; CA – carcinoma; lymph. – lymphoma; myx. – myxoma.

or more cardiac valves. Patients with NBTE often present with focal symptoms suggestive of a classic TIA or stroke (50–60%) but may have a more diffuse presentation consistent with encephalopathy or confusion (20–30%; see Figure 21.1). Approximately 25% of strokes in cancer patients are caused by NBTE.

Systemic symptoms such as fever, rash, bruising, or regions of swelling or pain are sought. A search for clues to the etiology of the cerebrovascular event, such as petechiae, heart murmur, nail bed splinter hemorrhages, or new swelling in the neck is undertaken. In patients with confusion or encephalopathy, cranial intravascular coagulation, NBTE, sinus thrombosis, or subarachnoid hemorrhage should be suspected.

Management

Laboratory tests include CBC and platelets, coagulation studies, disseminated intravascular coagulation (DIC) panel (quantitative fibrinogen, thrombin time, fibrin degradation products, protamine sulfate gelation, and mixing studies), and cultures. If a coagulopathy is present, initial treatment is instituted with vitamin K, fresh frozen plasma, or platelets as indicated. Neurological stabilization is often

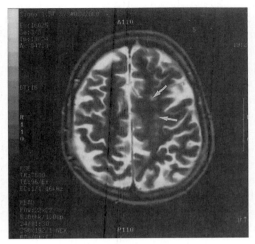 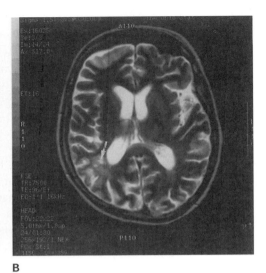

A   B

Figure 21.1. MRI scans of a 57-year-old woman with a history of non-Hodgkin's lymphoma who developed neurological symptoms and signs consistent with impaired short-term memory, dyscalculia, and other cognitive abilities. (A) and (B) On T2-weighted MRI, there are multifocal regions of high signal consistent with embolic infarct or leptomeningeal tumor involvement (white arrows). Lumbar punctures were unrevealing. Transesophageal echocardiography revealed vegetations on the mitral and aortic valves consistent with NBTE.

achieved in patients with DIC and NBTE with administration of heparin. Transesophageal echocardiography can be diagnostic in some cases of NBTE. A cranial CT is useful to screen for intratumoral, parenchymal, subdural, and venous infarction-related hemorrhage. Patients with a documented hemorrhage with significant edema and mass effect receive intravenous dexamethasone.

N-ONC Disorders Associated with Focal Neurological Deficits

Focal neurological signs and symptoms are common in patients with brain tumors and other forms of neuro-oncologic disease. Greater than 50% of patients with primary brain tumors have hemiparesis, cranial nerve palsies, or papilledema on initial evaluation. Patients with metastatic tumors are also likely to develop focal signs and symptoms. Focal deficits are also common with cerebrovascular emergencies, leptomeningeal metastases, and treatment-related toxicities. For patients with an established diagnosis of neuro-oncologic disease, focal neurologic signs can often worsen with tumor progression or recurrence and with altered metabolic status.

Evaluation and Differential Diagnosis

For patients with a known diagnosis of brain tumor, the differential diagnosis includes tumor progression, exacerbation of edema without tumor enlargement, hemorrhage, leptomeningeal spread, infection, and metabolic alterations. Leptomeningeal spread of tumor often presents with myelopathy, radicular pain or sensory loss, or a cauda equina syndrome. Patients with infection usually have a history of fever, malaise, and other signs of systemic illness. Metabolic alterations can cause exacerbation of fixed neurologic deficits and include medication toxicity (e.g., anticonvulsants), hyponatremia, hypoglycemia, dehydration, and hyperammonemia. In cancer patients without a known brain tumor, focal neurologic deficits are caused by cerebrovascular complications of cancer, new brain metastases, leptomeningeal tumor, spinal metastases (see next section), infection, or neurotoxicity from cancer therapy.

Management

For patients with a known brain tumor, CT or MRI with and without contrast determine the presence of tumor enlargement, tumor spread, exacerbation of edema, or intratumoral hemorrhage. Patients with a known spinal cord tumor undergo neuro-imaging with MRI. Patients with a cerebrovascular emergency or spinal cord compression are managed as outlined elsewhere in this chapter. When the evaluation discloses tumor progression of the brain or spinal cord, dexamethasone (a bolus of 10–20 mg given intravenously, followed by 4–6 mg given intravenously every 4–6 hours) is administered. When leptomeningeal tumor is suspected, an MRI with gadolinium enhancement may be diagnostic. However, the gold standard for diagnosis remains a lumbar puncture with cytological examination.

N-ONC Disorders Associated with Back Pain and Spinal Cord Compression

In patients with systemic or CNS cancer, back pain is often the first sign of a more virulent underlying neurological process. The structural components of the spinal column are the most common site for bony metastases. Back pain caused by epidural spinal cord compression (ESCC) arises from metastatic deposits to the vertebral column (85% of cases), paravertebral spaces (10–12%), or the epidural space (1–3%). ESCC is relatively common, occurring in 5–14% of patients with systemic cancer. Each year approximately 20,000 cancer patients are at risk for ESCC because of metastatic deposits in and around the spinal column (see Table 21.4). ESCC can be the first manifestation of cancer in up to one-quarter of patients. After the development of back pain, neurological deterioration can be rapid. Without proper treatment, ESCC will inexorably result in paraplegia, loss of lower extremity sensation, and incontinence. (See Chapter 26.)

Evaluation and Differential Diagnosis

The differential diagnosis of back pain is extremely broad. In addition to ESCC, herniated disk, degenerative joint disease, muscle sprain, epidural abscess, spinal osteomyelitis, primary spinal cord tumor, leptomeningeal tumor, facet syndrome, spondylolisthesis, spinal stenosis, and other less common entities are considered when evaluating back pain in a patient with cancer. In most patients, pain is the initial symptom and typically develops in the thoracic region. The pain is mild at first but is always progressive and is often described as a steady, deep ache that can be axial or radicular (i.e., radiating down a limb or around the ribcage anteriorly). Movement, Valsalva maneuvers, straight leg raising, and neck flexion often exacerbate the pain. Weakness is usually symmetric and involves the legs but

Table 21.4. Common Primary and Metastatic Spinal Cord Tumors

Primary Tumors	Metastatic Tumors
Extramedullary (89%)	Breast (22%)
Neurofibroma (29%)	Lung (15%)
Meningioma (25%)	Prostate (10%)
Sarcoma (12%)	Lymphoma (10%)
Other (10–15%)	Sarcoma (9%)
Dermoid	Kidney (7%)
Epidermoid	Gastrointestinal tract (5%)
Intramedullary (11%)	Melanoma (4%)
Ependymoma (55%)	Unknown primary (4%)
Astrocytoma (31%)	Head and neck (3%)
Vascular tumors (4%)	
Other (5–10%)	
Mixed glioma	
Oligodendroglioma	

can occasionally affect the arms. Autonomic dysfunction manifests as painless urinary retention in most patients. Sensory complaints usually involve numbness and paresthesias that start in the feet and extend proximally over time. Fever is suggestive of epidural abscess, discitis, osteomyelitis, or some other infectious process.

The general physical examination often demonstrates localized pain to percussion over the involved vertebral bodies. The tender areas are usually in the thoracic region; this differs from the pain of degenerative spine disease, which is more commonly cervical or lumbosacral. A rectal examination is performed to assess ESCC of the conus medullaris or cauda equina. On neurological examination, leg weakness is the most common finding. Initial findings may be mild, demonstrating proximal leg weakness and slightly exaggerated reflexes. Progression of ESCC reveals myelopathy, with severe upper motor neuron pattern weakness and hyperactive reflexes in the lower extremities, spasticity, and Babinski signs. In patients with ESCC of the lumbar vertebrae, the cauda equina is affected instead of the spinal cord, producing a lower motor neuron pattern characterized by lower extremity hypotonia, areflexia, atrophy, and muscle fasciculations. Sensory findings range from mild decrease in distal vibratory and proprioceptive sensation, to a complete sensory level.

Management

Initial management consists of pain control and diagnostic evaluation. The pain of ESCC is often severe and requires liberal use of parenteral narcotic analgesics for adequate control. With a history of fever, blood cultures and sedimentation rate are performed to screen for epidural abscess, discitis, osteomyelitis, and other infectious processes. Plain radiographs of the spine can identify an abnormality in 85–90% of patients with ESCC from solid tumors, demonstrating vertebral body erosion and collapse, subluxation, and pedicle erosion. Recently, MRI has replaced myelography as the most sensitive and specific imaging technique for evaluation of epidural tumor. An enhanced MRI scan of the complete spine will demonstrate epidural or paravertebral masses, ESCC, primary spinal cord tumors, most cases of leptomeningeal tumor, as well as benign causes of back pain.

The evaluation of ESCC should be rapid, since the most important prognostic factor for posttreatment neurologic function is the level of function at the initiation of therapy. Eighty percent of patients who are ambulatory at the start of treatment will remain so after therapy, while only 45% of paraparetic patients and 5–10% of paraplegic patients will be ambulatory following treatment. Patients with proven or suspected ESCC should receive intravenous dexamethasone, which rapidly reduces spinal cord edema, improves neurologic function, and often alleviates back pain. The proper dosage of dexamethasone remains controversial; however, most authors would agree on a loading dose of 20–100 mg, followed by 4–24 mg four times a day. Definitive therapy (i.e., radiation theropy ± surgical decompression) should begin no more than 24 hours after administration of dexamethasone. The mainstay of therapy for most ESCC patients is external beam radiation therapy (RT), with or without decompressive surgery.

PEARLS AND PITFALLS

- Toxic encephalopathy from abnormal levels or overusage of various medications is the most common cause of mental status alterations in cancer patients.

- The best method to acutely lower elevated ICP in an obtunded or comatose patient is hyperventilation, which will rapidly lower P_{CO_2}, causing cerebral vasoconstriction and a reduction of cerebral blood flow and volume. The target P_{CO_2} is approximately 27–33 mmHg.

- The most common cause of seizures in brain tumor patients is nontherapeutic anticonvulsant levels because of noncompliance with medication.

- Some cerebrovascular emergencies (e.g., NBTE) present as encephalopathy or confusional states and not as acute focal deficits, as in more typical TIA or stroke.

- ESCC can be the first manifestation of cancer in up to 25% of patients and should be suspected in any patient with cancer and new back pain.

- The most important prognostic factor for ESCC is the level of neurological functioning at the time of diagnosis. Following treatment, 80% of patients who can walk at diagnosis remain ambulatory, while only 5–10% of patients who are paraplegic at diagnosis are ambulatory afterward.

SELECTED BIBLIOGRAPHY

Black PM. Brain tumors (First of two parts). *NEJM*. 1991;324:1471–6.

Byrne TN. Spinal cord compression from epidural metastases. *NEJM*. 1992;327:614–19.

Newton HB. Primary brain tumors: review of etiology, diagnosis, and treatment. *Am Fam Phys*. 1994;49:787–97.

Newton HB. Neurologic complications of systemic cancer. *Am Fam Phys*. 1999;59:878–86.

Newton HB, Newton CL, Gatens C, Hebert R, Pack R. Spinal cord tumors. Review of etiology, diagnosis, and multidisciplinary approach to treatment. *Cancer Practice.* 1995;3:207–18.

Patchell RA. Metastatic brain tumors. *Neurol Clin.* 1995;13:915–25.

Pollock IF. Brain tumors in children. *NEJM.* 1994;331:1500–7.

Posner JB. Spinal metastases. In: Posner JB, ed. *Neurologic Complications of Cancer.* Philadelphia, Pa: FA Davis, 1995;6:111–42.

Rogers LR. Cerebrovascular complications in cancer patients. *Oncol.* 1994;8:23–30.

Schiff D, Batchelor T, Wen PY. Neurologic emergencies in cancer patients. *Neurol Clin.* 1998;16:449–83.

Sorensen PS, Borgesesn SE, Rohde K, et al. Metastatic epidural spinal cord compression. Results of treatment and survival. *2 Cancer.* 65:1990;1502–8.

22 Neuropsychiatry

Craig A. Taylor

INTRODUCTION

Neuropsychiatry is a discipline that evaluates and treats a broad array of psychiatric or behavioral symptoms that result from a central nervous system (CNS) dysfunction. The psychiatric disorder can be one of behavior, mood, or cognition, or it can be a psychosis. It can be caused by or can coexist with an underlying neurological or medical problem. Despite the number of potential underlying disorders, the neuropsychiatric patient can be placed in one of two major categories: (1) the individual who presents with neuropsychiatric symptoms but no history of a CNS disturbance (this patient requires a thorough evaluation for an underlying disorder) and (2) the individual with a known CNS disorder who presents with neuropsychiatric symptoms as evidenced by behavioral change. This patient presents with a symptom complex based on an underlying medical or neurological disorder. The goals of the emergency evaluation are to (1) stabilize the agitated or aggressive patient in order to protect him or her and others; (2) establish a presumptive diagnosis or broadly determine whether the cause is medical, neurological, or psychiatric or a combination of causes; and (3) determine whether the patient requires inpatient medical, neurological, or psychiatric care or can be discharged from the emergency department with outpatient follow-up (Table 22.1).

Evaluation and Management

Similar to patients with general psychiatric emergencies, neuropsychiatric patients with underlying CNS disturbance can present to the emergency department because of a change in behavior. A detailed and accurate history is obtained from anyone who presents with a cognitive, behavioral, emotional, or other neuropsychiatric disturbance. It is important to remember that brain dysfunction affects the ability of the patient to give an accurate history and can modify the expression of symptoms and behavior. The psychiatric history and mental status examination can provide specific clues to neurobehavioral symptoms that can help localize the underlying abnormalities of brain function.

236

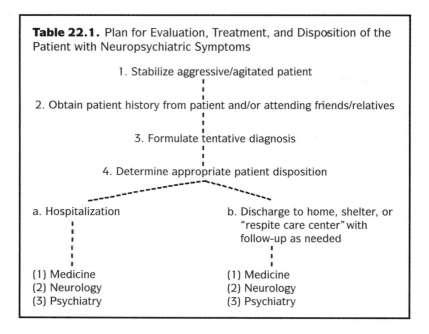

Table 22.1. Plan for Evaluation, Treatment, and Disposition of the Patient with Neuropsychiatric Symptoms

1. Stabilize aggressive/agitated patient

2. Obtain patient history from patient and/or attending friends/relatives

3. Formulate tentative diagnosis

4. Determine appropriate patient disposition

a. Hospitalization

(1) Medicine
(2) Neurology
(3) Psychiatry

b. Discharge to home, shelter, or "respite care center" with follow-up as needed

(1) Medicine
(2) Neurology
(3) Psychiatry

Patient History

Knowledge of a current or past neurological disorder can help determine whether the symptoms fit a particular pattern. Table 22.2 lists the key issues that are addressed in taking the history of a patient exhibiting neuropsychiatric symptoms. Because many of these patients are unable or unwilling to give complete (or any) descriptions, it is common practice for family members or friends to assist in providing relevant details of the patient's history. Medications the patient has in his or her possession can provide clues about the source of the presenting problem and the name of the prescribing physician, who can be contacted for additional information.

General Physical and Neurological Examination

A complete general physical and neurological examination helps differentiate medical and neurological conditions that may be contributing to the

Table 22.2. Medical History of the Neuropsychiatric Patient: Key Questions to Ask

What are the patient's symptoms?
When did the symptoms begin, and have they been continuous?
If not, how long did they last?
What stressors, events, or conditions are related to the symptoms?
What makes the symptoms better or worse?
Is the patient currently taking medication?
Have any changes occurred in medication dosage, or the time or route of their administration?
Have any changes occurred in the baseline medical or neurological condition?
Is there a history of illicit drug or alcohol use?

neurobehavioral presentation. Particular attention to the patient's appearance and behavior can be revealing and can substitute for part of the formal examination when the patient is uncooperative. The neurological examination is essential in neuropsychiatric evaluation because it can often help localize the site of neurological dysfunction. However, it can have limited value in discerning the neurological basis of a specific neurobehavioral disturbance, and results can be normal in a patient with gross brain disease.

In neuropsychiatric evaluation, the mental status examination is of paramount importance. It is structured and sufficiently detailed to (1) serve as a baseline for future comparisons; (2) give evidence of underlying neurological disturbance; and (3) detect confusional states. The mental status examination focuses on assessing the patient's level of arousal, attention, concentration, language function, memory, constructions, abstractions, insight, judgment, and praxis. Additionally, observations of appearance, motor behavior, affect, mood, verbal output, thought structure and content, and perceptions of the patient are documented. The patient is evaluated for the presence of depression, anxiety, mania, and thought disorders. These can occur as problems unrelated to a neurological disorder, or they can be the result of a stable or progressive neurological disorder. The presence of these symptoms in a "neurologically stable" or "non-acute" patient requires psychiatric intervention. The possibility of alcohol or illicit drug use is investigated thoroughly in any patient who presents with acute mental status or behavioral changes.

Diagnosis and Disposition

Neuropsychiatric symptoms can be difficult to diagnose under any circumstance. Patients with neurological disorders can present with a wide array of neurobehavioral disturbances (Table 22.3). Aberrant behavior in these patients can be the result of several different processes, each of which may require a separate treatment plan. Symptoms are determined to be acute, subacute, or chronic. Acute symptoms may be caused by worsening of a neurological or medical condition or by another underlying neuropsychiatric condition. Chronic neuropsychiatric symptoms that worsen are commonly associated with psychosocial stressors and a related adjustment disorder. Although the cause of a particular neuropsychiatric presentation may not be diagnosed in the emergency department, it is important to determine the nature and extent of the clinical condition so that appropriate disposition can be made.

Certain conditions of a psychiatric nature – including destructiveness, disorganization, depression, disorientation due to severe organic mental disturbances, and conditions requiring detoxification – require psychiatric hospitalization, whether or not the patient has an underlying CNS disturbance. However, not all patients who present with psychiatric symptoms require admission to a psychiatric unit. In patients with known brain injury, it is important to determine whether there is an exacerbation of an underlying medical or neurological condition that presents with neuropsychiatric symptoms. When neuropsychiatric symptoms are due to a change in a medical or an underlying neurological condition, only stabilization of those conditions will result in improvement in the neuropsychiatric symptoms. Neuropsychiatric evaluation is recommended

Table 22.3. Neuropsychiatric Symptoms Associated with Selected CNS Disorders

Disorder	Symptoms
Alzheimer's disease	Apathy, agitation, anxiety, irritability, depression, disinhibition, delusions
Frontotemporal dementias	Apathy, aberrant motor activity, disinhibition, agitation, anxiety, euphoria, depression, irritability
Parkinson's disease	Depression, anxiety, apathy, agitation, mania, irritability, euphoria, executive dysfunction, dementia
Progressive supranuclear palsy	Apathy, disinhibition, irritability, depression
Huntington's disease	Depression, apathy, psychosis, irritability, emotional instability, change in social conduct, executive dysfunction, dementia
Traumatic brain injury	Apathy, impulsivity, distractibility, indifference, poor anger control, rage, poor social skills, irritability, decreased concentration, decreased abstraction, depression, mania
Epilepsy	Mood disorders, irritability, impulsivity, schizophreniform disorder, anxiety, pseudoseizures, personality changes, amnesia-confusion
Cerebrovascular disease	Catastrophic reaction, anxiety, frustration, aggression when presented with cognitive tasks, anosognosia, apathy, depression, poor expression of emotional prosody, poor comprehension of emotion in others, pathological crying/laughing, mania
Brain tumors	
Frontal lobe tumors	Personality changes, impulsivity, disinhibition, emotional instability, poor judgment and insight, distractibility, apathy, indifference, psychomotor retardation, motor perseveration
Temporal lobe tumors	Mood swings; visual, olfactory, tactile, auditory hallucinations, dreamlike or dazed feeling, depression, instability, mania, personality changes, anxiety; verbal and nonverbal memory impairments
Parietal tumors	Depression, apathy, cognitive changes
Occipital tumors	Personality and behavioral changes, visual hallucinations
Diencephalic tumors	Emotional incontinence, psychosis, depression, hyperphagia, hypersomnia
HIV-AIDS	Cognitive impairment, depression, psychosis
Multiple sclerosis	Dementia, euphoria, depression, emotional dysregulation (pseudobulbar affect)

(1) when the underlying neurological condition is adequately controlled, (2) in the absence of active medical illness, and (3) when medications are not considered to be responsible for the symptoms. When major depression, manic episode, or psychosis significantly interferes with the patient's ability to function, inpatient evaluation and treatment are required. Immediate emergency department intervention may be necessary for the acutely agitated or aggressive patient (Table 22.4) including use of medications (Table 22.5).

Table 22.4. Steps to Take in the Control of the Agitated or Aggressive Neuropsychiatric Patient

1. Move the patient to a quiet, secure room and minimize stimuli. The room should not be isolated and should be equipped with an alarm or panic button. It should not be possible to lock the door from the inside.
2. Obtain information about the patient's acute change in behavior or mental status from friends, relatives, or available documentation.
3. Attempt to talk to and/or reason with the patient. Ask relatives or friends to talk to the patient.
4. Obtain a history from the patient, when possible.
5. Administer a sedative or tranquilizer when the patient poses an immediate threat to self or others.
6. Apply physical restraints when the patient is not controlled by medication and poses an immediate threat to self or others.
7. Generate a differential diagnosis.
8. Treat and make appropriate disposition to psychiatry, neurology, or general medicine department. Recommend inpatient or output status evaluation. When the patient responds to treatment in the emergency department and can be discharged, release with appropriate follow-up arrangements.

The acuity of symptoms and their relationship to psychosocial factors determine the need for either hospitalization or discharge to the previous living arrangement with appropriate follow-up. Typically, patients with conditions that appear to be psychosocially mediated (i.e., behavioral or mood disturbances that arise as a consequence of environmental stressors) are discharged from the emergency department to the home setting with follow-up by counselors or psychiatrists. A strategic plan with necessary support is arranged in case the patient's symptoms worsen.

Table 22.5. Psychotropics That Can Be Used To Calm the Agitated or Aggressive Patient

State	Possible Medication
Mildly to moderately agitated/aggressive	Lorazepam, 1–2 mg orally (Rarely, benzodiazepines can paradoxically disinhibit; avoid use in patient with a history of CNS depressant abuse or benzodiazepine-induced disinhibition. Haloperiodol, liquid, 5 mg orally, can be used as an alternative.)
Severely agitated/aggressive	Lorazepam, 1–2 mg intramuscularly, or haloperiodol, 5 mg intramuscularly, may be repeated in 20–30 minutes. For extreme agitation, a combination of lorazepam and haloperiodol may be given intramuscularly.

PEARLS AND PITFALLS

■ A patient with altered behavior and cognition may have an underlying organic illness.

■ Iatrogenic factors can be potential causes or contributors to emotional, behavioral, and cognitive disturbances; patients are evaluated for the presence of alcohol or illicit drugs.

■ Patients with CNS disturbances can have poor insight and understanding, and can inaccurately describe relevant history and their symptoms; patient information is obtained from family or friends when possible.

■ Grossly normal neurological and mental status examinations do not exclude the possibility of a CNS disturbance as the cause of behavioral and psychiatric symptoms.

■ Neuropsychiatric patients may require hospitalization on a medical or neurological unit, rather than a psychiatric unit.

SELECTED BIBLIOGRAPHY

Hyman SE. The violent patient. In: Hyman SE, Tesar GE, eds. *Manual of Psychiatric Emergencies*, 3rd ed. Boston, Mass: Little, Brown and Co; 1994:28–37.

Mueller J, Fogel BS. Neuropsychiatric examination. In: Fogel BS, Schiffer RB, Rao SM, eds. *Neuropsychiatry*. Baltimore, Md: Williams & Wilkins; 1996.

Popkin MK. Syndromes of brain dysfunction presenting with cognitive impairment or behavioral disturbance: delirium, dementia, and mental disorders due to a general medical condition. In: Winokur G, Clayton PJ, eds. *The Medical Basis of Psychiatry*, 2nd ed. Philadelphia, Pa: WB Saunders; 1994:17–37.

Roberts GW, Leigh PN, Weinberger DR. *Neuropsychiatric Disorders*. London: M Wolfe; 1993.

Strub RI, Black FW. *The Mental Status Examination in Neurology*, 3rd ed. Philadelphia, Pa: FA Davis; 1993.

Strub RL, Wise MG. Differential diagnosis in neuropsychiatry. In: Yudofsky SC, Hales RE, eds. *Textbook of Neuropsychiatry*. Washington, DC: American Psychiatric Press; 1992.

Taylor C, Price TP. Neuropsychiatric assessment. In: Silver JM, Yudofsky SC, Hales RE, eds. *Neuropsychiatry of Traumatic Brain Injury*. Washington, DC: APA Press; 1994: 81–132.

23 Increased Intracranial Pressure and Herniation Syndromes

Amy Blasen and Sid M. Shah

INTRODUCTION

Several distinct pathological processes follow a common pathway that leads to increased intracranial pressure (ICP). These varied disorders include traumatic brain injury (TBI) and space-occupying intracranial lesions, among many others. Initial identification and management of patients at risk for developing increased ICP commonly occurs in the emergency department. Traditional therapies for treatment of increased ICP have changed in several ways. Routine hyperventilation is no longer recommended. Controlled ventilation with adequate oxygenation and a Pa_{CO_2} within the normally defined range is the therapy of choice. Mannitol continues to be the preferred pharmacological treatment of increased ICP. Corticosteroids have no role in the treatment of increased ICP caused by trauma but are beneficial in the reduction of edema caused by tumors and abscesses. The use of barbiturate coma is limited to those patients with increased ICP who do not respond adequately to other ICP-lowering measures. Advances in the understanding of the pathophysiology of increased ICP and new strategies for its early detection and treatment continue to emerge with ongoing studies. Table 23.1 provides guidelines for prehospital care.

ICP Values

Resting ICP in the normal adult and child over 7 years of age is 0–10 mm Hg; 15 mm Hg is the upper limit of a normal ICP. In young children, the upper limit of normal ICP is 0–5 mm Hg; in neonates, the normal ICP is 0–2 mm Hg. Current data support the lowering of ICP when it is equal to or higher than 20–25 mm Hg. When the ICP is elevated to 40 mm Hg in the adult, the mortality rate is 65%. At ICPs of 60 mm Hg or higher, the mortality is virtually 100%. Brain herniation can occur at ICPs less than 20–25 mm Hg; therefore, an absolute ICP threshold for instituting treatment is not uniform. The likelihood of brain herniation depends on the location of the intracranial mass lesion.

Normalizing ICP does not ensure a good clinical result as a result of the presence of cerebral injury caused by the traumatic event or by prior high ICP. ICP

Table 23.1. Prehospital Care for Patients with Suspected Increased ICP

1. Aggressive airway management for controlled ventilation with adequate oxygenation and normalization of Pa_{CO_2}
2. Immobilization of the cervical spine when indicated
3. Assessment of the neurological deficits
4. Establishment of an initial Glagow Coma Scale score
5. Elevation of head to 30 degrees
6. Correction of hypotension due to possible extracranial injuries

---

due to generalized cerebral edema or hydrocephalus is much better tolerated than increased ICP caused by a focal mass lesion. In addition, an insidious rise in ICP occurring over a prolonged period is much better tolerated than an abrupt increase in ICP.

Evaluation

Primary survey of a patient suspected of having an increased ICP consists of a brief neurological examination and establishment of a Glasgow Coma Scale (GCS) score. The secondary survey includes a detailed history from family and the prehospital care providers, a more detailed and specific physical, and neurological examinations.

Examination of the eyes is singularly useful in patients with suspected increased ICP. Papilledema is the only reliable clinical sign of increased ICP. In the acute phase, TBI rarely causes papilledema, which may take several hours or days to develop. Other findings associated with an initial rise in ICP include a sixth nerve palsy. Papilledema, nuchal rigidity, and subhyaloid hemorrhage occur with subarachnoid hemorrhage (SAH). Pupils are examined for size, symmetry, and reactivity. Pupillary responses are associated with the immediate clinical condition and have little or no predictive value of subsequent clinical course or outcome.

➤A unilateral dilated pupil can give evidence of increased ICP, with a lesion typically ipsilateral to the pupillary dilatation.
➤Pupillary constriction can occur initially in response to an expanding supratentorial mass, followed by unilateral dilatation.
➤Bilaterally fixed, dilated pupils can indicate brain death.
➤Bilaterally dilated and poorly responsive pupils can be caused by sympathetic overactivity from a variety of catecholamines or from anticholinergic medications such as atropine sulfate.
➤Midposition and fixed pupils reflect sympathetic and parasympathetic failure at the midbrain level.
➤Extremely miotic pupils are characteristic of either a narcotic overdose or a pontine lesion.

Visual field defects can occur with postchiasmal hemispheric lesions, including ischemia in the distribution of the posterior cerebral artery, which can cause cortical blindness when bilateral.

Emergent evaluation for suspected increased ICP requires an immediate unenhanced computerized tomography (CT) imaging of the brain. Ancillary laboratory

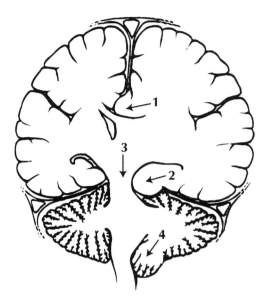

Figure 23.1. Patterns of brain herniation: (1) cingulate herniation under the falx; (2) uncal herniation through the tentorial incisura; (3) central transtentorial herniation through the incisural notch; (4) cerebellar tonsillar herniation through the foramen magnum (from Wilkins RH, Rengochary SS, eds. *Neurosurgery*, 2nd ed. New York, NY: McGraw-Hill; 1996:349. Used with permission.)

testing can help define clinical conditions causing raised ICP but does not supplant the need for an immediate CT imaging.

Common findings on unenhanced CT of the brain suggesting increased ICP:

➤ Cerebral edema. CT findings of diffuse cerebral edema include compression of the ventricular system and effacement of cortical sulci, basal cisterns, and the junction of gray and white matter.
➤ Focal brain lesions such as hematoma or neoplasm. When focal areas of edema are present, a mass effect can cause midline shift of structures or deviation of the posterior fossa structures.
➤ Midline shift of structures.

Brain Herniation

Brain herniation, an end-stage manifestation of increased ICP, refers to displacement of brain tissue from one intracranial compartment to another through an opening in the dural sheath (uncal herniation through a tentorial notch; tonsillar herniation through the foramen magnum) or beneath edges (falx cerebri herniation) of the dural sheath. This causes hemorrhagic necrosis, direct vascular injury, and lateral compression of vital structures. Several herniation syndromes are described in Figure 23.1.

A herniation syndrome is a neurosurgical emergency. When immediate intervention is not taken, death can ensue rapidly. Initial therapy is aimed at lowering ICP while determining and treating the underlying cause.

Cingulate herniation is also referred to as subfalcine or supracallosal herniation. It occurs when an expanding hemispheric mass forces all or part of the cingulate gyrus beneath the free edge of the falx, which causes compression of the anterior cerebral artery with resultant ischemia. Cingulate herniation may not produce any significant clinical symptoms in the initial stage and is frequently identified only on neuroimaging.

Uncal herniation is associated with supratentorial masses and masses in the temporal fossa. An expanding mass can cause the medial portion of the temporal lobe (uncus) to displace over the tentorial notch, causing compression of the ipsilateral oculomotor nerve and displacement of the brainstem. Compression of the ipsilateral posterior cerebral artery can also occur. An early clinical sign is dilatation of the ipsilateral pupil with loss of light reflex and the development of ptosis of the ipsilateral eyelid. Pupillary changes are typically followed by contralateral hemiparesis caused by compression of the contralateral cerebral peduncle against the free edge of the tentorium. Consciousness is depressed with these events and can be accompanied by respiratory changes and bradycardia. However, systemic vital signs may not change until just prior to fatal herniation.

Central transtentorial herniation results from lesions of the frontal, parietal, and occipital lobes. This occurs when there is downward movement of the diencephalon and rostral midbrain through the tentorial notch. Clinically, this displacement results in impairment of cognitive function and can result in loss of upward gaze secondary to midbrain compression. When central herniation is severe, bilateral pupillary dilatation occurs. Vital signs do not change until late in the clinical course, which underscores the importance of serial mental status evaluations in a patient with suspected increased ICP. Cerebellar tonsillar herniation typically is observed in the setting of posterior fossa mass lesions but can occur with supratentorial lesions. The most severe cases are seen when a sudden pressure gradient develops, as in the sudden release of CSF in the presence of raised ICP. When this herniation syndrome occurs, the cerebellar tonsils are displaced through the foramen magnum. Respiratory arrest occurs because of compression of the respiratory centers in the medulla oblongata. Blood pressure falls, pupils dilate, and coma ensues. These signs can occur precipitously. Once the medulla is severely compressed, death is virtually inevitable.

Differential Diagnosis

Common conditions resulting in increased ICP include TBI, cerebrovascular events, hydrocephalus, brain tumor, CNS infections, metabolic and hypoxic encephalopathies, and status epilepticus (see Table 23.2). The common factor linking the development of increased ICP in these various conditions appears to be the production of cerebral edema. Cerebral edema is categorized into vasogenic, cytotoxic, and interstitial types depending upon the pathogenesis, location of edema, fluid composition, extracellular fluid volume, and effects on the blood–brain barrier (see Table 23.3). This specific classification helps dictate appropriate management.

Vasogenic edema is characterized by an increase in vascular permeability. This allows exudative plasma fluid to be extracted into gray and white matter, accumulating predominantly in white matter. Common causes of vasogenic edema include TBI, neoplasm, abscess, meningitis, cerebral infarct, and hemorrhage.

Cytotoxic edema occurs with an intact blood–brain barrier and is likely the result of "cell membrane pump failure," causing intracellular swelling of neurons and endothelial cells with an overall reduction in the extracellular fluid volume. Gray and white matter are generally affected. Although hypoxia is classically

Table 23.2. Differential Diagnosis of Increased Intracranial Pressure

Condition	Pathogenesis
Traumatic brain Injury	Intracerebral hematoma
	Brain contusion and swelling
Cerebrovascular accidents	Subarachnoid hemorrhage
	Intracerebral hematoma
	Cerebral infarct
	Cerebral venous thrombosis
Hydrocephalus	Obstructive
	Communicating
Brain tumor	
CNS infection	Meningitis
	Abscess
	Encephalitis
Metabolic encephalopathy	Hepatic coma
	Hypoxic encephalopathy
	Reye's syndrome
	Diabetic ketoacidosis
	Hyponatremia
Status epilepticus	

Source: Adapted from Pickard JD, Czosnka M. Management of raised intracranial pressure. *J Neuro Neurosurg and Psychiatry*. 1993;56:845–58.

associated with cytotoxic edema, other conditions such as diabetic ketoacidosis, Reye's syndrome, water intoxication, and many "toxic encephalopathies" are associated with cytotoxic edema.

Interstitial edema occurs with an intact blood–brain barrier and generally involves the periventricular white matter. The edema results from an increased amount of CSF resulting from blocked CSF absorption, as in hydrocephalus.

Table 23.3. Types of Cerebral Edema

Type of Edema	Mechanism	Blood–Brain Barrier	Fluid	Pathological Examples
Cytotoxic	Impaired cellular membrane permeability	Mostly intact	Water/NaCl	Diabetic coma, Reye's syndrome, hypoxia, stroke
Vasogenic	Increased capillary permeability leading to disruption of microvasculature	Disrupted	Plasma filtrate and proteins	Traumatic brain injury, CNS neoplasm, CNS abscess, meningitis
Interstitial	Impaired CSF absorption and circulation	Mostly intact	Cerebrospinal fluid	Obstructive hydrocephalus, hemorrhage
Hydrostatic	Impaired brain/plasma osmotic gradient	Mostly intact	Water/NaCl	Water intoxication, hemodialysis, SIADH*

* Syndrome of inappropriate secretion of antidiuretic hormone.

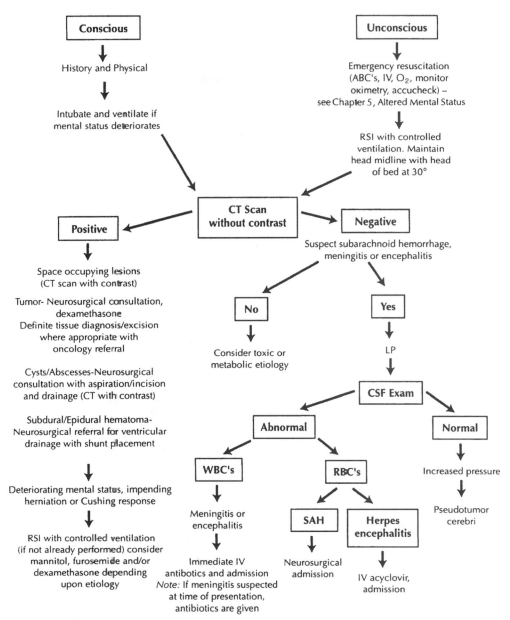

Figure 23.2. Management of patient with suspected raised intracranial pressure. ABCs = airway, breathing, and circulation; CSF = cerebrospinal fluid; CT = computerized tomography; IV = intravenous; LP = lumbar puncture; RBCs = red blood cells; RSI = rapid sequence intubation; SAH = subarachnoid hemorrhage; WBCs = white bood cells.

Management

An immediate attention to airway, breathing, and circulation is mandatory (see Figure 23.2). The goals of airway management are protection of the airway and controlled ventilation. Rapid-sequence intubation (RSI) is the preferred method of securing the airway in order to prevent laryngeal spasm, which can raise the ICP.

Maintenance of Adequate Systemic Blood Pressure

Since systemic hypotension can exacerbate brain injury via cellular hypoxia and cerebral edema, maintenance of adequate systemic blood pressure (BP) (systolic BP > 90 mm Hg) is of paramount importance. Adequate fluid resuscitation is carried out using either lactated Ringer's solution or normal saline. Recently, the use of hypertonic saline solution in fluid resuscitation has been shown to result in less cerebral edema and lower ICP values than isotonic saline in patients with traumatic brain injury. More comprehensive clinical trials studying the use of hypertonic saline in patients with increased ICP are needed. *Cushing's phenomenon* refers to profound increases in ICP associated with hypertension and bradycardia that precedes brain herniation and death. Spinal injuries above T1 can cause hypotension and bradycardia, which are treated with inotropic support. An increase in ICP associated with TBI (except for concomitant heavy blood loss from scalp injuries) does not cause hypotension and shock.

Role of Hyperventilation

Hyperventilation has been used traditionally to lower ICP by decreasing the Pa_{CO_2}, resulting in vasoconstriction and decreased cerebral blood flow (CBF). However, recent evidence suggests that the prophylactic use of hyperventilation to achieve a Pa_{CO_2} of less than 35 mm Hg during the first 24 hours after severe brain injury can compromise cerebral perfusion during a time when CBF is reduced; therefore, it is not performed.

Routine use of hyperventilation to "prevent" increased ICP is no longer recommended. Controlled hyperventilation with maintenance of Pa_{CO_2} levels between 25 and 40 mm Hg and Pa_{CO_2} levels at or above 80 mm Hg for a short duration is recommended when intracranial hypertension is refractory to sedation, paralysis, cerebrospinal fluid (CSF) drainage, or the use of osmotic diuretics. Chronic prophylactic hyperventilation is avoided in the first 5 days after severe TBI and particularly during the first 24 hours because CBF measurements in patients with severe TBI demonstrate a "low" CBF state. Hyperventilation reduces CBF further, does not consistently lower ICP, and can contribute to a loss of autoregulation.

Role of Diuretics

Mannitol, an osmotic diuretic, is currently the diuretic of choice for treating increased ICP. There is an initial rapid fall in ICP after the administration of mannitol due to reflex vasoconstriction that results from its ability to increase flow velocity in cerebral vessels. Following this, mannitol gradually causes dehydration of areas of brain where the blood–brain barrier is intact. Mannitol has the capacity to diffuse across injured areas of the brain and, in some instances, can increase edema in focally injured areas of the brain. When mannitol is given in therapeutic doses, significant diuresis results, which requires close monitoring of the volume status and serum osmolality. Hyperosmotic states (>320 mOsm/dl) are avoided. The dosage of mannitol is 1 g/kg given over a period of 10–20 minutes, followed by smaller doses of approximately 0.25–0.50 g/kg every 4–6 hours. Furosemide, a loop diuretic, is also effective in lowering ICP. It can have a synergistic effect when used with mannitol. The adverse effect associated with combined therapy is accelerated electrolyte loss.

Role of Corticosteroids

Recent studies have not shown a beneficial effect of corticosteroid use in the management of patients with increased ICP resulting from trauma. Corticosteroids are effective in reducing vasogenic edema caused by abscesses and by primary or metastatic neoplasms of the brain. Although the edema surrounding brain hemorrhage is known to be vasogenic, corticosteroids typically are not recommended. Dexamethasone, at an initial dose of 10 mg followed by 4 mg every 6 hours, is used when indicated. When the cause of increased ICP is uncertain, and a neurodiagnostic test is not immediately available, a single dose of corticosteroids does not adversely affect the outcome.

Role of Barbiturate Coma

Barbiturate therapy is effective in lowering ICP in a select subset of patients such as those with persistently high ICP despite aggressive management. Therapy is usually begun with pentobarbital in a dose of 3–5 mg/kg given over several minutes. A change in ICP is noted in about 15 minutes. When the response is favorable, treatment is continued at a dose of 1–2 mg/kg per hour. Serum pentobarbital levels are followed and should not exceed 4 mg/dL. The complications of pentobarbital coma often preclude its use. Hypotension is the most common and serious complication; typically it occurs when pentobarbital levels exceed 4 mg/dL. The use of barbiturates for prophylactic management of patients with increased ICP is not indicated.

Miscellaneous Management Points

Patients with suspected ICP, particularly patients with TBI, should have the heads of their beds elevated to 30 degrees. The heads are positioned in the midline to augment venous drainage. Endotracheal suctioning causes a transient but significant rise in ICP that cannot be ameliorated with preoxygenation. Some patients actually show a cumulative increase in ICP based on the number of suction catheter passes. Therefore, it is recommended to pretreat patients with lidocaine, 1 mg/kg given intravenously, and to limit the number of suction catheter passes to two per procedure. Seizures increase ICP by increasing metabolic and electrical activity within the brain and are managed aggressively and prevented when possible. Generalized seizures in a patient with an elevated ICP can be life-threatening. High fever is treated aggressively in patients with elevated ICP because it increases cerebral metabolism and CBF. Mild hypothermia of a few degrees has been shown to be beneficial, for unknown reasons.

Monitoring Techniques

There is no reliable clinical sign of increasing ICP. A high index of suspicion of its presence is based on the clinical presentation and guides the evaluation of

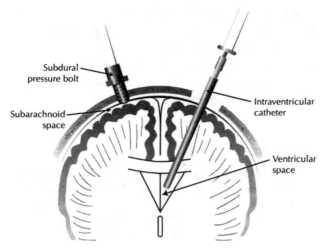

Figure 23.3. Schematic representation of a subdural pressure bolt (*left*) and an intraventricular catheter (*right*). Both systems are connected by nonexpansile tubing to a pressure transducer (from McGillicuddy JE, Cerebral protection: pathophysiology and treatment of increased intracranial pressure. Chest. 1985;87:85–93. Used with permission).

an underlying cause. Of the several noninvasive methods of measuring ICP on an emergency basis, transcranial Doppler examination and tympanic membrane displacement are commonly advocated but are not practiced routinely. The most widely used method to monitor ICP continuously is an invasive procedure of intraventricular catheter placement (see Figure 23.3). It also provides a potential route for the drainage of CSF in instances of refractory increases of ICP. Other methods include a fiberoptic system, with placement of the monitor in an intraparenchymal or subdural location.

PEARLS AND PITFALLS

- Increasing ICP cannot be reliably detected clinically. Increased ICP is considered in patients with TBI, known brain tumor, or central nervous system infection.

- Adequate oxygenation with controlled ventilation is required in the treatment of patients with increasing ICP either out-of-hospital or in the emergency department.

- Maintenance of a normal arterial blood pressure is critical in a patient with increased ICP. Fluid resuscitation, vasoactive agents, or antihypertensives are used as indicated.

- Keep the head of the bed at 30 degrees to augment venous drainage in patients with elevated ICP.

- Seizures are prevented or treated rigorously when present.

- Prophylactic hyperventilation is not indicated in the management of patients with increased ICP.

- The absence of papilledema does not exclude the diagnosis of increased ICP.

- A repeat CT scan of the brain is considered in a patient with declining mental status despite aggressive management.

SELECTED BIBLIOGRAPHY

Bingaman WV, Frank JI. Malignant cerebral edema and intracranial hypertension. *Neurol Clin.* 1995;13:479–509.

Duncan CC, Ment LR. Central nervous system: head injury. In: Toulorian RJ, ed. *Pediatric Trauma*, 2nd ed. Philadelphia, Pa: CV Mosby; 1990.

Fink ME. Emergency management of the head-injured patient. *Emerg Med Clin North Am.* 1987;5:783–95.

Hareri RJ. Cerebral edema. *Neurosurg Clin N Am.* 1994;5:687–706.

McGillicuddy JE. Cerebral protection: pathophysiology and treatment of increased intracranial pressure. *Chest.* 1985;87:85–93.

Pickard JD, Czosnyka M. Raised intracranial pressure. In: Hughes RAC, ed. *Neurological Emergencies*, 1st ed. London: BMG, 1994:150–86.

Wilkins RH, Rengochary SS, eds. *Neurosurgery*, 2nd ed. New York, NY: McGraw-Hill; 1996:349.

Wilkinson HA. Intracranial pressure. In: Youmans JR, ed. *Neurosurgery*. Philadelphia, Pa: WB Saunders; 1990:661–91.

24 Idiopathic Intracranial Hypertension

Eric R. Eggenberger and Sid M. Shah

INTRODUCTION

Idiopathic intracranial hypertension (IIH) and pseudotumor cerebri (PTC) are the terms applied to a clinical syndrome resulting from increased intracranial pressure (ICP) without a known pathophysiology. The major permanent sequela of IIH is visual loss.

IIH typically is a rare disease of obese young females: over 90% of IIH patients are overweight and over 90% are women with a mean age of 30 years at diagnosis. Pediatric cases of IIH are uncommon. The pathophysiology of IIH remains enigmatic. The epidemiology of IIH suggests a relationship to hormonal alterations; however, the exact association remains unknown. Recent hypotheses suggest that cerebral venous outflow obstructions are related to the final common pathway, leading to increased ICP (see Table 24.1).

Evaluation

Typically, the patient with IIH is a young, obese, white female with a headache (see Table 24.2). The headache typically is worse on awakening or in the mornings and may be aggravated by straining or coughing. Transient visual obscurations occur in association with optic disc edema and are characterized by brief episodes (seconds to minutes) of marked diminution, blackout, graying, or complete visual loss often precipitated by postural changes in straining. Commonly, patients do not report pulsatile tinnitus unless asked specifically. Diplopia can result from either unilateral or bilateral abducens nerve palsies, a potential consequence of increased ICP.

The clinical signs of IIH are generally limited to the visual and ocular motor systems, and examination of patients with suspected IIH focuses on visual acuity, visual fields, eye movements, and funduscopy (see Figure 24.1A–D). Bilateral papilledema is present in the vast majority of patients with IIH.

The rate of vision loss in patients with IIH is variable, but typically it is slow and characterized by peripheral visual field defects that develop long before central vision is affected, as measured by Snellen visual acuity.

Table 24.1. Conditions Associated with IIH

1. Medications
       Tetracycline
       Vit A
       Retinoic acid
       Nalidixic acid
       Indomethacin
       Lithium
       Anabolic corticosteroids
       Amiodarone
       Nitrofurantoin
       Cyclosporin
       Levonorgestrel implant
       Psychotropic agents
2. Guillain-Barré syndrome
3. Systemic lupus erythromatosus (SLE)
4. Pregnancy
5. Renal failure
6. Iron deficiency anemia

Table 24.2. Common Symptoms of IIH[a]

Headache
Transient visual obscuration
Pulsatile intracranial noises
Photopsia
Retrobulbar pain
Diplopia
Visual loss

[a] Listing in order of decreasing incidence.

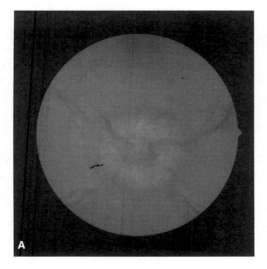

Figure 24.1. A 25-year-old obese female presented with increasing headache and diplopia. (A) Initial examination revealed 20/20 vision in each eye with normal color vision and pupils: chronic-appearing fully developed disc edema was present in each eye. [Right eye shown] (B) Even with this degree of papilledema, the afferent visual examination revealed only an enlarged blind spot in each eye. Neuroimaging was unremarkable, and lumbar puncture revealed OP 458 mm H_2O. With the addition of acetazolamide, headaches and diplopia resolved. Follow-up examination 3 months after presentation revealed resolution of (C) disc edema and (D) enlarged blind spots.

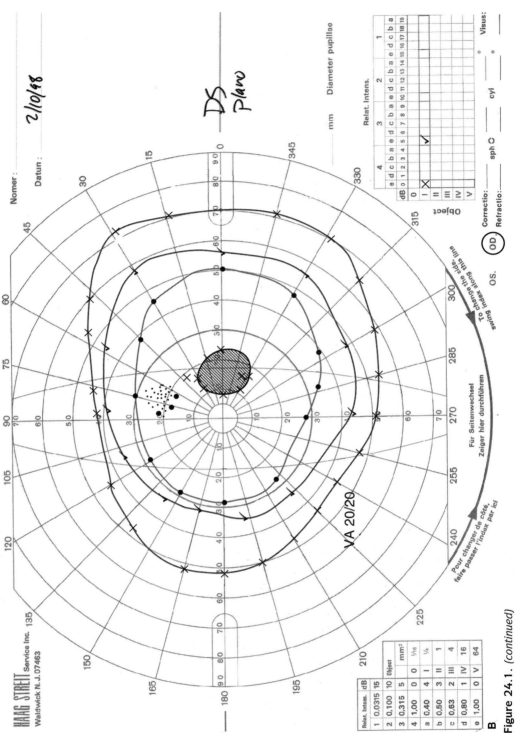

Figure 24.1. *(continued)*

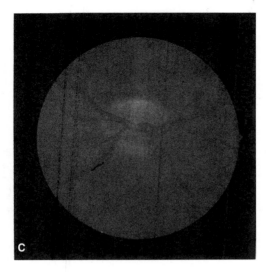

Figure 24.1. *(continued)*

Clinical Features

IIH is considered when evaluating a young patient with symptoms such as headache, transient visual obscuration or finding of palliedema. IIH is a diagnosis of exclusion. See Table 24.3 for diagnostic criteria.

Contrast-enhanced neuroimaging is essential to exclude other causes of increased ICP. Magnetic resonance imaging (MRI) is the diagnostic study of choice. Several subtle imaging signs are common accompaniments of IIH; they include posterior scleral flattening (80%), empty sella (70%), optic nerve sheath distention (45%), prelaminar enhancement of the optic nerve (50%), and vertical tortuosity of the optic nerve (40%).

Lumbar puncture (LP) with opening pressure recording and cerebrospinal fluid (CSF) examination are required in patients with suspected IIH. ICP is measured. Patients with IIH can have large variations in ICP, but rarely will a single measurement of ICP be normal. Serial LPs may be necessary to document intracranial hypertension. A diagnosis of IIH requires a completely normal CSF analysis.

Differential Diagnosis

Pathological conditions that resemble IIH clinically include cerebral mass lesions, hypertensive encephalopathy, hydrocephalus, and dural sinus thrombosis. Dural sinus thrombosis can cause increased ICP with cephalgia and papilledema. Superior sagittal thrombosis often occurs in patients with hypercoagulable disorders. Seizures, hemorrhagic venous infarcts, and bloody CSF are often present in patients with dural sinus thrombosis. Although findings on computerized tomography (CT) of the brain may suggest the diagnosis of dural sinus thrombosis

---

Table 24.3. Characteristic Diagnostic Criteria for IIH

1. Increased ICP
2. Normal cerebrospinal fluid
3. No evidence of central nervous system mass lesion or hydrocephalus
4. Nonfocal neurological examination

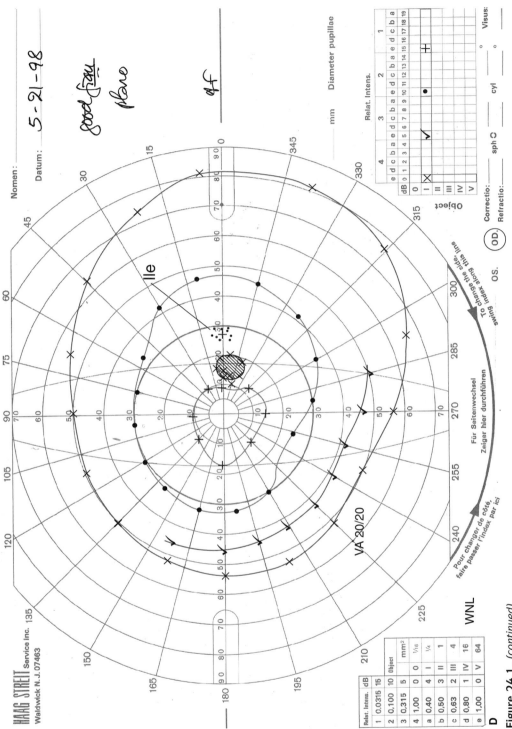

Figure 24.1. *(continued)*

> **Table 24.4.** Modalities Used To Lower ICP
>
> Medications: Lasix, Diamox
> Surgical: lumboperitoneal shunt, optic nerve sheath fenestration

(the "delta" sign of blood clot within the sagittal sinus), MRI is a more sensitive test to detect this condition (sagittal T1-weighted images and magnetic resonance angiography sequences are very useful). Chronic forms of meningitis such as cryptococcal meningitis can resemble IIH initially because of headache and papilledema. CSF results are diagnostic with a positive cryptococcal antigen and cellular reaction. Rarely, certain tumors can cause symptoms and signs suggestive of IIH, especially early in the clinical course. These include gliomatosis cerebri (diffuse neoplasia involving astrocytes) and soft tissue tumor seeding of the CSF. The patient is evaluated for associated medical conditions that can cause or aggravate IIH. Particular attention is paid to medication use, especially in those who do not fit the profile typical of patients with IIH, such as nonobese males.

Management

Treatment is individualized according to the clinical setting and the condition of the patient. Visual field testing and stereoscopic fundus photographs guide follow-up care and treatment decisions. Changes in visual acuity or visual-evoked potentials are signs of end-stage IIH-related optic nerve injury.

Weight loss has been documented to improve the symptoms and signs of IIH but is often difficult to accomplish. In the absence of optic neuropathy, headaches are treated with analgesics.

Headaches from increased ICP can improve with medications that lower ICP such as acetazolamide. Patients with refractory, incapacitating headache, despite the absence of abnormal visual symptoms and signs, require surgical lowering of increased ICP.

Systemic steroid therapy is generally avoided because of concomitant fluid retention, weight gain, systemic and intraocular hypertension, and multiple long-term adverse effects. However, corticosteroids may be a final medical treatment option prior to surgical intervention. Serial lumbar punctures may be used to lower ICP, but this treatment is often unsuccessful and over time is associated with the suboptimal patient follow-up. Other medical options are limited by serious side effects. Corticosteroids are only rarely used in the treatment of IIH and should never be used for prolonged periods (see Table 24.4).

The majority of patients with IIH are managed successfully with medical therapy alone; relatively few require more aggressive therapy. The existence of a significant optic neuropathy at the initial presentation of the patient or the development or progression of optic neuropathy despite optimal medical therapy requires surgical intervention before severe, and possibly, permanent visual dysfunction occurs.

Placement of a Silastic lumboperitoneal shunt is currently the definitive procedure for restoring normal ICP in patients with IIH. Reports indicate that 65–100% of patients with IIH experience resolution of their symptoms, including stabilization or improvement of visual function, following this procedure. Optic nerve sheath fenestration (ONSF) has been performed for the treatment of papilledema.

ONSF creates one or more openings in the dural sheath of the orbital portion of the optic nerve just posterior to the globe. The exact mechanism of the success of ONSF in the treatment of papilledema is controversial.

Because swollen optic nerves require increased perfusion pressures, prophylactic surgical intervention is considered in certain circumstances such as in anticipation of potential hypotensive episodes (e.g., dialysis or the administration of medications with antihypertensive effects). Similarly, protective surgical intervention is considered when accurate monitoring of the patient's visual function is not possible.

IIH associated with evidence of severe or rapidly progressive optic neuropathy is a neuro-ophthalmological emergency. When untreated, these patients can become blind in a matter of days, and lost visual function can be regained rarely. Treatment in these situations is the immediate reduction of ICP, especially surrounding the optic nerves, and can include the use of mannitol and furosemide given intravenously, lumbar puncture, or lumbar drain. Attention is directed at minimizing coexisting risk factors for visual loss in IIH and avoiding extremes of blood pressure and intravascular volume. Although these measures may be appropriate for the short-term treatment of patients with acute loss of visual function, lumboperitoneal shunting or ONSF is performed within 24–48 hours after it has been determined that urgent treatment of IIH is required.

Disposition

Hospitalization is required when rapid visual loss or serious complications of IIH are suspected. Consultation with a neurologist, ophthalmologist, and neurosurgeon is indicated according to the severity of symptoms and the current treatment. When mild, recurrent symptoms of IIH – particularly headache – result in numerous evaluations in the emergency department, referral is given to the appropriate outpatient setting.

PEARLS AND PITFALLS

- IIH is suspected in an obese female patient of childbearing age who presents with headache, visual obscuration, or papilledema.
- Over 90% of patients with IIH are overweight; over 90% are females.
- In a patient with IIH, headaches frequently are worse on awakening or in the morning. Headaches can be aggravated by straining or coughing.
- Transient visual disturbances occur in association with optic disc edema and are characterized by brief episodes of diminished vision, blackout, or complete vision loss precipitated by postural changes or straining.
- Because 20% of normal individuals lack spontaneous venous pulsations on funduscopy, absence of venous pulsations cannot reliably confirm the presence of increased ICP.
- Because only 13% of patients with IIH demonstrate Snellen visual acuity less than 20/20 upon initial evaluation, visual acuity cannot be relied on to document visual loss associated with IIH.
- Hospitalization of a patient with IIH associated with rapid vision loss is prudent.

SELECTED BIBLIOGRAPHY

Durcan FJ, Corbett JJ, Wall M. The incidence of pseudotumor cerebri. Population studies in Iowa and Louisiana. *Arch Neurol.* 1998;45:875–7.

Eggenberger ER, Miller NR, Vitale S. Lumboperitoneal shunt for the treatment of pseudotumor cerebri. *Neurology.* 1996;46:1524–30.

Giuseffi V, Wall M, Siegel PZ, Rojas PB. Symptoms and disease associations in idiopathic intracranial hypertension: a case-control study. *Neurology.* 1991;41:239–44.

Goh KY, Schatz NJ, Glaser JS. Optic nerve sheath fenestration for pseudotumor cerebri. *J Neuroophthalmol.* 1997;17:86–91.

Karahalios DG, Rekate HL, Khayata MH, et al. Elevated intracranial venous pressure as a universal mechanism in pseudotumor cerebri of varying etiologies. *Neurology.* 1996;46:198–202.

Kupersmith ML, Gamell L, Turbin R, et al. Effects of weight loss on the course of idiopathic intracranial hypertension in women. *Neurology.* 1998;50:1094–8.

Radhakrishnan K, Ahlskog JE, Garrity JA, Kurland LT. Idiopathic intracranial hypertension. *Mayo Clin Proc.* 1994;69:169–80.

Vaphiades MS, Brodsky MC. Neuroimaging signs of elevated intracranial pressure. Presented at North American Neuro-ophthalmologic Society, Orlando, Fla, March 1998.

Wall M, George D. Idiopathic intracranial hypertension (pseudotumor cerebri): a prospective study of 50 patients. *Brain.* 1991;114:155–80.

25 Normal Pressure Hydrocephalus

Oliver W. Hayes and Lara Kunscher

INTRODUCTION

Normal pressure hydrocephalus (NPH) is a syndrome of dementia, gait disturbance, and urinary incontinence associated with ventriculomegaly and normal cerebrospinal fluid (CSF) pressure that occurs in the elderly.

The mechanism(s) that cause NPH remain unclear because the connection between ventriculomegaly with normal CSF pressure and the symptoms of NPH has not been fully explained. Isotope cisternographic studies of patients with NPH demonstrate a communicating hydrocephalus due to partial obliteration of the subarachnoid space with defective reabsorption of CSF.

At the time of definitive diagnosis, most patients with NPH have normal or slightly increased CSF pressures suggesting that increased CSF pressures initiated the hydrocephalus antecedently. Continuous monitoring of CSF pressure in NPH patients has shown intermittent elevation of CSF pressures above normal. Although NPH can occur after head injury, subarachnoid hemorrhage, or meningoencephalitis, the etiology is not known in most patients.

Evaluation

NPH is a clinical syndrome of dementia, gait disturbance, and urinary incontinence that progresses over a period of weeks to years. Patient examination reveals confusion, apraxic gait, increased tone and hyperactive tendon jerk reflexes of the legs, and extensor plantar reflexes. Gait disturbance is commonly the first symptom of NPH, an important clinical feature that distinguishes NPH from other dementias. The severity of gait disturbance is also the best predictor of clinical improvement following ventriculoperitoneal shunting. A broad-based stance, hesitant initiation of walking (apraxia), and frequent falling characterize the gait abnormalities.

The dementia of NPH presents with lack of judgment and insight followed by impairment of immediate and recent recall. Initiative and spontaneity are decreased and is described by the family as disinterested, apathetic, or lethargic.

The dementia of NPH is less severe and less rapidly progressive than that of Alzheimer's disease.

Urinary incontinence, a late symptom, occurs in less than 50% of patients. Incontinence is accompanied by a lack of concern by the patient. If untreated, NPH progresses resulting in an inability to stand, akinetic rigidity, and withdrawn behavior.

Differential Diagnosis

The differential diagnosis includes Parkinson's disease, bifrontal brain disease due to tumor, metastases, cerebral infarction, aqueductal stenosis, metabolic encephalopathy, and Alzheimer's disease.

Ancillary Testing

When NPH is suspected clinically, computerized tomography (with contrast enhancement) reveals ventriculomegaly, minimal or absence of cortical atrophy, periventricular lucencies, and nearly normal-sized subarachnoid space. Magnetic resonance imaging (MRI) is the study of choice to evaluate ventriculomegaly and functional imaging of CSF flow.

Lumbar puncture, rarely indicated in the emergency department unless other disease processes are suspected, reveals CSF pressure readings from 80 to 150 mm of water (H_2O) and normal CSF analysis. Some patients with NPH experience temporary improvement in gait disturbance and cognitive functioning following removal of 20–50 ml of CSF (CSF tap test).

Management

When progressive dementia and gait disturbance are accompanied by ventriculomegaly and normal CSF pressure, surgical correction with ventriculoperitoneal shunting benefits between 40% and 70% of patients. The role of the emergency physician is to consider the diagnosis of NPH in patients with dementia and gait disturbance and to initiate appropriate referral.

PEARLS AND PITFALLS

- NPH is a clinical syndrome of progressive dementia, gait disturbance, and urinary incontinence.
- NPH is associated with enlarged ventricles and normal CSF pressure.
- It is important to differentiate the dementia of NPH from that of other neurodegenerative processes.

SELECTED BIBLIOGRAPHY

Adams RD, Fisher CM, Hakim S, Ojemann RG, Sweet WH. Symptomatic occult hydrocephalus with "normal" cerebrospinal fluid pressure: a treatable syndrome. *N Engl J Med.* 1965;273:117–26.

Malm J, Kristensen B, Karlson T, Fagerlund M, Elfvevson J, Ekstedt J. The predictive value of cerebrospinal fluid dynamic tests in patients with idiopathic adult hydrocephalus syndrome. *Arch Neurol*. 1995;52:783–9.

Ojemann RG, Black PM. Evaluation of the patient with dementia and treatment of normal pressure hydrocephalus. *Neurosurgery*. 1985;1:312–21.

Sahuqullo J, Rubio E, Codina A, et al. Reappraisal of the intracranial pressure and cerebrospinal fluid dynamics in patients with so-called "normal pressure hydrocephalus" syndrome. *Acta Neurochir*. 1991;112:50–61.

Sorenson PS, Jansen EC, Gjerris F. Motor disturbances in normal pressure hydrocephalus, special reference to stance and gait. *Arch Neurol*. 1986;43:34–8.

Vanneste J, Augustijn P, Tan WF, Dirven C. Shunting normal pressure hydrocephalus: the predictive value of combined clinical and CT data. *J Neurol Neurosurg Psychiatry*. 1993;56:251–6.

26 Nontraumatic Spinal Cord Emergencies

Michael G. Millin, Sid M. Shah, and David G. Wright

> **INTRODUCTION**
>
> It is important to maintain a high index of suspicion in evaluating a patient with intractable back pain. Back pain may be the only symptom of patients presenting with a variety of spinal emergencies. Nontraumatic spinal emergencies can be caused by a wide spectrum of conditions including infection, hemorrhage, and neoplasm.

Presentation

The five most common findings in patients with spinal emergencies are pain, motor deficits, sensory deficits, abnormal reflexes, and urinary dysfunction. In organizing the history and physical examination around these five symptoms and signs, one can narrow the differential diagnosis to a few conditions.

Back Pain

A 70% lifetime incidence makes back pain one of the more common complaints of the ED population. Location, radiation, and temporal progression are important considerations. Because the spinal cord ends at the L1–L2 level, back pain in spinal cord emergencies is unlikely to localize in the lower lumbar region. Unless the patient is asked to localize back pain, all too frequently the lumbar spine becomes the focus of radiologic investigations with potentially negative and falsely reassuring results. Local pain can be due to lesions pressing on the structures surrounding the cord. Radicular pain results from compression of the nerve roots or a diffuse destruction of spinal cord pain pathways. Radiation of pain in a girdling distribution around the chest or abdomen is a useful symptom of thoracic root compression and may signify vertebral body or pedicle collapse. Subacute pain that develops over weeks to months is common with an epidural abscess. Chronic pain can result from tumors. Acute back pain can be the only symptom of catastrophic spinal emergencies such as spinal hemorrhage or infection.

Motor Deficits

Virtually all patients with significant spinal cord emergencies have some form of motor weakness. Sudden paralysis can result from trauma, cord infarction, or hemorrhage. Progressive weakness can be due to epidural disease, tumors, or inflammatory conditions such as transverse myelitis. Slowly evolving motor deficits are common with multiple sclerosis.

Sensory Deficits

Even though a thorough sensory examination in the emergency department is often difficult and unreliable, seven complexes of sensory and motor abnormalities are helpful. These complexes are (a) *central cord syndrome* – quadriparesis with weakness greater in the upper extremities than in the lower extremities and with some associated loss of pain and temperature sensation; (b) *anterior cord syndrome* – complete paralysis below the lesion and loss of pain and temperature sensation with preservation of position and vibratory sensation; (c) *dorsal cord syndrome* – loss of position and vibratory sensation with preservation of pain and temperature sensation and minimal motor loss; (d) *Brown-Séquard syndrome* (*hemicord syndrome*) – ipsilateral spastic paresis and loss of position and vibratory sensation with contralateral loss of pain and temperature sensation; (e) *thoracic cord lesion* – bilateral loss of position and vibratory sensation in the feet with an identifiable level of pinprick loss on the abdomen or chest; (f) *intramedullary* or *anterior extramedullary cord compression* – loss of pinprick sensation over the legs and trunk with normal sensation in the perianal area; (g) *conus medullaris or cauda-equina syndrome* – loss of pinprick sensation in the perianal area and in the posterior thighs with flaccid paralysis of the lower extremities.

Deep Tendon Reflex Abnormalities

As a result of the anatomical distribution of upper and lower motor neurons, acute spinal cord lesions almost always present with hyperreflexia. Deep tendon reflexes (DTR) help distinguish upper from lower motor neuron disease and, once identified as upper motor neuron disease, the location of the lesion. The isolation of a level of hyperactive reflexes versus normal reflexes is particularly useful. The exception to this rule is cord compression from cauda-equina syndrome, in which the patient will have bilateral hypoactive reflexes of the lower extremities.

Bowel and Bladder Dysfunction

The mechanism of urinary incontinence depends on the type of lesion. Compression of the cauda-equina causes bladder paralysis with urinary retention and overflow incontinence. Progressive myelopathies result in a hyperactive detrusor with associated spasticity and incontinence from decreased compliance.

Ancillary Tests

Laboratory

Because urogenital pathology is often referred to the back, a urinalysis to test for infection is useful. Complete blood count (CBC) and erythrocyte sedimentation rate (ESR) are helpful in certain conditions. Leukocytosis can indicate infectious and inflammatory causes of back pain. Examination of cerebral spinal fluid assists in diagnosing infectious causes of back pain as well as some inflammatory causes such as multiple sclerosis and sarcoidosis.

Radiography

Patients with back pain who have been involved in significant trauma (not simple lifting) are candidates for plain radiographs to identify acute fractures. Plain radiographs in patients who are greater than 50 years old have approximately a 75% sensitivity and 70% specificity for tumors based on age criteria alone. (See Chapter 17, "Musculoskeletal and Neurogenic Pain") Plain radiographs may be helpful in identifying infections of greater than 10 weeks, mass effects in the soft tissues surrounding the cord, or disruption of the bones from congenital and inflammatory conditions. Plain radiographs of the spine are useful in evaluating patients with fevers, unresolved pain greater than 6 weeks, or a history of inflammatory disorders and cancers.

Computerized tomography (CT) of the back provides sharper resolution of the bony components and the ability to examine the vertebra from multiple angles. Cord compression by bony elements can be determined by accurate measurement of the size of the spinal canal with CT. CT is accurate at examining the paravertebral soft tissues for masses and calcifications. The major limitation to CT is that it does not provide an accurate assessment of the spinal cord.

Myelography with CT is an imaging modality in which radiographic dye is injected into the subdural space followed by examination of the spine with CT. Myelography assesses the spinal cord by observing for blockage of the dye caused by cord compression or mass effects. Myelography is useful in assessing the spinal cord when magnetic resonance imaging (MRI) is either not available or is contraindicated.

MRI is the imaging modality of choice for assessment of the spinal cord. The relatively few indications for emergent MRI are listed in Chapter 2, "Neuroradiology." Acute spinal cord compression, which often requires emergent surgical decompression, is best visualized with MRI. MRI is limited in its ability to accurately evaluate the bony vertebrae compared to CT.

Differential Diagnosis and Management

Spinal Cord Infections

Spinal Meningitis
Spinal meningitis is an inflammatory infectious process involving the membranes that cover the spinal cord. Spinal meningitis rarely exists isolated from the brain; thus, patients have a constellation of symptoms and signs related to the entire neuraxis including brain and spinal cord. See Chapter 11, "Central Nervous System Infections in Adults."

Infectious Spondylitis
Infectious spondylitis describes any infection involving the vertebral bodies, intervertebral discs, epidural spaces, posterior elements, and/or paraspinal soft

tissues. Osteomyelitis of the spine and acute discitis are separate entities, but they typically coexist in the adult population. The most common route of infection is hematogenous spread from a separate infectious source. Other routes of infection include extension from adjoining soft tissues (retroperitoneal, intraabdominal, or deep abscess) and primary infection (penetrating trauma, open wounds, surgical instrumentation).

Infectious spondylitis most commonly affects the lumbar spine (50% of cases), followed by the thoracic (35%) and cervical (<10%) spine. Pertinent risk factors are blunt trauma, alcoholism, corticosteroid therapy, an immunocompromised state, diabetes, intravenous drug abuse, and previous back surgery.

Greater than 90% of patients with infectious spondylitis have back pain. The focus of infection can often be localized by the examiner using the thumb to press on each spinous process from cervical to lumbar levels until the exquisitely tender level is found. Other clinical findings are found in less than 50% of patients. These include sudden onset of pain, age greater than 50, fever (50% of patients are unaware of fever; the primary source is the genitourinary tract), and neurological abnormalities (meningismus, radiculopathy, neurogenic bladder, paraparesis, paraplegia).

Erythrocyte sedimentation rate is elevated (20–80 mm/hr) in greater than 90% of patients. However, fewer than 50% of patients will have leukocytosis.

In patients who have been symptomatic for 8–10 weeks, plain radiographs of the spine can show loss in disc-space height with erosion of the vertebral endplates and demineralization of subchondral bone. A paravertebral soft tissue mass may also be identified. CT can identify bony demineralization and destruction associated with infectious spondylitis. The presence of gas and destruction of the bone or disc with paravertebral soft tissue masses is highly specific for infectious spondylitis. Depending on the primary site of infection, many different organisms are implicated in the development of infectious spondylitis. While *Staphylococcus aureus* is the most common infectious agent, *Eschericia coli*, *Pseudomonas aeruginosa*, *Streptococcus*, and *Salmonella* are also frequently found. Polymicrobial and anaerobic infections are uncommon. Therapy is initiated with broad-spectrum antibiotics, eventually narrowing to organism-specific antibiotics. Surgery is required at times to drain or decompress drug-resistant infection or abscess for persistent back pain.

Tuberculosis of the Spine

Tuberculosis of the spine begins with hematogenous seeding of the vascular vertebral metaphysis from a separate primary source of infection. The disease follows a relatively slow progression. Infection of the vertebrae develops into spondylitis with extension to the subligamentous spaces, progressing to paraspinal abscesses and eventual seeding of the leptomeninges. A drawn out clinical course includes fever, malaise, and back pain. Up to 20% of patients with tuberculous spondylitis have a negative purified protein derivative (PPD) test; an elevated ESR is infrequent. Isolation of organisms on culture and acid-fast stain is positive in less than 50% of patients. Plain radiographs can reveal erosion of the vertebral column. Findings of soft tissue calcifications with paraspinal abscess on CT are specific for tuberculosis of the spine. The treatment of tuberculosis spondylitis begins with a regimen of isoniazid, ethambutol, rifampin, and streptomycin.

Deterioration of neurological status with associated paraspinal abscess mandates surgical intervention.

Spinal Epidural Abscess

Spinal epidural abscess is an uncommon disease that is often not diagnosed in the early stages. In hospitalized patients, the national incidence in tertiary care hospitals is less than 0.01%. Because outcome is directly related to clinical status at the time of presentation, early diagnosis is important. Any patient with back pain and fever is evaluated for possible spinal epidural abscess. Most patients have other co-morbid diseases, most commonly, diabetes. Other associated diseases include alcoholism, cirrhosis, and recent infections (urinary, pneumonia, dental abscess, pharyngitis, pelvic inflammatory disease, skin, and soft tissue infection). A history of trauma, intravenous drug use, or recent back surgery increases clinical suspicion of an epidural abscess.

An ESR has a high sensitivity for detecting epidural abscess, but leukocytosis is only about 70% sensitive. Plain radiographs of the thoracic spine occasionally demonstrate a soft tissue mass extending into the chest cavity. CT is helpful, but it can fail to delineate the abscess. Myelography with CT identifies the abscess by a blockage in the flow of dye, compression of the thecal sac, and a mass in the epidural space. On gadolinium-enhanced T1-weighted MRI, a mass in the epidural space appears as a low signal intensity within a contrast-enhancing ring. Treatment is surgical drainage with intravenous antibiotics. Urgent surgical drainage is associated with a higher rate of favorable outcome.

Noninfectious, Inflammatory Spinal Emergencies

Transverse Myelitis

Transverse myelitis describes any inflammatory condition that involves the entire cross-sectional area of the spinal cord at a particular level. The complete transection of the spinal cord disrupts all motor and sensory nerves that extend beyond the level of the lesion. The exact pathophysiological mechanism that leads to the development of transverse myelitis is unknown. The associated conditions believed to contribute to the development of transverse myelitis include collagen vascular diseases (specifically systemic lupus erythematosus), acquired immune deficiency syndrome, sarcoidosis, and multiple sclerosis. Transverse myelitis is a diagnosis of exclusion. Other considerations include neoplasm, spinal infarction, multiple sclerosis, infectious spondylitis, and spinal cord compression. The diagnosis is considered in a patient with acute sensory and motor deficits in a transverse distribution without evidence of spinal cord compression or any other known neurologic disease. Myelography with CT demonstrates spinal cord enlargement. MRI with gadolinium demonstrates spinal cord edema associated with enhancement in the area of the inflamed region. The management of transverse myelitis consists of supportive care and the use of corticosteroids.

Multiple Sclerosis

See Chapter 19, "Multiple Sclerosis."

Multiple sclerosis (MS) is a chronic inflammatory disease of the white matter in the brain and spinal cord. The inflammatory process forms plaques that

Table 26.1. Clinical Findings in Multiple Sclerosis

1. Acute monocular visual disturbance
2. Limb weakness
3. Urinary dysfunction
4. Lhermitte's sign – shooting pains in the neck and arms with neck flexion
5. Brown-Séquard – ipsilateral motor deficits with contralateral pain and temperature deficit
6. Devic's syndrome – transverse myelitis with optic neuritis

degrade myelin proteins. The plaques preferentially form in the periventricular white matter of the brain and brainstem, the spinal cord, and the optic nerves. The most common site of involvement in the spinal cord is in the cervical region. Some of the common clinical findings in MS are listed in Table 26.1.

The MRI findings of MS in the spinal cord are elongated areas of hyperintense signal affecting the posterior and lateral columns, best seen on the T2-weighted images. Chronic inflammatory plaques are sharply demarcated without signs of edema. Acute lesions have associated cord edema. Therapy for acute relapsing episodes of MS includes corticosteroids, immunosuppressive therapy, and plasmapharesis. The diagnosis of new onset MS is rarely made in the emergency department.

Spinal Sarcoidosis

Sarcoidosis is a chronic multisystem inflammatory disorder with derangements of normal tissue caused by the formation of noncaseating epithelioid granulomas. The lungs are the most commonly affected organs, and approximately 5% of cases involve the central nervous system. Sarcoidosis of the spine is rare and primarily affects the cervical cord. The granulomas are located within the cord parenchyma and the leptomenignes. The clinical effect of sarcoidosis of the spine is a nonspecific myelopathy that ranges from a mild unilateral weakness to severe plegias.

Funduscopic examination can reveal retinal granulomas. Chest radiographs and CT imaging are useful in diagnosing sarcoidosis. Sarcoid granulomas of the spine are identified on MRI by spinal cord enlargement with increase in signal intensity on T2-weighted images. The enhanced areas are usually asymmetric and may be nodular, linear, or multifocal. Magnetic resonance imaging findings are nonspecific and can also be identified with MS, transverse myelitis, tumors, and tuberculosis. Leptomeningeal involvement often results in CSF abnormalities – pleocytosis (70%), elevated protein (70%), and decreased glucose (18%). Definitive diagnosis is made by biopsy. Treatment of spinal sarcoidosis is systemic corticosteroids and supportive therapy. Surgical resection of granulomatous lesions can result in increased morbidity and a worsening of neurological deficits.

Rheumatoid Arthritis

Rheumatoid arthritis (RA) is a chronic multisystem inflammatory disease characterized by a persistent synovitis. The inflammatory process of RA can affect any joint in the body including the joints of the spine. The most common area

Table 26.2. Clinical Presentations of Cervical Spine Rheumatoid Arthritis

Syndrome	Clinical Findings	Radiographic Findings
1. Anterior and posterior atlantoaxial subluxation	a. Occipitocervical pain with a "clunking" sensation on neck flexsion b. Ataxia c. Vertigo d. Dysarthria e. Nystagmus	Separation between the anterior odontoid and the posterior inferior tubercle of C1 by more than 2.5 mm in women and 3.0 mm in men
2. Vertical subluxation "cranial settling"	a. Myelopathy b. Dysphagia c. Dysphonia d. Diplopia e. Facial numbness f. Death	Projection of the odontoid more than 4.5 mm superior to the line formed by the most caudal point of the occipital curve of the skull to the dorsal margin of the hard palate
3. Lateral and rotation subluxation	a. Neck and shoulder pain b. Limited head rotation	Lateral masses of C1 are displaced more than 2 mm lateral to the masses of C2
4. Subaxial subluxation	a. Radicular pain b. Paresthesia c. Muscular weakness d. Diminished deep tendon reflexes e. Atrophy	Serial staircase patterns of the vertebral bodies

affected is the cervical spine at the atlantoaxial joint. Patients complain of dull aching pain in the neck or an occipital headache. Rheumatoid arthritis of the cervical spine presents as distinct syndromes as listed in Table 26.2.

Management of RA of the cervical spine is supportive. An unstable cervical spine requires stabilization of the neck and neurosurgical consultation for definitive treatment.

Spinal Vascular Emergencies

Spinal Cord Infarction

Due to the anatomical distribution of spinal arteries, most infarcts affect the anterior spinal cord. Neurologic deficits from spinal cord infarction develop abruptly over minutes to hours. Profound weakness or paralysis with sensory loss involving the spinothalamic tract (touch and temperature) occurs. Posterior columns (joint position and vibratory sensation) are spared. Significant bladder or bowel dysfunction is common.

The pathophysiologic mechanisms of spinal cord infarction are hypoperfusion (cardiovascular collapse), thrombosis, or embolism. Associated clinical events include major vessel arterial dissection, trauma, aortic atherosclerosis, spondylosis, vasculitis, embolism from cardiac source, hypercoagulable states, thrombosis of a spinal arteriovenous malformation, and disc disease. Spinal cord infarction can also result from iatrogenic causes primarily related to surgery. Surgical procedures most commonly associated with infarction include repairs of abdominal aortic aneurysms, thoracotomy for resection of lung tissue, and scoliosis repair.

CT is sensitive in identifying the cord edema that develops in the latter stages of the disease; however, CT is inferior to MRI in identifying the specific patterns of contrast enhancement of cord infarction. The initial areas affected with anterior spinal artery syndrome are the anterior horns, which appear on MRI as "owls eyes."

The therapy of spinal cord infarction, like ischemic cerebral stroke, is mainly supportive. Current literature does not support the use of antithrombotics or anticoagulants in the setting of spinal cord infarction.

Intraspinal Hemorrhage

Intraspinal hemorrhages occur in one of four anatomic locations – the epidural space, the subdural space, the subarachnoid space, and the spinal cord parenchyma. The pathophysiology includes transmission of increased vascular pressure from the intraabdominal venous system, spontaneous rupture of branching arteries under high pressure, intraspinal tumors, collagen vascular diseases, anticoagulation therapy, and trauma (including iatrogenic trauma from surgical intervention, placement of epidural space catheters, and lumbar puncture).

Acute onset of severe, stabbing back pain is the classic presentation. The onset of back pain is quickly followed by profound neurological deficits with paralysis that develops over minutes to hours. CT identifies acute intraspinal hemorrhages by an area of focal hyperdensity within either the spinal cord or the spinal canal.

Treatment of intraspinal hemorrhage depends on its severity. Patients with minimal back pain and no neurological deficit are observed closely without intervention if the hematoma resolves spontaneously. For patients with moderate to severe back pain and minimal neurological deficit, aspiration of the hematoma is an alternative approach to neurosurgical intervention. Patients with severe pain and profound neurological deficits need emergent surgical intervention for decompression of the hematoma.

Spinal Tumors

The most common complaint of patients with spinal cord tumors is pain. (See Chapter 21, "Brain Tumors and other Neuro-Oncological Emergencies.") Back pain secondary to tumors is usually localized to the area of the lesion and persistent despite limitation of activity, rest, and analgesics. Primary tumors can be intra- or extramedullary. Metastatic tumors are most common in the vertebral bodies. Metastases to the vertebrae are located in the thoracic spine in 70% of patients, followed by the lumbosacral and cervical areas. Up to 86% of patients have multilevel lesions. Complications of spinal cord tumors are typically related to compression of the cord. Compression occurs either directly by the tumor or secondary to instability of the vertebral column. Patients with cord compression secondary to tumors have weakness of the lower extremities. Urinary retention is a late finding. Common primary and metastatic tumors are listed here.

Primary Tumors	Metastatic Tumors

Extramedullary
   Neurofibroma, meningioma, sarcoma
Intramedullary
   Ependymoma, astrocytoma, vascular, gliomas
	Breast, lung, prostate, lymphoma, sarcoma, kidney, gastrointestinal, melanoma, neck, unknown

Patients with suspected spinal tumors are initially evaluated with plain radiographs. Common findings include disruption of the pedicles, compression of the vertebral bodies, or soft tissue mass. CT or MRI further evaluates suspicious findings.

Treatment of spinal tumors is a four-step approach. Adequate analgesia is provided. The spine is stabilized as necessary – a cervical collar or other appropriate device. Neurosurgical consultation is obtained for stabilization and possible debulking of the tumor. Radiation therapy is provided on an emergent basis when neurosurgical intervention is not indicated.

Special Challenges in Diagnosis

Spinal cord emergencies frequently go unrecognized initially or are misdiagnosed even with such obvious symptoms as the inability to walk or failure of bladder function. Diagnostic focus can be compromised after early placement of a urinary catheter and alleviation of patient discomfort. The patient's behavior can also be misleading. Many patients take ambulation for granted and are in denial or even indifferent when this function is lost. They may assume that leg function is easily regained when their overall health returns. This can easily be misinterpreted as "la belle indifference" of hysteria. In fact, hysterical paralysis is quite rare compared to spinal cord pathology, and this diagnosis should not be made in the emergency department. A period of inpatient observation and neurological or neurosurgical consultation is indicated for any patient with unexplained paraparesis.

Paradoxical findings can also lead to a mistaken impression of hysteria or malingering. A patient may complain of being unable to feel or move the legs yet demonstrate a forceful flexion of the legs when touched with a pin. This is a triple flexion reflex, a spastic reaction to a noxious stimulus similar to the Babinski sign. Another paradox is the flaccidity and hyporeflexia seen with spinal shock, a physiological condition that can persist for days to weeks. This can be confusing to the examiner who is looking for hyperreflexia as a sign of spinal cord pathology. Finally, one must remember the somatotopic layering in the spinal cord in which the motor and sensory pathways for the legs are outermost. This can result in an ascending sensory or motor level with the legs being involved earliest in a cervical spinal cord compression. For the physician who is accustomed to evaluating nerve root problems and who associates leg symptoms with the low back and arm symptoms with the neck, this paradox can be confusing. Negative radiographic studies of the lumbar or thoracic spine may give false reassurance in a patient with cervical cord compression.

PEARLS AND PITFALLS

- Back pain can be the only symptom of a very serious underlying condition.

- Radiation of back pain in a girdling distribution around the chest or abdomen can indicate thoracic root compression and may signify vertebral body or pedicle collapse.

- Urinary dysfunction caused by spinal cord emergencies depends on the type of lesion. Compression of cauda euina can present with urinary retention, and progressive myelopathies can result in urinary incontinence.

- One can never rely on absence of leucocytosis or elevated ESR to diagnose infectious or inflammatory causes of back pain.

- Emergent MRI is the study of choice when spinal cord compression is suspected.

- Vascular emergencies (causing spinal cord infarction) mostly affect the anterior spinal cord as a result of the anatomic distribution of spinal arteries.

- Back pain is the most common complaint of patients with spinal cord tumor.

- Spinal cord emergencies are frequently unrecognized or misdiagnosed.

SELECTED BIBLIOGRAPHY

Adams RD, Victor M. Diseases of the spinal cord. In: *Principles of Neurology*, 5th ed. New York, NY: McGraw-Hill; 1993.

Amour TES, Hodge SC, et al., eds. *Epidural Abscess, in MRI of the Spine*. New York, NY: Raven Press, 1994.

Andersson GBJ. The epidemiology of spinal disorders. In: Frymoyer JW, et al, eds. *The Adult Spine*, 2nd ed. Philadelphia, Pa: Lippincott-Raven; 1997.

Andersson GBJ, Deyo RA. Sensitivity, specificity, and predictive value: a general issue in screeing for disease and in the interpretation of diagnostic studies in spinal disorders. In: Frymoyer JW, et al., eds. *The Adult Spine*, 2nd ed. Philadelphia, Pa: Lippincott-Raven; 1997.

Campana BA: Soft tissue spine injuries and back pain. In: Rosen P, Barkin R, et al., eds. *Emergency Medicine – Concepts and Clinical Practice*, 4th ed. St. Louis, Mo: Mosby; 1998.

Quint DJ: Indications for emergent MRI of the central nervous system. *JAMA*. 283:7;2000.

Schwartz DT, Reisdorff EJ, eds. Introduction to emergency radiology. In: *Emergency Radiology*. New York, NY: McGraw-Hill; 2000.

Woolsey RM, Young RR. The clinical diagnosis of disorders of the spinal cord. *Neurologic Clinics*. 1991;9:3.

27 Sleep Disorders

A. Sinan Baran

INTRODUCTION

Injury can be a result of excessive daytime sleepiness (EDS) or behaviors during sleep (parasomnias). Obstructive sleep apnea can cause or contribute to cardiovascular disorders observed in the emergency department. Cataplexy, an auxiliary symptom of narcolepsy characterized by sudden muscle weakness, can be mistaken for other acute medical problems. Sleep-related panic attacks can occur in patients without daytime panic attacks and may mimic acute cardiovascular symptoms. Insomnia (difficulty falling asleep or staying asleep) due to various causes, including primary sleep disorders or primary medical/psychiatric disorders, can compromise daytime functioning and predispose to trauma. Underlying sleep-related breathing disturbances may predispose a patient to complications of sedating medications administered in the emergency department.

Sleep Disorders That Predispose to Trauma

Disorders Associated with Excessive Daytime Sleepiness

Many automobile and occupational accidents are thought to be at least partially due to sleepiness and associated impairment of vigilance. Although insufficient sleep is the leading cause of EDS, sleep disorders can also cause sleepiness either by disrupting nocturnal sleep or, in the case of narcolepsy, by as yet uncharacterized neurological mechanisms. Table 27.1 lists features of sleep disorders pertinent to evaluation in the emergency department. Table 27.2 lists general treatment approaches to sleep disorders.

Obstructive Sleep Apnea and Upper Airway Resistance Syndrome

Loud snoring is the hallmark of obstructive sleep apnea (OSA), which is caused by the instability of the upper airway during sleep. OSA can occur at any age, but most patients come to medical attention between the ages of 40 and 60 years.

Table 27.1. Features of Sleep Disorders Pertinent to Emergency Medicine

	EDS[a]	Behaviors During Sleep[a]	Associated Medical Conditions	Mimic Other Medical Problems
Obstructive sleep apnea/upper airways resistance syndrome	X		X	
Periodic limb movement disorder	X			
Narcolepsy	X			X
Recurrent hypersomnia	X			
Sleep terrors		X		
Sleepwalking		X		
REM sleep behavior disorder		X	X	
Sleep panic attacks				X

[a] Potential for trauma.

Factors that can contribute to upper airway collapse include adipose infiltration of the parapharyngeal structures (due to obesity), mass effect of an enlarged neck, and nasal or oropharyngeal obstruction from any cause. OSA can also occur in association with neurological disorders that cause abnormal control of pharyngeal muscles.

Upper Airway Resistance Syndrome

Upper airway resistance syndrome (UARS) is a variant of OSA. Mild to moderately increased upper airway resistance as a result of the narrowing of the upper airway during sleep may be overcome by increased respiratory effort, without a significant reduction in airflow. The increased resistance requiring increased effort can nevertheless result in an arousal that fragments sleep. In most cases, the patient with UARS may have EDS without evidence of an obvious respiratory disturbance other than snoring.

Periodic Limb Movement Disorder

Previously known as nocturnal myoclonus, this disorder of periodic and highly stereotyped involuntary movements of the limbs during sleep can cause sleep

Table 27.2. Typical Treatment Approaches to Sleep Disorders

Disorder	Treatment
Obstructive sleep apnea/upper airway resistance syndrome	CPAP/ENT surgery/oral appliances
Periodic limb movement disorder/RLS	Benzodiazepines/dopamine agonists/opiates
Narcolepsy	Stimulants (for EDS) and tricyclic antidepressants (for cataplexy)
Sleep terrors/sleepwalking	Benzodiazepines/tricyclic antidepressants
REM sleep behavior disorder	Benzodiazepines (clonazepam)

fragmentation and resultant EDS. Onset is usually during middle adulthood, with a tendency to progress with advancing age. Rare cases occur during childhood. The prevalence is unknown. Periodic limb movements typically occur in the legs but may also involve the arms. The leg movements involve extension of the great toe, along with partial flexion of the ankle, knee, and occasionally the hip. Both legs are usually affected, and movements can occur in intervals lasting minutes to hours, or throughout the sleep period. Sleep disruption is associated with periodic limb movements.

Narcolepsy

Narcolepsy is characterized by the so-called narcoleptic tetrad: excessive daytime sleepiness, cataplexy, sleep paralysis, and hypnagogic hallucinations. EDS is the hallmark of narcolepsy, and the other three symptoms (the auxiliary symptoms) are not necessary for the diagnosis of this disorder. All three auxiliary symptoms are thought to be rapid eye movement (REM) sleep-related phenomena.

Cataplexy

Cataplexy is a sudden loss of voluntary muscle tone typically precipitated by emotional excitement, particularly laughter. The duration is usually several seconds or minutes but may be longer. Severity can range from a subtle, barely noticeable sagging of facial muscles or slurring of speech to a generalized and profound weakness resulting in a collapse to the floor. Cataplexy should be distinguished from syncope, transient ischemic attacks, and partial seizures. Consciousness is fully intact during cataplexy although patients may sleep following an episode. A history of emotional excitement as a precipitant of the events, EDS, and other auxiliary symptoms of narcolepsy help to clarify the diagnosis.

Sleep Paralysis and Hypnagogic Hallucinations

Sleep paralysis and hypnagogic hallucinations are other REM sleep-related phenomena that the narcoleptic patient may experience. Sleep paralysis is the occurrence of atonia during the transition from wakefulness to REM sleep (during a sleep-onset REM episode) or from REM sleep to wakefulness. Typically, the patient reports a transient inability to move (lasting no longer than several minutes) as he or she is falling asleep or awakening, and this may be particularly frightening the first time it occurs. Hypnagogic hallucinations are dreamlike images or sounds that may occur at sleep onset, as the patient is entering REM sleep. Hypnapompic hallucinations are their counterpart experienced while awakening from REM sleep. Hypnagogic or hypnapompic hallucinations may accompany sleep paralysis, adding to the frightening nature of the occurrence. Hypnagogic and hypnapompic hallucinations are not symptoms of psychosis. Sleep paralysis and hypnagogic/hypnapompic hallucinations can occur in normal individuals, especially during an irregular sleep schedule or REM sleep rebound caused by sleep deprivation or withdrawal from a REM sleep-suppressing agent.

Disorders Associated with Behaviors while Asleep (Parasomnias)

Injury can result from behaviors that occur during sleep. The patient's ability to recall the episode depends partly on the type of the parasomnia (occurrence during non-REM versus REM sleep).

Sleep Terrors and Sleepwalking

Sleep terrors and sleepwalking are both non-REM sleep phenomena that specifically occur during stage 3 or 4 sleep (slow-wave sleep). Because the majority of slow-wave sleep occurs in the first third of the night, sleep terrors and sleepwalking are most likely to occur at that time. Patients may demonstrate dangerous behaviors, including jumping through a closed window in an attempt to escape a perceived threat or danger, leading to significant injury. Both sleep terrors and sleepwalking are common during childhood and usually resolve during adolescence.

REM Sleep Behavior Disorder

The atonia of skeletal muscles during REM sleep may be conceptualized as a protective mechanism that prevents the physical enactment of dreams. When atonia is abolished, movements become possible and are dictated by the content of dreams. Patients with REM sleep behavior disorder (RBD) have intermittent loss of REM atonia and, as a result, may engage in various behaviors, with a potential for injury to themselves or their bed partners. RBD typically occurs in men over the age of 50, but it may occur in both sexes and begin at any age. Sixty percent of cases are idiopathic.

Other Sleep Disorders

Recurrent Hypersomnia

Kleine-Levin syndrome, a disorder thought to be due to hypothalamic dysfunction, is characterized by recurrent hypersomnia and disinhibited behaviors. Cases involve recurrent episodes of hypersomnia and hyperphagia that typically begin in adolescent males and resolve by adulthood. The syndrome occurs less commonly at a later age and in women. Episodes occur 2 to 12 times per year and may last several days to weeks. During an episode, patients may sleep up to 20 hours per day, with awakenings to eat and void.

Insomnia

Insomnia is characterized by difficulty falling asleep or staying asleep. Although patients with insomnia typically do not complain of EDS, they can nevertheless have impaired daytime functioning that can increase their risk for accidents and injury. Insomnia can result from multiple causes including psychiatric or general medical disorders, medication effects, substance abuse, and other sleep disorders.

Restless legs syndrome (RLS) is another important cause of insomnia. RLS is thought to be related to periodic limb movement disorder and is characterized by lower extremity dysesthesias that occur at rest and are particularly bothersome as patients lie in bed at bedtime. The discomfort is relieved transiently by movement, and patients are compelled to keep their legs active, sometimes requiring them to get up and walk. As a result, sleep onset is delayed until the symptoms subside, sometimes taking hours in severe cases. Most cases are idiopathic.

PEARLS AND PITFALLS

- Excessive daytime sleepiness, regardless of its etiology, can lead to trauma.
- Patients may underestimate and minimize the severity of their daytime sleepiness.
- Patients with obstructive sleep apnea may experience respiratory compromise when given sedating medications.
- Not all patients with sleep-disordered breathing (upper airway resistance syndrome and obstructive sleep apnea) are obese.
- Cataplexy, an auxiliary symptom of narcolepsy, may be mistaken for syncope, transient ischemic attacks, and partial seizures.

SELECTED BIBLIOGRAPHY

Chokroverty S. *Sleep Disorders Medicine: Basic Science, Technical Considerations, and Clinical Aspects.* Boston, Mass: Butterworth-Heinemann; 1994.

Kryger M, Roth T, Dement W. *Principles and Practice of Sleep Medicine*, 2nd ed. Philadelphia, Pa: WB Saunders; 1994.

28 Traumatic Brain Injury

Christopher Carpenter, Kevin Gingrich,
James E. Wilberger, Jr., Lee Warren, and Sid M. Shah

INTRODUCTION

Traumatic brain injuries (TBI) account for 25% of all traumatic deaths in the United States where 500,000 patients require admission annually, with 40% of these admissions for moderate to severe injury. The incidence of TBI peaks in adolescence and again in the elderly. Males are three times more likely to sustain TBI as females. Up to half of TBI patients are intoxicated, and 75% have injuries to other organ systems. Almost 34,000 patients die each year before emergency department (ED) arrival. Of those surviving to reach the ED, 80% have minor head trauma (defined on the Glasgow Coma Scale as GCS 13–15), 10% have moderate head trauma (GCS 9–12), and 10% have severe head trauma (GCS 3–8). More than 50% of serious TBI patients have multiple injuries; on presentation to the ED, 30% are hypoxic and 15% are hypotensive. Benefits of an emergent airway are weighed against the risks of increasing ICP, cervical spine injury and aspiration. The prompt pre-hospital and ED diagnosis and management of TBI and associated injuries can improve outcomes.

Pathophysiology

Head injury refers to an injury that presents with physical findings such as ecchymosis, soft tissue swelling, lacerations, or CSF leakage. Traumatic brain injury refers to primary brain injury that is not always clinically apparent. Patients with mild TBI can have normal neurological and physical examinations.

Primary brain injury is caused by mechanical force resulting in functional and physical disruption of brain tissue. Secondary brain injury occurs when post-injury factors such as hypotension, hypoxia, anemia, hyperthermia, hypercapnea, hypocapnea, electrolyte imbalances, hyperglycemia, hypoglycemia, acid-base abnormalities, intracranial hypertension (ICH), mass lesions, cerebral edema, vasospasm, hydrocephalus, infection, and seizures adversely affect the injured brain. Secondary brain injury is the leading cause of significant morbidity and brain death. Interventions in the ED can greatly influence the ultimate outcome by preventing secondary brain injury. Increased intracranial pressure is reviewed in Chapter 23, "Increased Intracranial Pressure and Herniation Syndromes."

Subdural hematoma (SDH) results from tearing of the veins or cortical arterioles in acceleration/deceleration injuries such as motor vehicle collisions or falls. Acute SDH appears as a crescent-shaped heterogeneous density between the dura and parenchyma on computerized tomography (CT) of the brain. The typical patient presents with event-related loss of consciousness (LOC), initial improvement, then deterioration. Findings range from complaints of a headache to profound altered mental status with unilateral pupillary dilatation. Though patients with isolated SDH less than 3 mm can be observed on a neurosurgical service, removal of small SDHs can markedly decrease elevated intracranial pressures (ICP) and improve outcomes.

Epidural hematomas (EDH) result from direct trauma to the skull, either with or without associated skull fractures. The incidence of EDH peaks in the second and third decades of life and is rare in infancy and the elderly. EDHs form a lenticulate homogenous hyperdense image on the brain surface (usually temporal) on CT. After an initial LOC, patients may experience a "lucid interval" followed by rapid deterioration. Timely surgical evacuation in the immediate postinjury period allows excellent recovery.

Diffuse axonal injury (DAI) is likely the primary reason for persistent coma following TBI. DAI can be found scattered throughout the brain and results from widespread injury to the axonal fibers particularly in the area of internal capsule and brainstem. In mild to moderate injury, axons may regenerate.

Cerebral contusions and intraparenchymal hemorrhage are hemorrhages within brain parenchyma, typically occurring where brain is injured by bone, although they can also occur from shear strain and rotational stresses. They can be associated with edema, shift, and herniation.

Concussive syndromes are transient alterations in neural functioning with several different interpretations. According to the summary and agreement statement of the first international conference on concussion in sport, held in Vienna in 2001, concussion is defined as a complex pathophysiological process affecting the brain, induced by traumatic biomechanical forces. Several common features that incorporate clinical, pathological, and biomechanical injury constructs that may be used in defining the nature of a concussive head injury include:

1. Concussion may be caused by a direct blow to the head, face, neck, or elsewhere on the body with an "impulsive" force transmitted to the head.
2. Concussion typically results in the rapid onset of short-lived impairment of neurological function that resolves spontaneously.
3. Concussion may result in neuropathological changes, but the acute clinical symptoms largely reflect a functional disturbance rather than structural injury.
4. Concussion results in a graded set of clinical syndromes that may or may not involve loss of consciousness. Resolution of the clinical and cognitive symptoms typically follows a sequential course.
5. Concussion is typically associated with grossly normal structural neuroimaging studies.

Table 28.1. Indications for Emergent CT Scan in TBI

Low Risk	High Risk
Asymptomatic at time of evaluation	Focal neurologic findings
No focal findings	Asymmetric pupils
Pupils normal	Skull fracture
No other injuries	Multiple traumas
Level of consciousness normal	Painful, detracting injuries
Intact orientation/memory	LOC (>2 min)
Initial GCS > 13	GCS ≤ 13
Accurate history	Amnesia/confusion
Trivial mechanism	Worsening headache
Injury > 24 hours ago	Vomiting
Reliable home observers	Posttraumatic seizure
	Coagulopathy
	Intoxication
	Unreliable history
	Suspected child abuse
	Age > 60, < 2 years old

Adapted from Biros MH, Heegaard W. Head. In: Rosen P. et al., eds. *Emergency Medicine: Concepts and Clinical Practice*, 5th ed. St. Louis: Mosby; 2002:298.

Patients with concussion can present with or without LOC for up to 6 hours. More severe syndromes involve retrograde and anterograde amnesia as well as subtle cognitive changes very similar to EDHs. Persistent focal neurological findings imply more severe injury than a concussion. Skull fractures of significance include those predisposing to EDH (overlying a major dural sinus), those underlying a scalp laceration, those associated with intracranial air, those depressed below the level of the inner skull table, and basilar skull fractures.

Mild traumatic brain injury is not always clinically apparent. Findings include (1) any period of loss of consciousness, (2) amnesia of the event, and (3) change in mental status such as feeling dizzy or disoriented. Mild TBI is commonly encountered in the ED with highest incidence among those 15 to 24 years of age and those older than 75 years. The incidence of pathological conditions requiring neurosurgical intervention in this group is small. Whether patients with mild TBI require neuroimaging is a matter of controversy. See Table 28.1 for risk stratification of TBI patients. All patients in the high-risk category must be evaluated with a CT scan of the brain. Clinical findings in sports-injury-related concussion are listed in Table 28.2.

Evaluation

While adequate IV access is obtained, the primary survey ascertains adequacy of airway and oxygenation as well as initial GCS. Vital signs are monitored closely and appropriately corrected. Next, the secondary survey includes an inspection for depressed skull fractures, facial deformities, and lacerations. An otoscopic evaluation notes the presence of hemotympanum, cerebral spinal fluid leakage, or bleeding from the ears. The neurological examination assesses mental status,

Table 28.2. Clinical Findings in Sports-Injury-Related Concussion

Cognitive features	Unware of the time – period, opposition, score of game, confusion; amnesia; loss of consciousness; unware of time, date, place
Typical symptoms	Headache; dizziness; nausea; unsteadiness/loss of balance; feeling "dinged" or stunned or "dazed," "having my bell rung"; seeing stars of flashing lights; running in the ears; double vision
Physical signs	Loss of consciousness/impaired conscious state; poor coordination or balance; concussive convulsion/impact seizure; gait unsteadiness/loss of balance; slow to answer questions or follow directions; easily distracted, poor concentration; displaying unusual or inapproapriate emotions such as laughing or crying; nausea/vomiting; vacant stare/glassy eyed; slurred speech; personality changes; inappropriate playing behavior – for example, running in the wrong direction; appreciably decreased playing ability

Adapted from Aubry M, Cantu R, Dvorak J, Graf-Baumann T, Johnston K, Kelly J, Lovell M, McCrory P, Meeuwisse W, Schamasch P. *British Journal of Sports Medicine*. Summary and agreement statement of the first international conference on concussion in sport, Vienna 2001: Recommendations for the improvement of safety and health of athletes who may suffer concussive injuries (concussion in sport). 2002;36:1–6.

pupillary function, and motor and sensory function. Serial exams are imperative in TBI because the neurological exam can change rapidly.

Hypotension, hemorrhage, hypoglycemia, hypoxia, drug or alcohol intoxication, or ICH is a potentially correctable causes of altered mental status. Pupillary assessment includes pupil size and reactivity, including oculocephalic and oculovestibular reflexes in patients with severe brainstem injury. Focal motor findings in the unconscious patient with TBI can localize intracranial lesions or spinal cord injuries.

Imaging

Noncontrast computerized tomography (CT) scans of the brain are done as soon as possible in patients with GCS of 13 or less, or in patients with a higher GCS, but persistent altered mental status or focal neurologic findings. Although CT scanning is limited in defining nonhemorrhagic injuries such as DAI, it does provide useful anatomical and pathological information regarding the location, extent, and nature of the TBI within minutes. Up to 14% of patients with blunt head trauma and GCS less than 6 have a fracture of the first two cervical vertebrate, so CT should extend to visualize these injuries in appropriate patients. Xenon-enhanced CT or positron emission tomography provides information on blood flow and metabolic function of the brain.

Universally accepted guidelines to study mild TBI with CT imaging does not exist. There are many studies for and against CT imaging of the brain in "low-risk patients." A simple decision algorithm to identify those with potentially positive CT scans does not exist. However, variables such as the length of LOC or degree of altered mental status, location of injury, intoxication, age greater than 55 years,

Table 28.3. Rapid Sequence Intubation for TBI Patients

Preparation
➤ Optimize systemic blood pressure
➤ Equipment: suction, laryngoscopes, endotracheal tubes and cricothyroidotomy setup

Preoxygenate
➤ Apply cricoid pressure
➤ 100% oxygen by bag mask for 5 minutes or four vital capacity breaths

Pretreatment
➤ Vecuronium (0.01 mg/kg)
➤ Lidocaine (1.5 mg/kg)
➤ Fentanyl (1–2 mcg/kg if not hypotensive)
➤ In-line axial cervical spine stabilization
➤ Wait 2–3 minutes if possible

Unconsciousness and paralysis
➤ Thiopental (3–5 mg/kg or 0.5–1 mg/kg if hypotensive) OR etomidate (0.1–0.2 mg/kg if hypotensive)
➤ Succinylcholine (1.5 mg/kg)

Direct laryngoscopy and endotracheal intubation
➤ Release cricoid pressure
➤ Confirm placement using breath sounds and expired CO_2 monitor
➤ Cricothyroidotomy if unsuccessful endotracheal intubation

Mechanical ventilation
➤ Tidal volume 10 cc/kg
➤ Rate 8–12 breaths/min
➤ $Pa_{O_2} > 80$ mm Hg
➤ Pa_{CO_2} 35–45 mm Hg

repeated vomiting, or evidence of skull fracture are considered when deciding whether to obtain CT scan of the brain. See Table 28.1.

Managment

The Brain Trauma Foundation published "Guidelines for the Management of Severe Head Injury" in 1995 with a focus on adult head trauma victims with a GCS less than 9. These guidelines may be accessed at www.braintrauma.org. This document divides interventions into *standards*, *guidelines*, and *options*. All patients with severe head injury require immediate neurosurgical consultation.

Apnea or cyanois in the field or a PaO_2 less than 60 mmHg is corrected immediately. However, endotracheal intubation of patients with intracranial injury has a number of additional risks: exacerbation of cervical spinal cord injury, aspiration and increased ICH by inducing systemic hypertension. Therefore, the technique of rapid sequence intubation (RSI) is critical. See Table 28.3. The inherently difficult airway of the trauma patient makes a thorough evaluation and individualized approach, as well as a backup plan, essential for success. During periods of acute neurological deterioration, hyperventilation may be necessary, but in routine hyperventilation is avoided. See Chapter 23, "Increased Intracranial Pressure and Herniation Syndromes."

A single systolic blood pressure of less than 90 mm Hg doubles mortality. A hematocrit of 30–33% optimizes rheological considerations, while higher hematocrit favor the use of crystalloid. Though normal saline and lactated ringers are the current mainstays, mounting evidence supports the prehospital and ED use of hypertonic saline (7.5% hypertonic saline) to decrease edema and ICP while increasing CPP and oxygen delivery. Evidence of shock includes tachycardia, low urine output, metabolic acidosis, altered mental status, pallor, and cool, mottled extremities. Fluid resuscitation is carried out in order to maintain the MAP above 90 mm Hg.

ICP monitoring is appropriate in patients with severe head injury and an abnormal ED CT (hematomas, contusions, edema, compressed basal cisterns). If the admission CT is normal, ICP monitoring is appropriate in severe head injury if two or more of the following are present: age above 40, motor posturing, or hypotension. ICP monitoring can guide therapy and may lower mortality.

Intermittent boluses of mannitol of 0.25–1 g/kg every 4 hours for control of elevated ICP may be effective. With 30 minutes of administration, mannitol increases plasma volume, cerebral blood flow, and oxygen delivery. Volume resuscitation should occur before mannitol therapy because osmotic diuretics can otherwise cause hemodynamic deterioration. In the absence of ICP monitoring, mannitol is utilized only in the setting of acute or impending herniation.

Opiate analgesics are used on an individual basis to avoid agitation and elevated ICP. Neuromuscular blockage results in longer intensive care unit stays and a higher incidence of pneumonia without improvement in outcomes. Steroids do not reduce ICP or improve outcomes and are avoided.

Although available evidence does not show that prevention of early posttraumatic seizures improves outcomes following TBI, anticonvulsants are an option in patients at high risk for seizures following head injury (GCS < 9, cortical contusion, SDH, depressed skull fracture, EDH, ICH, penetrating head injury, seizure within first 24 hours). Anticonvulsant therapy for longer than 7 days postinjury, however, is not recommended.

Pediatric TBI

TBI is the cause of death in approximately 40% of childhood injuries and occurs more frequently in males and infants or adolescents. Infants have a thin, pliable skull and immature cerebral autoregulatory mechanisms and hence have a poorer TBI prognosis. Child abuse must be suspected in any TBI patient under 2 years old. Other warning signs include histories, which are either inconsistent between observers or discordant with clinical findings. Recognition of two physiologic principles unique to childhood TBI are important: isolated head trauma can cause hypovolemic shock in children, and children have a steep intracranial pressure-volume curve when compared to adults. An ICP monitor is therefore indicated in those with GCS less than 5 or in those with a GCS of less than 8 with CT evidence of an intracranial injury. Otherwise, the ED approach to pediatric head injury parallels that of adult TBI with prevention of secondary brain injury by meticulous management of the ABCs of resuscitation and frequent neurological assessments.

PEARLS AND PITFALLS

■ Primary brain injury is caused by functional and physical disruption of the brain tissue; secondary brain injury occurs when postinjury factors such as hypoxia and hypotension further adversely affect the injured brain.

■ DAI is likely the primary reason for persistent coma following TBI.

■ Patients with TBI can be intoxicated, confounding the presentation of TBI.

■ Sports-injury-related concussion may be caused by a direct blow to the head, face, neck, or elsewhere on the body with an "impulsive" force transmitted to the head.

■ Concussion is typically associated with grossly normal structural neuroimaging studies.

■ Concussion largely reflects a functional disturbance rather than structural brain injury.

■ Hyperventilation is not routinely performed in a patient with TBI, except when there is evidence of acute herniation or neurological deterioration.

SELECTED BIBLIOGRAPHY

Aubry M, Cantu R, Dvorak J, Graf-Baumann T, Johnston K, Kelly J, Lovell M, McCrory P, Meeuwisse W, Schamasch P. Summary and agreement statement of the first international conference on concussion in sport, Vienna 2001: Recommendations for the improvement of safety and health of athletes who may suffer concussive injuries. (concussion in sport). *British Journal of Sports Medicine*. Feb 2002;36:1–6.

Biros MH, Heegaard W. Head. In: Rosen P. et al., eds. *Emergency Medicine: Concepts and Clinical Practice*, 5th ed. St. Louis: Mosby; 2002:298.

29 Spinal Cord Injuries

Charles H. Bill II and Vanessa L. Harkins

INTRODUCTION

Injury of the spine and spinal cord is one of the most common causes of disability and death following trauma. The incidence of spinal cord injury is highest in the 15- to 30-year age group, with a male-to-female ratio of 4:1. The most common causes of spinal cord injury are motor vehicle accidents (approximately 50%), falls (21%), and violence (15%).

Evaluation

Prehospital and emergency department (ED) evaluation is directed toward careful assessment of current neurological and hemodynamic status and preventing secondary injury. Secondary injury results from further injury to an unstable spine, hypoperfusion of the injured spinal cord (frequently due to systemic hypotension), and other conditions such as hypoxia and metabolic abnormalities. A trauma patient with impaired consciousness due to intoxication is treated as if there is an unstable spinal injury and head injury. Hemodynamic instability can occur due to not only ongoing blood loss but also sympathectomy-induced reduction in blood pressure, pulse, cardiac contractility, and cardiac output. Vigorous fluid resuscitation in a patient with spinal shock can be hazardous because of compromised cardiac output. The use of vasopressors such as dopamine may be required to correct hypotension in patients with spinal shock.

It is critical to document the initial neurological assessment and vital signs when EMS providers arrive at the scene. Any deterioration in the clinical condition is carefully documented and communicated to the receiving physician. Paralysis can ascend over a short period of time secondary to intraspinal hemorrhage. Rapid recognition of rapidly progressive clinical conditions requires urgent radiographic evaluation and immediate surgical evaluation.

Fifty percent of spinal cord-injured patients have multisystem involvement, and spinal cord injury may not be the most life-threatening event. The primary survey consists of assessing airway, breathing, circulation, disability (assessment of neurological status), and exposure (patient is fully undressed for examination). When exposing the trauma patient during the initial survey, patients with spinal cord injury at or above the T8 level are at higher risk for hypothermia.

Spinal cord injuries at or above the C4 level can result in respiratory compromise. When the level of injury is just below the origins of the phrenic nerves, intercostal muscle function is lost, the patient can be completely dependent on diaphragmatic contraction for respiration. Signs of respiratory fatigue require immediate ventilatory support. Tracheal intubation is accomplished by the oral route and in-line support of the head and neck, or nasotracheally with fiberoptic visualization. Cervical traction is *not* used because it can result in inadvertent spinal cord injury, especially in the very young patient.

Determination of neurological level of a patient with spinal cord injury includes assessment of both sensory and motor function. Intoxication and other alterations in level of consciousness interfere with accurate determination of the level of injury. A standardized scoring sheet, such as that prepared by the American Spinal Cord Injury Association (International Standards for Neurological Classification of Spinal Cord Injury) can be used (Figure 29.1).

Determination of Neurological Level

It is important to establish the spinal cord level of dysfunction when spinal cord injury is suspected on initial evaluation. Accurate description of the clinical findings of spinal cord injury is assisted by several definitions:

1. *Neurological level* refers to the most caudal level of the spinal cord with normal function.
2. *Zone of partial preservation* refers to the partially innervated segments below the neurological level.
3. *Complete spinal cord injury* refers to the absence of any motor or sensory function in sacral segments S4–S5.

Both sensory and motor components are evaluated to determine their respective neurological levels. It may be helpful to draw a line on both sides of the patient's body for future comparison of neurological level.

Sensory function is evaluated by testing pinprick and light touch bilaterally for each dermatome starting at insensate levels and moving rostrally. Sensory function is graded as follows: 0 = absent, 1 = impaired, 2 = normal. Posterior column function is assessed by applying deep pressure to extremities, testing with a tuning fork over bony prominences, and testing position sense in a distal to proximal fashion. (See Chapter 1, "Neurological Examination.")

Motor function is evaluated by testing strength of various muscle groups as follows:

Levels of Motor Function
- C5 = Elbow flexors
- C6 = Wrist extensors
- C7 = Elbow extensors
- C8 = Finger flexors (check the distal phalanx of the middle finger)
- T1 = Finger abductors (check the little finger)

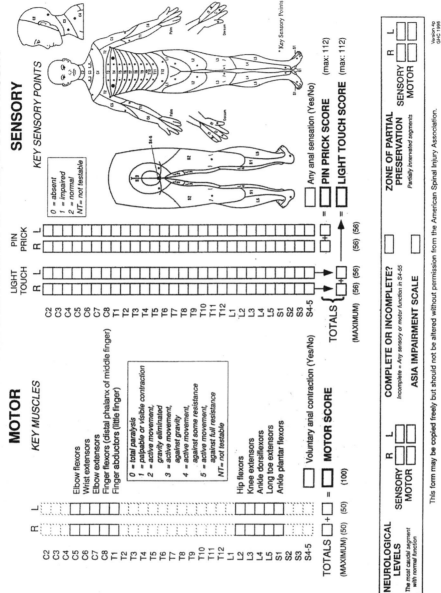

Figure 29.1. Standard score sheet for classification of spinal cord injury (from *International Standards for Neurological and Functional Classification of Spinal Cord Injury*. Revised 1996. American Spinal Injury Association/International Medical Society of Paraplegia, Chicago, Ill. Reprinted by permission.).

L2 = Hip flexors

L3 = Knee extensors

L4 = Ankle dorsiflexors

L5 = Long toe extensors

S1 = Ankle plantar flexors

S4–55 = Voluntary anal contraction

Patients with suspected hysterical paralysis or weakness require a focused neurological examination, followed occasionally by radiographic evaluation. Generally the hysterical patient presents with a profound motor deficit, typically in the lower extremities, with normal reflexes and normal rectal tone. These patients are hospitalized until the paralysis resolves and further evaluation takes place.

Spinal Shock

Various degrees of transient neurological disability may occur as a result of a phenomenon known as spinal shock. Spinal shock results from physiological transection of the spinal cord, which commonly lasts 24–48 hours. During this time, flaccid paralysis occurs below the level of spinal cord injury, and all reflexes below this level are absent. In the spinal cord-injured patient inadequate spinal cord perfusion results from a diastolic blood pressure of less than 70 mm Hg. Continuous infusion of vasopressors may be required to maintain diastolic blood pressure at or above 70 mm Hg.

Following recovery from spinal shock, return of reflex arcs below the level of injury (such as the bulbocavernosus reflex and the "anal wink") occurs. These reflexes are checked with sequential examinations. The presence of one or more of these findings indicates that complete spinal cord injury is no longer present:

➤ Bulbocavernosus reflex (S3–4) is elicited by pulling on glans penis or clitoris (or tug on inserted Foley catheter) and noting contraction of the anal sphincter.
➤ Anal wink (S2–4) refers to noting a contraction of the anal sphincter by stroking the skin of the perianal area.
➤ "Sacral sparing" is demonstrated clinically by voluntary anal contraction and retained perianal sensation. This indicates an incomplete spinal cord injury, and a more favorable prognosis.

Patients with continued paralysis after the return of reflex arcs following spinal shock have a poor prognosis. A clinical transition occurs 6–12 weeks after complete spinal cord injuries. Flaccid extremities become spastic, hyperactive deep tendon reflexes develop, and extensor plantar reflexes are present.

Categories of Spine Injury

    I. Soft tissue injuries
    II. Dislocations and vertebral bony injuries.

    I. Soft tissue injuries include:
      A. Acute cervical strain

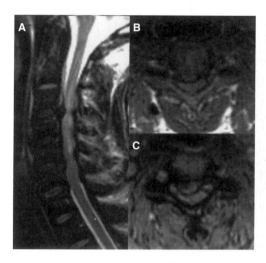

Figure 29.2. Traumatic cervical disc herniation in a 38-year-old unrestrained man who lost control of his car and and struck a tree. (A) T2 sagittal MRI showing the C3–4 disc herniation stripping the posterior longitudinal ligament from the vertebral bodies. Compression of the spinal cord and increased signal in the spinal cord are observed. (B, C) T1 and gradient refocused images.

B. Vascular injuries: (i) arterial injuries (resulting in stroke or spinal cord infarction) and (ii) venous injuries, which can cause epidural hematoma.

C. Nervous System Injuries: (i) nerve root injuries, (ii) complete and incomplete spinal cord injuries, and (iii) spinal cord syndromes.

II. Vertebral bony injuries include the dislocations and fractures of the spine.

Soft Tissue Injuries

Acute Cervical Strain

Acute cervical strain is the most common injury following a vehicular accident. The typical mechanism is hyperflexion-hyperextension of the neck with or without concomitant head injury. There is partial tearing of ligaments, muscle, connective tissue (fascia), discs, and joint capsules, but most the fibers remain intact. Radiographs are typically normal. Treatment is supportive. The term "whiplash" does not describe a pathological condition, and its use is avoided. Disc herniation can result from trauma. (See Figure 29.2.) A nerve root syndrome (radiculopathy) resulting from mechanical pressure on a single nerve is the typical presentation.

Vascular Injuries

Over 90% of carotid artery injuries in the United States result from penetrating injuries. Injuries to the carotid and vertebral arteries and jugular veins are commonly associated with spinal cord injuries caused by gun shot wounds. Blunt "seat belt" injury to the neck from a motor vehicle accident can cause dissection of the carotid artery; the presentation is typically consistent with stroke involving the opposite side of the body. Vertebral arteries are most commonly compressed at the C6 level. Degenerative osteophytes can compromise the vessels from the C2 to the C5 level. Although magnetic resonance angiography (MRA) and duplex studies reveal the diagnosis in most cases, angiography is the definite study. Epidural hemorrhage can result from venous injuries in the same location. Patients with ankylosing spondylitis are at an increased risk of developing epidural hemorrhage following spinal fractures. (See Figure 29.3.)

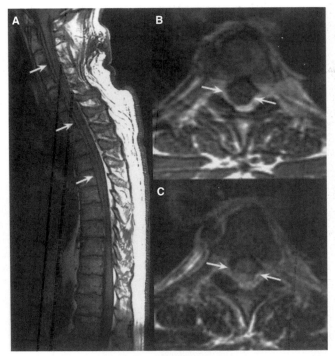

Figure 29.3. Spinal epidural hematoma in a 57-year-old man who had a minor fall and presented with progressive quadriplegia and neck and back pain. He was taking coumadin for a prosthetic mitral value. (A) T1 sagittal MRI. Arrows outline the epidural hematoma, which is anterior to the spinal cord with which it is isointense. (B, C) T1 and T2 axial images. Arrows demarcate the cleft between the hematoma and the posteriorly displaced spinal cord. The increased signal in the spinal cord is observed on T2 imaging (C).

Nervous System Injuries

Nerve Root Injuries. Compression of a nerve root by a disc or bone can result in loss of sensory innervation of dermatome, motor innervation of a myotome, or both. Isolated nerve root irritation without spinal cord injury can occur with cervical sprains when there is significant spondylosis, traumatic disc herniation, or subluxations associated with significant disc disruption as in unilateral facet dislocation. More commonly, these accompany spinal cord injury at the level of disruption.

Complete and Incomplete Spinal Cord Injuries. Clinical features were reviewed in the previous section entitled, "Determination of Neurological Level."

Spinal Cord Syndromes. There are several spinal cord syndromes. Each syndrome is manifested by a constellation of unique clinical findings based on a specific injury pattern of the spinal cord. The ability to recognize each of these syndromes will facilitate rapid, accurate diagnosis of the specific cord injury. Patients with preexisting spondylosis can develop new nerve root or spinal cord syndromes (i.e., central cord syndrome) without soft tissue injury or fracture. Patients with spondylosis due to rheumatoid arthritis can have preexisting C1–2 ligamentous instability predisposing these patients to spinal cord injury. Magnetic resonance

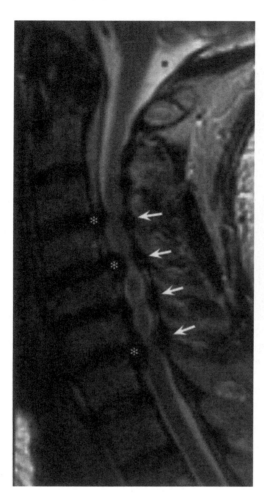

Figure 29.4. Cervical stenosis in a 78-year-old man who fell forward, striking his forehead on the sidewalk. He presented with a central cord syndrome. T2 sagittal MRI. Asterisks indicate disc herniations that are chronic (degenerative spondylosis). Arrows indicate buckling of ligamenta flava from the loss of disc height.

imaging (MRI) usually demonstrates evidence of injury at the corresponding spinal cord level.

1. *Central cord syndrome* is the most common spinal cord syndrome. This results from injury to the medially located corticospinal tracts of the upper extremity. The mechanism of injury is hyperextension of the neck, which induces a shearing-type injury. This is commonly observed in elderly patients when the ligamentum flavum buckles from loss of disc height (Figure 29.4). Clinical findings follow:
   ➤ Disproportionately greater weakness in upper extremities compared with the lower extremities
   ➤ Upper extremity hypesthesia, dysesthesia, hyperesthesia
   ➤ Initial bowel, bladder, and sexual dysfunction with gradual limited improvement
   There is a 75% probability of functional recovery following central cord syndrome. Treatment is generally supportive with immobilization using the hard cervical collar. Surgical decompression is controversial.
2. *Anterior cord syndrome* is caused by an isolated injury to the anterior half of the spinal cord following axial loading or flexion injury that causes dislodgement

of bone fragments or disc into the anterior spinal cord. The clinical findings are complete motor deficit beginning at the level of injury and loss of pain and temperature sensation starting a few levels below that of the motor loss. There is a 10–20% probability of functional recovery. Surgical intervention to stabilize the spine is generally required.

3. *Brown-Séquard syndrome* results from spinal cord hemisection. This rare syndrome is manifested by *ipsilateral* motor paralysis, *ipsilateral* dorsal column injury (loss of two-point discrimination, proprioception, vibration, and deep pressure), and *contralateral* loss of pain and temperature starting two levels below the level of injury. Functional recovery is common.

4. *Conus medullaris syndrome* involves T11–L1 spinal level. This results from thoracolumbar spinal injury causing bone or disc fragments to be thrust into the caudal end of the spinal cord. Clinical findings are early urinary dysfunction and *symmetrical* saddle-type anesthesia. Early pain is *uncommon*. Neurological examination reveals components of both nerve root and cauda equina injury.

5. *Cauda equina syndrome* results when the level of injury is below the termination of the spinal cord (i.e., L1–2 level). Clinical findings are *asymmetrical* sensory loss and urinary dysfunction, and weakness or flaccid paralysis of the lower extremities. As opposed to the conus Medullaris syndrome, early pain is *common* with the cauda equina syndrome.

6. *Posterior cord syndrome* results from selective injury to the posterior spinal columns. The clinical findings of this rare condition are loss of deep pressure and pain, vibration sense, and proprioception.

Dislocations and Vertebral Bony Injuries

Cervical Spine Injuries

Fractures of the cervical spine have an associated 39% incidence of spinal cord injury; 10–15% of patients with a spinal fracture have a second noncontiguous spinal fracture. The most important radiological components of spinal fractures are alignment, displacement, and extent of canal compromise. Each type of cervical spine fracture has a unique mechanism of injury, fracture pattern, and associated neurological findings.

Atlanto-Occipital Dislocation. Ligamentous damage at the atlanto-occipital joint is the cause of atlanto-occipital dislocation. The mechanism of injury is distraction forces, typically seen in a pedestrian struck by a vehicle. Severe neurological compromise is common and is usually fatal before the patient reaches the hospital.

Radiographic findings on lateral cervical spine films, indicate that there is increased distance between tip of odontoid and end of the clivus (basion). A Power's Ratio > 1.0 suggests atlanto-occipital dislocation.

$$\text{Powers ratio} = \frac{\text{Distance from basion to posterior arch of the atlas}}{\text{Distance from opisthion to anterior arch of the atlas}}$$

False negative ratios may occur with posterior dislocations. A Power's ratio is not valid if the atlas is fractured or if congenital abnormalities of the skull base exist.

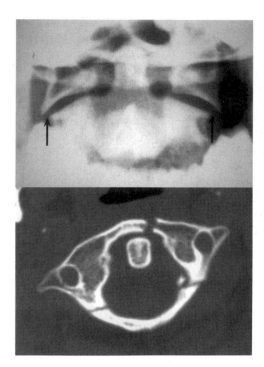

Figure 29.5. Jefferson fracture in an 18-year-old unrestrained backseat passenger who struck the top of his head on the dashboard. (A) Openmouth odontoid view reveals overhanging of the lateral masses of C1 with respect to the articular facets of C2 bilaterally. (B) Expanded ring of C1 is observed on axial CT image. The three breaks in the ring are observed.

Atlas Fractures. There are four basic patterns of Atlas fractures. (1) Posterior arch fractures result from arch hyperextension–compression; they rarely causes neurological deficits. (2) Lateral mass fractures result from axial loading and are treated conservatively with cervical collar when there is minimal displacement. (3) Jefferson fractures occur when the ring of C1 is broken (Figure 29.5). The transverse ligament is assumed to be disrupted when the lateral masses are displaced at least 7 mm on open mouth view radiograph. Bone fragments tend to move away from spinal cord. (4) The fourth pattern includes atlas fracture and either C2 lateral mass fractures or occipital condyle fractures.

Axis Fractures (Odontoid Fractures). Type I fracture involves the tip of the odontoid process and results from an avulsion injury by the alar ligament. This is rare and of minimal clinical significance. Type II fracture, a potentially fatal and the most common type of odontoid fracture, involves the base of the odontoid process. This can be easily missed on plain radiographs. A computerized tomography (CT) scan with contiguous 1-mm slices with reconstruction may be required to visualize the fracture (Figure 29.6). This is considered to be a unstable fracture and requires immobilization with halo placement, and possibly fusion or screw placement. Type III fracture, also a potentially fatal fracture, involves the body of C2 and separates the odontoid process and part of the body of C2 from the rest of C2. This is an unstable fracture that requires immobilization with a halo placement.

"Hangman's Fracture." Traumatic spondylolisthesis or hangman's fracture results from bilateral fractures through the pedicles or pars interarticularis with

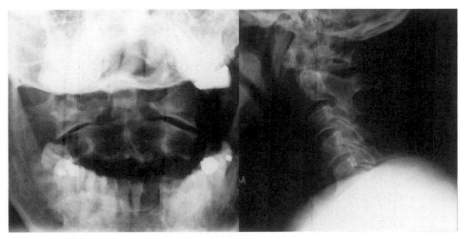

Figure 29.6. Type II odontoid fracture in a 48-year-old man who was involved in a roll-over accident and presented to the emergency department with high cervical neck pain. (A) Open-mouth odontoid radiograph. (B) Lateral radiograph. The fracture is seen only on the open-mouth view.

ligamentous disruption between C2 and C3 vertebrae. The mechanism of injury is hyperextension of the neck. Clinical findings range from minimal neurological findings in minor variants to fatal injuries from cord transection. Lateral cervical spine films demonstrate bilateral fractures of the posterior elements of C2 disrupting the neural arch. This condition is unstable and requires traction and immobilization with halo or surgical intervention depending on the extent of injury.

Vertebral Body Fractures. *Compression fracture* results from a structural failure of the anterior aspect of the vertebral body with associated posterior ligament disruption. The mechanism of injury is flexion and axial loading. The clinical findings are usually limited to pain in the involved area and neurological deficit is rare. Lateral cervical spine films demonstrate loss of anterior height of the vertebral body. There may be increased distance of the interspinous space at the level of damage due to corresponding ligamentous disruption. This is generally considered to be a stable fracture but confirmation of ligamentous stability with flexion/extension cervical spine views is prudent.

Burst fracture refers to the structural failure of both anterior and posterior aspects of the vertebral body. Axial loading is the mechanism of injury. Significant spinal cord injury ensues from retropulsion of bony fragments into the spinal cord. Quadriplegia or anterior cord syndrome can result. Lateral cervical spine films demonstrate loss of height of the entire vertebral body.

Teardrop fracture refers to a displaced large triangular bony fragment from the anterior inferior aspect of the vertebral body. This is associated with complete disruption of ligaments, intervertebral disc, and bilateral facets. Mechanism of injury is hyperflexion. The neck usually appears to be in a flexed position with soft tissue swelling anteriorly. Clinically, this is associated with anterior cord syndrome. Lateral radiographs demonstrate a large triangular fragment displaced from the anterior inferior aspect of the vertebral body. Treatment consists of reduction and stabilization with spinal fusion.

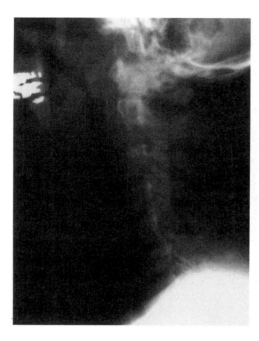

Figure 29.7. Unilateral facet dislocation in a 58-year-old man who was rear-ended while driving his pickup truck. He presented with arm and neck pain. The subluxation at C5–6 is less than 50% of the vertebral body anteroposterior diameter.

Facet Disorders. *Unilateral facet dislocation*, also called "jumped facet" syndrome, consists of unilateral dislocation of an articular facet. Mechanism of injury is flexion and rotation injury. Clinical findings vary from minimum neurological deficits to incomplete quadriparesis or nerve root compression. Lateral neck radiographs demonstrate an anterolisthesis of less than 50% of the anteroposterior (AP) diameter of vertebral body. Treatment consists of tong traction alone or with surgical reduction and stabilization (Figures 29.7 and 29.8).

Bilateral facet dislocation involves disruption of all posterior ligaments, the facet joints, intervertebral disc, and occasionally the anterior longitudinal ligament. This can result in anterior dislocation of vertebrae and its facets with respect to the vertebra immediately inferior to it. Hyperflexion is the usual mechanism of injury and is commonly associated with complete spinal cord injury. Lateral radiographs of the cervical spine demonstrate anterior translation of the upper vertebral body of 50% or more. Angular (kyphotic) deformity can be large. This highly unstable condition is treated with realignment of the cervical spine via tong traction and surgical stabilization.

Perched facets syndrome refers to a lesion when facet rides up but not over the superior facet of the vertebrae below with associated incomplete ligamentous injury. Hyperflexion is the mechanism of injury. Clinical findings vary from incomplete quadriparesis to nerve root compression. Lateral cervical radiographs demonstrate subluxation of the superior facets anteriorly, but only partially anterior to the inferior vertebra's facets. Persistent neurological deficits or significant neck pain after closed reduction mandates a CT scan to evaluate possible facet fracture or MRI to evaluate soft tissue injury.

"Clay Shoveler's Fracture." The fracture of spinous process of C7 (most frequently), C6, or T1 (least frequently) is called the clay shoveler's fracture. Mechanism of injury is forceful flexion, such as with shoveling clay or coal

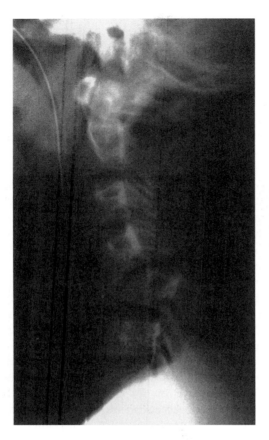

Figure 29.8. Bilateral facet dislocation in a young man who was in a high-speed motor vehicle accident. He presented with a complete quadriplegia. Near-complete subluxation of C4 anterior to C5 is observed.

overhead (or from a direct blow to the spinous process itself). Neurological deficits are rare. Lateral cervical spine radiographs demonstrate isolated fracture of the spinous process of C6, C7, or T1. Treatment remains supportive.

Hyperextension Dislocation Injuries. Hyperextension dislocation injuries occur after forceful hyperextension of the neck and can result in ligamentous disruption of the anterior longitudinal ligament, disc, joint capsules, and posterior ligament complexes. This can occur with or without concomitant spine fracture. Clinical findings are often consistent with central cord syndrome. Disruption of the anterior longitudinal ligament with or without fracture results in diffuse anterior soft tissue swelling observed on a lateral radiograph. The normal prevertebral soft tissue width observed on lateral radiograph is approximately 5 mm at C1 and C2, 2–7 mm at C3 and C4, and approximately 10–20 mm at C6 and C7.

Spinal alignment typically returns to normal after posterior dislocation and radiographs are normal, making this diagnosis difficult. This injury is suggested by a soft tissue injury to the face or forehead, neurological findings typical of central cord syndrome, and diffuse prevertebral soft tissue swelling on lateral radiographs with normal alignment. CT can define facet fractures; MRI can identify disruptions of ligaments and discs, and spinal cord contusion.

Thoracic Spine Injuries

Patients with thoracic spine fractures have a 10% incidence of associated spinal cord injury. Similar to cervical spine fractures, thoracic spine fractures have characteristic mechanisms of injury, fracture pattern, and neurological findings.

Thoracic Compression Fracture. Thoracic compression fractures occur with structural failure of the anterior aspect of the vertebral body and associated posterior ligament disruption. Flexion with axial loading is the usual mechanism of injury. Clinical findings are usually limited to pain in the involved area. Neurological injury is rare. Lateral cervical spine films demonstrate loss of anterior height of the vertebral body. There may be increased distance of the interspinous space at the level of injury due to corresponding ligamentous disruption. This is generally a stable fracture but ligamentous stability must be confirmed with flexion/extension views of the spine. When anterior vertebral height is reduced by 50% or more, there is an increased probability of injury to the anterior and middle columns, which can compromise spinal stability.

Thoracic Burst Fracture. Thoracic burst fractures occur with structural failure of both anterior and posterior aspects of vertebral body, which can result in retropulsion of bony fragments into the spinal cord. The mechanism of injury is axial loading. This serious injury is associated with quadriplegia or anterior cord syndrome. Radiographic findings are comminution of the vertebral body, increase of the interpedicular distance (can see spreading of pedicles on AP view), vertical fracture of the lamina, retropulsion of the fractured posterior vertebral body into the canal, and the loss of height of entire vertebral body (Figure 29.9). This is a highly unstable condition that requires decompression and internal fixation.

Thoracic Fracture-Dislocation Injuries. Thoracic fracture-dislocation injuries cause the failure of all three spinal columns. The mechanism of injury is axial torsion, usually from a high-speed motor vehicle accident. This usually results in complete spinal cord injury. On plain radiographs of the spine, misalignment of the vertebrae is readily apparent.

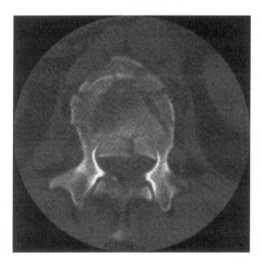

Figure 29.9. Burst fracture in a 40-year-old man who fell out of a deer stand. He sustained a complete spinal cord injury at the T11 level. Comminution of the vertebral body and the retropulsed bony fragments are observed. The latter compromise the spinal canal by about 50% of the anteroposterior diameter.

Thoracolumbar Junction (T11–LI) and Lumbar Spine Fractures. During axial loading, the thoracic spine deforms in kyphosis while the lumbar spine deforms in lordosis. Subsequently, the thoracolumbar region is exposed to significant compression. In addition, the thoracolumbar junction is uniquely susceptible to rotational forces, making dislocations more likely in this area. Wedge compression fracture, burst fractures, seat belt injuries, and fracture dislocations are more likely to occur at the thoracolumbar junction. Lumbar fractures below the L1–2 junction spare the conus medullaris but can result in cauda equina injuries.

Sacral Fractures

When a sacral fracture is suspected, two radiographic views are obtained: (1) an AP sacral radiograph performed with the radiation beam directed 30° rostrally (Ferguson's view) and (2) a lateral sacral radiograph including the coccyx.

Sacral fractures are suspected when the following findings are present on radiographs:

1. Fracture of lower lumbar transverse process
2. Significant anterior pelvic ring fracture without an identifiable posterior pelvic lesion
3. Asymmetry of the sacral notch
4. Clouding of the radiating trabecular pattern in the lateral sacral mass
5. Irregularity of the arcuate lines of the upper three sacral foramina

Sacral fractures are divided into three anatomical zones.

➤ *Zone I fractures* usually result from a vehicular-pedestrian accident. The fracture occurs through the ala of the sacrum without injuring the foramina or the spinal canal. This is a stable condition that rarely results in neurological injury. With severe injury, the L5 nerve root can be involved.
➤ *Zone II fractures* involve one or more sacral foramina but not the central canal. This can also involve fractures in zone I but may not involve zone III. The mechanism of injury is usually vertical shear force causing fractures from high-speed motor vehicle accidents. Neurological injury occurs in 28–54% patients with zone II fractures and commonly involves the S1 nerve root.
➤ *Zone III fractures* involve the sacral canal medial to the foramina and can also involve fractures in zones I and II. The mechanism of injury includes vertical shear injuries, high and low transverse fractures, and traumatic lumbosacral fracture-dislocations. Cauda equina syndrome can result.

Management

The Third National Acute Spinal Cord Injury Randomized Controlled Trial (NASCIS III) concluded that high-dose methylprednisolone administration is associated with improved neurological outcome in spinal cord-injured patients, compared with placebo or tirilazad mesylate. Methylprednisolone is administered as a loading dose of 30 mg/kg given intravenously over 1 hour, followed by a constant infusion of 5.4 mg/kg per hour for the next 23 hours when started within the first 3 hours of the injury or for the next 47 hours when the injury occurred 3–8 hours from the time of onset of therapy. Beyond 8 hours, the initiation of corticosteroids is contraindicated because the second trial showed a poorer outcome in this delayed drug treatment group. An H_2 blocker is included in the medical regimen for gastrointestinal prophylaxis in these patients.

Despite widespread use of the methylprednisolone protocol, its scientific basis has been brought into question. Recently published articles include critical reviews of the data from the NASCIS II and III studies and outline concerns with the original conclusions of the NASCIS II and III trials. The central issue involves the criticism that the trials, "failed to demonstrate improvement in primary outcome measures as a result of the administration of methylprednisolone." The commonly referenced outcome difference between the treatment group and the control group in the original NASCIS trials was a result derived from a subset of data that excluded 70% of the study population. However, when the entire study population of both trials was analyzed, there was no statistical difference between the population that was treated with methylprednisolone and those that were not. In addition, issues have been raised regarding the clinical relevance of the outcome measures that were used as end points. Methylprednisolone administration also carries inherent risks. The NASCIS III trial demonstrated a worsened outcome due to respiratory complications that equaled a sixfold higher mortality in those treated with methylprednisolone. In summary, the methylprednisolone protocol that was rapidly adapted after the NASCIS trials were first published is now being carefully reassessed for its evidence-based risks and benefits.

Pediatric Spinal Injuries

Spinal cord injuries are rare in patients under 17 years old. In newborns, elasticity of the spine and supporting ligaments allows for up to 2 inches of longitudinal distraction. However, the spinal cord stretches only a quarter of an inch before failing. The combination of large head and ligamentous laxity contributes to the high incidence of upper cervical spine and craniovertebral junction injuries in children up to 3 years of age. In the 0–9 years of age group, pedestrian-motor vehicle accidents and falls account for more than 75% of the injuries. In older children, accidents due to motor vehicles and sport-related activities are more common.

Special measures must be taken when immobilizing patients younger than 8 years of age. In this age group, the difference between head and chest circumference results in cervical kyphosis when the child is placed on a backboard. Therefore, when immobilizing children up to 8 years of age, the body from the shoulders down should be propped up on folded blankets.

Injuries in children older than 8 years of age tend to be avulsions, epiphyseal separations, and fractures of the growth plate (not true fractures). When interpreting pediatric cervical spine radiographs, knowledge of timing of the ossification process is necessary to avoid misinterpreting ossification centers as fractures.

Normal Radiographic Variants of the Pediatric Cervical Spine

1. The atlanto-dens interval (measured between the posterior border of the anterior arch of the atlas and the anterior margin of the dens) can be greater than 3 mm in flexion in 20% of patients. The upper limit of normal in children is 5 mm.
2. The anterior arch of the atlas can override the unossified tip of the dens in extension, giving the appearance of odontoid hypoplasia.

3. Among children younger than 8 years of age, 40% have evidence of "physiological" anterior displacement of C2 on C3 that exceeds 3 mm.
4. Among children younger than 8 years of age, 14% can have a "physiological" anterior displacement of C3 on C4 that exceeds 3 mm.
5. Marked angulation at a single intervertebral space can be normal.
6. Absent cervical lordosis can occur in the neutral position.
7. Absence of a flexion curve can occur between the second and the seventh cervical vertebrae.

Special Pediatric Considerations of Upper Cervical Spine Injuries

Atlanto-occipital dislocation occurs usually after a car has struck the child. It is seen twice as often in the pediatric population as in the adult population. As with adults, this injury is usually fatal before the child reaches the ED.

Atlantoaxial rotary subluxation can occur due to trauma in children and adults. In addition, it has been associated with upper respiratory infections (Grisel's syndrome) and has occurred following surgical procedures such as repair of cleft lip and palate and removal of orthodontic devices. Clinical presentation tends to be a "cock-robin" appearance of the head (patient's head is turned in the opposite direction to the subluxation of the articular process of C1 with that of C2) creating a "jumped facet." The diagnosis is confirmed when the position of C1 vertebrae remains fixed with respect to C2 vertebrae on comparison CT scans obtained with the patient's head rotated in the extremes of both directions. (Figure 29.10). Neurological deficit is uncommon. This condition is usually treated with cervical traction for both reduction and immobilization.

Growth plates create a diagnostic challenge in children when evaluating the integrity of the C2 vertebra. In patients younger than 10 years old, odontoid

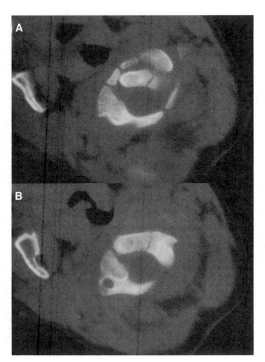

Figure 29.10. Atlantoaxial rotatory subluxation in a 2-year-old girl who was injured by her older brother. Allegedly, he twisted her head. She was taken to the emergency department on a back board with her head fixed in rotatory subluxation. The subluxation was reduced with in-line traction under sedation and direct fluoroscopy, and neck was immobilized in a cervical collar. (A, B) Axial views by CT, adjacent 3-mm cuts showing the counterclockwise rotation of C1 with respect to C2.

fractures generally occur as an epiphyseal separation of the growth plate at the base of the dens. Treatment is reduction and immobilization for 6–8 weeks.

SCIWORA

Spinal cord injury without radiographic abnormality (SCIWORA) is a traumatic myelopathy without identifiable fractures or subluxation on plain spine radiography, plain tomography, or CT scans. The mechanism of injury includes hyperextension, flexion, distraction, or spinal cord ischemia. SCIWORA can involve cervical, thoracic, or thoracolumbar spinal cord regions. Neurological deficits may be delayed in presentation from 30 minutes to 4 days after injury. Recurrent SCIWORA can occur with deficits manifesting up to 10 weeks following injury. Delayed presentation or recurrence of the syndrome suggests the possibility of ligamentous laxity and vulnerability of the spinal cord to further damage. Subsequently, these patients should be treated with 3 months in a hard cervical collar.

Five Patterns of Spinal Cord Injury in SCIWORA as Defined by MRI
1. Complete anatomical disruption of the spinal cord
2. Major hemorrhage observed in greater than 50% of the cross-sectional area of the spinal cord
3. Minor spinal cord hemorrhage
4. Edema only, without hemorrhage
5. A normal MRI

MRI can also identify vertebral endplate fractures or separations from the vertebral body (through the epiphysis), causing an associated increase in the disc height, and accompanied by adjacent bony fractures in older children.

The best predictor of long-term outcome in children with SCIWORA is the neurological status at presentation. Those with complete spinal cord lesions have the worst prognosis and rarely improve. Children who present with severe but incomplete lesions typically have limited improvement with time but rarely regain normal function. Patients with mild-to-moderate deficits on presentation are likely to have complete recovery.

PEARLS AND PITFALLS

- Of patients with a spinal fracture, 10–15% have a second noncontiguous spinal fracture.
- The most important factors of spinal injury are alignment, displacement, and extent of canal compromise.
- When CT evaluation of the spine is necessary, 3-mm slices must be utilized (5-mm cuts are inadequate to assess clinically significant spinal fractures).
- The decision to remove a hard collar and "clear the cervical spine" requires an awake, nonintoxicated patient with no neurological deficit or neck pain and no distracting injury.

SELECTED BIBLIOGRAPHY

Hurlbert RJ. Methylprednisolone for acute spinal cord injury: an inappropriate standard of care. *J Neurosurg.* 2000;93:1–7.

Nesathurai S. Steroids and spinal cord injury: revisiting the NASCIS 2 and NASCIS 3 trials. *J Trauma.* 1998;45:1088–93.

30 Peripheral Nerve Injuries and Compression Neuropathies

Patricia B. Jozefczyk and Mark Baratz

INTRODUCTION

Peripheral nerve injuries are one of three types. (1) Neuropraxia is a nerve injury in which there is a temporary ischemic insult. These injuries can occur with mild stretch or compression, and symptoms associated with a neuropraxia resolve within a short time. (2) Axonotmesis occurs when there is a separation of all or part of the axon, while the nerve sheath remains intact. Recovery from this type of injury requires regeneration of the axons and this may take up to three months. Finally, (3) neurotmesis is the complete disruption of all neural elements of the peripheral nerve, and recovery cannot occur without nerve repair.

Evaluation and Management

With complaint of loss of sensation in a limb, the possibility of a peripheral nerve or spinal cord injury is considered. Careful attention is paid to the vascular supply of the injured extremity. The neurological status is assessed quickly by testing sensation and motor function in the area of a suspected injured nerve (Table 30.1). Certain locations of fractures and dislocations suggest the possibility of a peripheral nerve injury. The nerves at risk with various fractures or dislocations are outlined (Table 30.2).

Penetrating Wounds

High-velocity firearm wounds create a concussive effect that damages a wide area of tissue. Immediate surgical treatment is advisable when a peripheral nerve injury is suspected with vascular compromise or an open fracture.

Laceration or stab wounds result in abnormal sensation when a nerve is transected. If the wound is clean, surgical exploration can be delayed for several weeks, and bleeding is controlled only with a pressure dressing. Coagulation and clamping may cause further nerve injury. An arteriogram is considered when nerve injury is associated with diminished peripheral pulse of the limb.

Table 30.1. "Short Form" Neurological Examination

Nerve	Sensation[a]	Motor Function[a]
Axillary	Lateral aspect of shoulder, several centimeters below acromium	Deltoid: shoulder flexion (palpate deltoid and feel contraction)
Radial	First web space	Wrist, finger, and thumb extension
Median	Tip of index finger	Thumb opposition: place tip of thumb on tip of small finger, feel contraction of thenar muscles
Ulnar	Tip of small finger,	Finger abduction: spread fingers apart; feel contraction of first dorsal interosseous muscle
Femoral	Anteromedial thigh and leg	Quadriceps
Sciatic	Posterior thigh, posterolateral leg	Hamstrings
Tibial	Sole of foot	Gastrocnemius and toe flexors
Common peroneal		
Superficial branch	Dorsum of foot	Foot eversion
Deep branch	First web space	Foot dorsiflexion

[a] This list of sensory regions and motor functions for each nerve is, in some cases, incomplete. However, testing these functions provides an adequate initial assessment of peripheral nerve function.

Table 30.2. Nerves at Risk with Various Fractures and Dislocations

Fracture or Dislocation	Nerve at Risk
Shoulder dislocation	Axillary
Proximal humerus fracture	Axillary
Humeral shaft (distal third)	Radial
Supracondylar humerus fracture in child	Median[a] or radial
Intraarticular distal humerus fracture in adult	Ulnar
Elbow dislocation	Ulnar
Proximal ulna fracture with radial head dislocation (Monteggia's fracture)	Radial
Distal radius fracture	Median
Carpal dislocation (especially lunate)	Median
Hip dislocation	Sciatic
Supracondylar femur fracture in child	Peroneal
Knee tibio-femoral dislocation	Peroneal

[a] Particularly the anterior interosseous portion of the median nerve, which controls "precision pinch" through the action of the flexor pollicis longus tendon in the thumb and the flexor digitorum profundus tendon to the index finger.

Blunt Trauma and Traction Injuries

Blunt trauma and traction injuries may cause nerve transection when associated with open fractures, but the majority result in neuropraxia or axonotmesis. Most traction injuries may be followed with serial examinations and nerve conduction studies after it has been determined that the limb is viable and there are no other associated injuries. Fractures and dislocations may be reduced with careful documentation of neurological and vascular status before and after any manipulation.

Compartment Syndrome

High-energy trauma to an extremity with or without a fracture may produce a compartment syndrome. Pain with passive motion of the joints adjacent to the compartment is the most common early symptom. Dysesthesias with muscle paralysis and vascular compromise may follow. Early surgery should be considered in a patient with neurological compromise and tense muscle compartments.

Electrical Injuries

Nerve injury does not usually result from a direct electrical source. Typically, the energy is dissipated throughout the soft tissues and the nerve injury resolves more commonly from surrounding soft tissue swelling. Management requires early detection and early decompression of a developing compartment syndrome.

Compression Neuropathies

Peripheral nerve compression may occur where the nerve passes through a "tunnel" and slides back and forth with joint flexion and extension. All points of compression with a limb should be considered. These syndromes may occur without a history of recent trauma. Chronic irritation to the nerve may result in nerve sensitivity on palpation during the examination or percussion over the nerve may produce local pain and dysesthesias in the sensory distribution of that nerve (Tinel's sign).

Upper Extremity Compression Neuropathies
See Figures 30.1 and 30.2, and Table 30.3.

Median Nerve: Pronator Syndrome. Compression occurs in the forearm as the median nerve passes between the two headaches of the pronator teres. Forearm pain is the primary symptom and increases with forearm pronation.

Median Nerve: Anterior Interosseous Syndrome. A nerve inflammation or neuritis may occur as the anterior interosseous portion of the median nerve is compressed by the edge of the flexor digitorum sublimus, deep head of the pronator teres, or the accessory head of the flexor pollicis longus. Midshaft fracture of the radius may also be the etiology. Tenderness may occur along the anterior aspect of the proximal forearm and examination shows weakness of the flexor pollicis longus or flexor digitorum profundus resulting in a weak pinch.

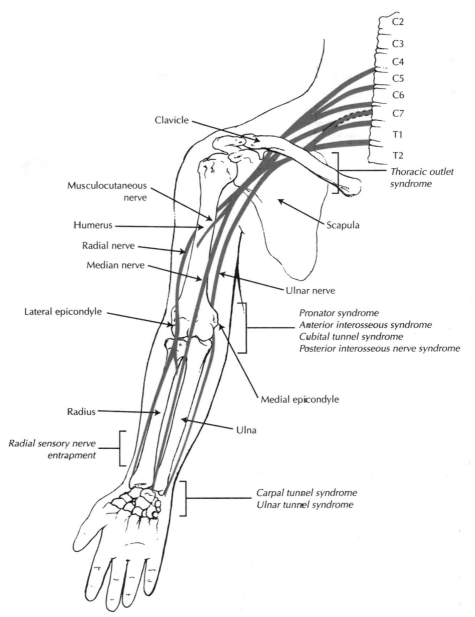

Figure 30.1. Anatomical areas of upper extremity peripheral nerve compression and resulting conditions.

Median Nerve: Carpal Tunnel Syndrome. Carpal tunnel syndrome is the most common form of median nerve compression that occurs at the wrist. This may be associated with a congenital small tunnel, rheumatoid arthritis, osteophytes, diabetes, pregnancy, amyloidosis, and thyroid dysfunction. Percussion may reproduce pain over the carpal tunnel, and examination may show thenar atrophy, weakness of thumb opposition, and numbness in the thumb and first finger.

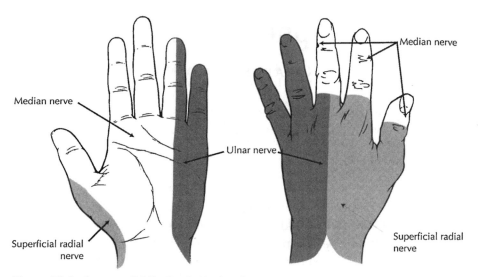

Figure 30.2. Sensory distribution in the hand.

Ulnar Nerve: Thoracic Outlet Syndrome. Thoracic outlet syndrome results in compression of the medial cord of the brachial plexus as it passes between the anterior and middle scalenes. Diffuse anterior shoulder pain may occur, as well as paresthesias in the fourth and fifth digits. Neurological examination is typically normal, although pain may be produced with extension of the shoulders or an overhead stress test.

Ulnar Nerve: Cubital Tunnel Syndrome. Cubital tunnel syndrome occurs with compression of the ulnar nerve at the elbow. Tinel's sign may be positive behind the medial epicondyle or distal humerus. Examination may show decreased sensation in the fourth and fifth fingers with intrinsic hand weakness and atrophy.

Table 30.3. Chronic Compression of the Median Nerve

Site of Compression	Incidence	Symptoms	Findings	Provocative Maneuvers
Pronator teres	Rare	Forearm pain; numbness absent or of secondary importance	Forearm tenderness	Pain with resisted forearm pronation
Neuritis of anterior interosseous nerve	Uncommon	Weak pinch	Weak flexor pollicis longus and/or flexor digitorum profundus to the index finger	Tinel's sign on anterior aspect of the proximal forearm
Carpal canal	Common	Finger numbness; wrist weakness and occassional arm pain	Dry fingers; ± thenar atrophy; increased 2-point discrimination	Phalen's and/or Tinel's sign at wrist flexion crease

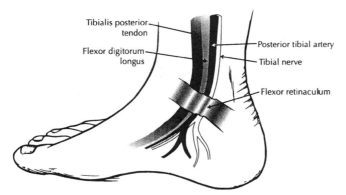

Tibialis posterior tendon

Flexor digitorum longus

Posterior tibial artery

Tibial nerve

Flexor retinaculum

Figure 30.3. Anatomical relationship of the tibial nerve at the ankle.

Ulnar Nerve: Guyon's Canal Syndrome. Guyon's canal syndrome occurs with ulnar nerve compression at the wrist. Typically pain occurs in the wrist along with paresthesias and decreased pinprick appreciation in the fourth and fifth fingers. Intrinsic hand muscle atrophy and weak grip may be present.

Radial Nerve: Posterior Interosseous Nerve Syndrome. Compression occurs from elbow synovitis or a mass in the proximal forearm on the posterior interosseous portion of the radial nerve. Signs include weakness of finger and wrist extension with radial deviation of the hand.

Radial Nerve: Radial Tunnel Syndrome. Radial tunnel syndrome occurs with compression of the radial nerve in the proximal forearm as it passes through the supinator muscle. Pain occurs in the proximal forearm and increases with forearm supination and/or middle finger extension.

Radial Nerve: Radial Sensory Nerve Entrapment. Also called cheiralgia paresthetica, this syndrome can be seen with compression of the radial sensory nerve in the distal forearm. Compression occurs as the nerve passes between the brachioradialis and extensor carpi radialis longus tendons. The patient may demonstrate tenderness in the distal forearm with decreased sensation in the first web space and over the dorsum of the hand. Radial nerve injuries may occur with direct compression such as handcuffs or tight plaster casts. Direct trauma and lacerations may also result in radial nerve compression.

Lower Extremity Compression Neuropathies
See Figures 30.3 and 30.4.

Posterior Tibial Nerve: Tarsal Tunnel Syndrome. Tarsal tunnel syndrome is the most common entrapment neuropathy of the posterior tibial nerve, which is compressed inferior to the medial malleolus as it passes under the flexor retinaculum of the ankle. Burning and numbness along the plantar aspect of the foot result, and Tinel's sign may be positive behind the medial malleolus. This can be a result of posttraumatic inflammation, soft tissue masses, or foot deformities.

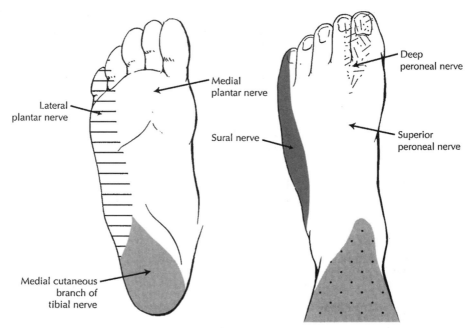

Figure 30.4. Sensory distribution in the foot.

Proximal Tibial Nerve. The tibial nerve is the continuation of the medial trunk of the sciatic nerve. It passes through the popliteal fossa and then deep to the two heads of the gastrocnemius muscle. Compression may occur with Baker's cysts or nerve sheath tumors. Clinical weakness of the plantar flexors and invertor muscles and intrinsic muscles of the foot characterize this neuropathy. The sensory loss is noted along the sole of the foot.

Saphenous Nerve. A saphenous neuropathy may occur from external compression related to knee-supporting stirrups or with lower extremity surgery such as varicose vein removal or harvesting an arterial graft. The saphenous nerve is the termination of the femoral nerve and passes from the femoral triangle to enter the subsartorial canal. Symptoms include sensory loss, pain, or paresthesias along the medial aspect of the knee radiating down the calf and into the medial aspect of the foot.

Femoral Nerve. The femoral nerve arises from the lumbar plexus and emerges from the lateral border of the psoas muscle and then passes under the inguinal ligament lateral to the femoral artery and vein. Compression may result from hematomas, intrapelvic or inguinal, and hip surgery. Numbness and paresthesias may be noted along the anterior thigh, and weakness of the quadriceps muscle results in buckling of the knee.

Deep Peroneal Nerve. The deep peroneal nerve descends in the leg lying between the extensor hallucis longus and the tibialis anterior muscles and tendons. Trauma to the dorsum of the foot, poorly fitted shoes, or casts may cause a compression neuropathy in this area. Abnormal sensation or paresthesias can occur in the web space between the first and second toes.

Superficial Peroneal Nerve. The superficial peroneal nerve divides from the common peroneal nerve at the fibular neck and then descends along the shaft of the upper third of the fibula. A twist of the ankle, excessive exercise, or habitual crossing of the ankles may result in this type of neuropathy. Sensory loss or burning may occur along the anterior aspect of the ankle and along the dorsum of the foot.

Common Peroneal Nerve. The common peroneal nerve is the most common peroneal compression neuropathy in the lower extremity. The common peroneal nerve is a continuation of the lateral trunk of the sciatic nerve and passes behind the fibular head. Compression can occur from coma, casts, leg crossing, or prolonged squatting. Numbness may be seen along the lateral aspect of the leg and foot and muscle weakness results in acute foot drop and weakness of eversion of the ankle.

Lateral Femoral Cutaneous Nerve of the Thigh. Meralgia paresthetica is a sensory abnormality involving varying degrees of numbness and hyperesthesia. This is noted over the lateral aspect of the thigh in a relatively stereotyped area. The lateral femoral cutaneous nerve at the thigh emerges from the lateral corner of the psoas muscle and runs down laterally in the pelvis on the iliacus muscle. It then passes either under or through the inguinal ligament, and compression typically occurs in this area. It may result from wearing tight clothing, wide belts, or leaning against the edge of a firm surface.

PEARLS AND PITFALLS

- Nerve status is documented prior to and after any manipulation of a wound or fracture.
- Attempts to coagulate or tie off bleeding vessels are not made in the emergency department particularly when the bleeding is associated with nerve injuries.
- Clavicle fracture with a brachial plexus injury portends a poor prognosis for recovery.
- Nerve compromise occurs in established compartment syndromes and requires prompt surgical decompression.

SELECTED BIBLIOGRAPHY

Adelaar RS, Foster WC, McDowell C. The treatment of the cubital tunnel syndrome. *J Hand Surg.* 1984;9:90–5.

Eaton CJ, Lister GD. Radial nerve compression. *Hand Clin.* 1992;2:345–57.

Hartz CR, Linscheid RL, Gramser RR, et al. The pronator teres syndrome. Compressive neuropathy of the median nerve. *J Bone Joint Surg.* 1981;63A:885–90.

Kihol LG, Nevin S. Isolated neuritis of the anterior interosseous nerve. *Br Med J.* 1952;1:850–1.

Leffert RD. Thoracic outlet syndrome. *Hand Clin.* 1992;2:285–97.

Moneim MS. Ulnar nerve compression at the wrist-ulnar tunnel syndrome. *Hand Clin.* 1992;2:337–44.

Pfeffer GB, Gelberman RH, Boyes JH, Rydevik B. The history of carpal tunnel syndrome. *J Hand Surg.* 1988;13:28–34.

Phalen GS. The carpal tunnel syndrome: clinical evaluation of 598 hands. *Clin Orthop.* 1972;83:29–40.

Tinel J. The tingling sign in peripheral nerve lesions. In: Spinner M, ed.; Kaplan EB, trans. *Injuries to the Major Branches of Peripheral Nerves of the Forearm*, 2nd ed. Philadelphia, Pa: WB Saunders; 1978:8–13.

31 Hydrocephalus and Shunts in Children

Stephen Guertin and Anthony Briningstool

INTRODUCTION
Due to the rapid and potentially lethal result of complete cerebrospinal fluid shunt failure, systematic identification of the shunt components, evaluation of shunt patency, recognition of peripheral shunt-related complications, and effective therapeutic measures proceed in tandem.

Almost all cerebrospinal fluid (CSF) shunt systems fail over time. On average, within 1 year of placement, 30–40% of shunts fail; 80–90% fail over a 10-year period. The greatest single risk of shunt failure is the age of the patient. Children under 2 years of age are at the highest risk for shunt obstruction. Approximately 10% of shunts become infected within the first year. The most common cause of shunt failure is occlusion of the ventricular tubing by cellular debris, fibrous tissue, choroid plexus, ventricular walls, and, in the case of catheter migration, the brain itself. Distal catheter blockage or migration of the catheter is the second most common cause.

With rare exception, shunt systems consist of several distinct components, and disconnections in the systems account for 15% of all shunt malfunctions. After the shunt system is compromised, the pace of clinical deterioration depends on the size of the ventricles and the age of the child. Children with large dilated ventricles have tremendous volume-buffering capacity and can tolerate large increases in volume with relatively small increases in intracranial pressure (ICP) compared to children with small ventricles. After a CSF shunt is in place, this volume-buffering capacity is lost. Intracranial compliance reverts to that of healthy children. In response to accumulating CSF, a child with normal-sized ventricles experiences greater increases in ICP more rapidly than an adult would. The rise in ICP is exacerbated after chronic shunting results in small "slit ventricles" where drained ventricular volume is compensated for by expanded brain volume, which fills the intracranial space.

Mechanical dysfunction of a CSF shunt system can cause either intracranial hypertension or intracranial hypotension. Shunt blockage is the chief concern when evaluating shunt dysfunction. However, life-threatening sudden "overdrainage" can cause a rapid drop in the ICP, potentially resulting in brainstem traction and shift, leading to immediate compromise of the hindbrain.

Evaluation and Differential Diagnosis

Symptoms and Signs of Shunt Dysfunction

Most children with CSF shunts who present with irritability, headache, vomiting, and fever are more likely to have a "viral illness" than a shunt malfunction. Fever makes the diagnosis of shunt dysfunction less likely; drowsiness or lethargy makes the diagnosis of shunt dysfunction more likely. Typically vague general complaints are offered, and these parental concerns must be considered seriously – especially if the family is concerned that the current symptoms are identical to those seen with a previous shunt failure. Unless a convincing finding exists to support a diagnosis of "viral" infection, CSF shunt dysfunction is assumed, particularly with changes in sensorium, autonomic instability, or cranial nerve findings. Symptoms and signs of elevated ICP due to shunt dysfunction include headache, changes in sensorium (lethargy, irritability, disorientation, coma), nausea, vomiting, and neck pain. Ominous changes include a precipitous change in sensorium, decerebrate posturing, pupillary changes, and components of Cushing's triad (hypertension, bradycardia, and respiratory ataxia). These changes suggest impending brain herniation. Exaggeration of preexisting neurological deficits, an enlarging or bulging fontanel, fluid extravasation along the shunt tract, upward gaze palsy, diplopia, dilated scalp veins, and increased muscle tone are the other findings of increasing ICP.

Neuro-ophthalmological signs of shunt dysfunction can precede findings on computerized tomography (CT) scanning. These include palsies of cranial nerves III, IV, and VI; anisocoria; dilated and slowly reactive pupils; upward gaze paresis; tonic downward eye deviation; and eyelid retraction. Any preexisting abnormality of movement or muscle tone is accentuated when ICP is increased. Asymmetrical dilatation of the ventricles can cause focal weakness and the signs of uncal herniation. Symptoms and signs of gradual ventricular enlargement from partial CSF shunt system dysfunction include gait disturbance, urinary incontinence, worsening of cerebral palsy, deteriorating school performance, visual deterioration, and hypothalamic signs.

Brainstem signs such as stridor, laryngospasm, syncope, disturbed consciousness, pallor, respiratory ataxia or arrest, opisthotonus, and a vacillating heart rate can result from high ICP as well as sudden "overdrainage" of CSF. Low ICP is suspected clinically by marked indentation of a cranial defect or collapse of the fontanel. This life-threatening condition can be ameliorated by placing the child into a Trendelenburg position and providing supportive ventilation.

Evaluation of Shunt Function

Almost all CSF shunt systems have intraventricular tubing, a valve apparatus, and distal tubing (Figure 31.1). When a separate reservoir is included in the system, it is located proximal to the valve. The most common reservoir used is seated in the skull with proximal connection to the ventricular tubing and distal connection to

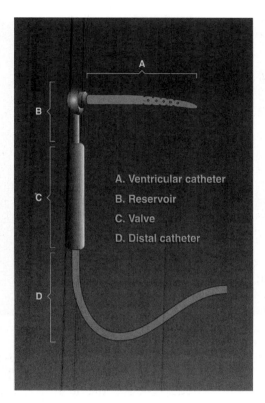

A. Ventricular catheter

B. Reservoir

C. Valve

D. Distal catheter

Figure 31.1. Basic shunt components.

the valve apparatus. The components and connections are identified and tracked (Figure 31.2). Valves are identified by inspection, palpation, and plain radiography as "tubular" or "domed" (Figures 31.3 and 31.4).

History obtained from the patient, the family, and medical records focuses on occurrence of a fall, the number of shunt systems, the pressure gradient and types of each of the shunt systems, which (if any) of the shunts are known to be not working, where the shunt systems terminate, and which system (when more than one) was the last shunt system to be revised.

Tubing that ends in the heart, the pleural space, or the peritoneal cavity can cause symptoms and signs referable to each location.

Inspection of the Shunt System

Distended scalp veins or bulging of the fontanel or a craniotomy site indicates high ICP. A sunken fontanel and sunken craniotomy site indicate low ICP. Unusual or recent swelling over the shunt site or any portion of the shunt system is considered diagnostic of shunt failure. Cellulitis, frank pus, or erosion of the scalp is associated with a high incidence of ventriculitis leading to mechanical dysfunction. The distal tubing usually can be tracked visually across the neck, chest, and abdomen on its way to the peritoneal space, pleural space, or heart. Swelling at the distal insertion site indicates fluid tracking up the catheter because of distal loculation (Figure 31.5).

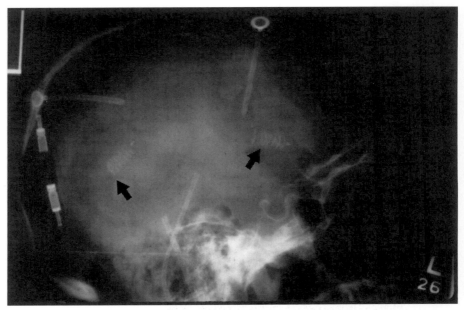

Figure 31.2. Superior: Domed shunt system consisting of intraventricular catheter. Rickham reservoir, dome valve, and distal tubing. The distal tubing is disconnected and separated from the valve by a long gap. Midfield: Two abandoned "flanged" ventricular catheters (arrows), left in place because they could not be extracted. The abandoned distal tubing has been left in place. Far left: Tubular shunt system consisting of intraventricular catheter, Rickham reservoir, tubular valve, and distal tubing. All connections are intact. This is the only functional system in this child's head.

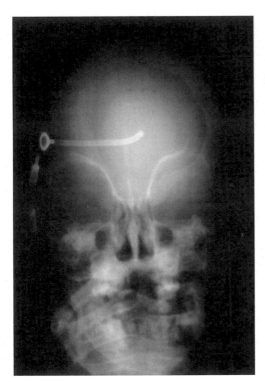

Figure 31.3. Tubular CSF shunt system consisting of intraventricular catheter, Rickham reservoir, tubular valve, and distal tubing. All connections are intact. The ventricular catheter is bent against the septum pellucidum.

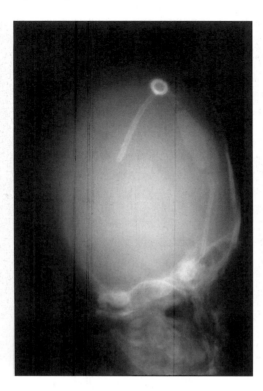

Figure 31.4. Domed CSF shunt system consisting of intraventricular catheter, Rickham reservoir, domed valve, and distal tubing. All connections are intact.

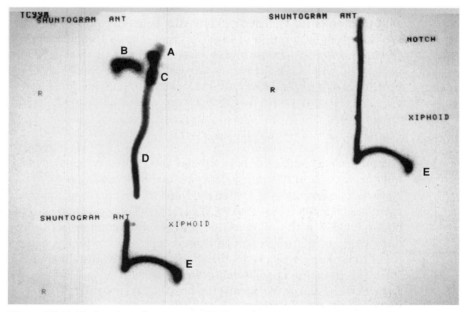

Figure 31.5. Technetium shuntogram. (A) The nuclide has been injected into the reservoir. (B) There is reflux into the lateral ventricle. (C) The technetium passes into a valve and (D) is carried through the distal tubing. (E) The technetium does not freely diffuse throughout the peritoneum but terminates in a distal loculation. This pseudocyst is the cause of the shunt obstruction.

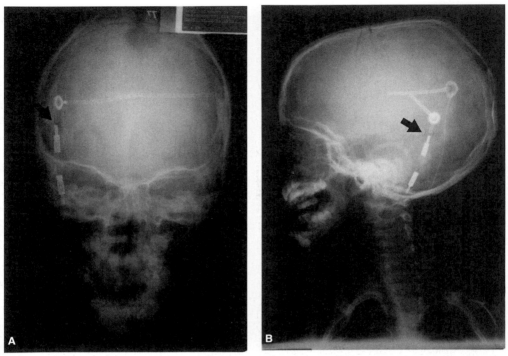

Figure 31.6. (A) A-P and (B) lateral skull radiographs. A close look painly reveals a gap and a misalignment between the reservoir and the valve of the "tubular" valve system (arrows). The valve is disconnected from the reservoir.

Palpation of the system checks for gaps between components and establishes the presence and location of reservoirs and pumping chambers. Palpation of a "floating reservoir" confirms both displacement of the Rickham reservoir from its position within the skull and a CSF leak upward around the reservoir and the ventricular tubing. Local warmth indicates an underlying infection.

Manual Evaluation to Test CSF Shunt Patency

The pumping chambers of both tubular and domed systems are designed to allow the assessment of shunt patency by manually testing the system. In domed systems, one occludes the system proximal to the pumping chamber. When the pumping chamber is depressed, CSF is ejected distally. When the chamber is released, it refills with CSF from the ventricle. Easy compression implies that the distal components are patent. Difficult compression or high resistance indicates that distal tubing is blocked, or that CSF is loculated distally and is under pressure. The pumping chamber allows refill within seconds. When the chamber remains depressed or fills slowly, the proximal (ventricular catheter) may be partially occluded. An audible "click" that occurs during valve compression or refill indicates an incompetent valve. Normal pumping and refill correctly predict a normally functioning shunt system about 80% of the time. In contrast, a delay in refill of the chamber is associated with an obstructed system only 20% of the time.

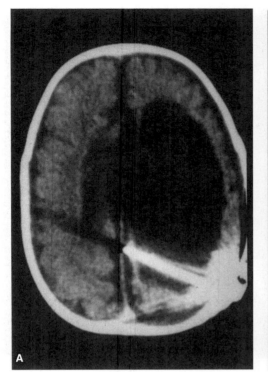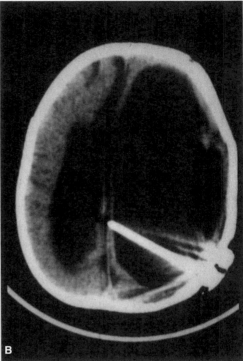

Figure 31.7. Comparison CT scans of a child with cerebral atrophy and ventriculomegaly. On the left, well-defined sulci and gyri and generous subarachnoid space are observed. Despite the marked ventriculomegaly, the child has normal ICP and a functioning shunt. On the right, the sulci and gyri are flattened against the cranial vault and ventricular expansion has occured. The shunt does not work, and the child is symptomatic.

Imaging Studies

The plain radiograph shunt survey includes anteroposterior (A-P) and lateral views of the skull and neck, and an A-P view of the chest. Lateral as well as right and left lateral decubitus views of the abdomen and pelvis are also obtained. Disconnection of the shunt components is generally obvious and can occur after minimal trauma (Figure 31.6), yet the fibrous sleeve around the shunt tubing often conducts CSF. In these cases, elevated ICP and death can occur rapidly. Right and left lateral decubitus films of the abdomen demonstrate the final destination of the ventricle-to-peritoneum tubing. The peritoneal catheter changes position with changes in body position, indicating that the peritoneal catheter is free-floating. Tube migration outside of the peritoneal cavity, fixed or stuck distal tubing, a curled catheter within the abdominal wall or within pseudocysts, and a kinked or defective tube itself can be seen. Fusiform swelling of the distal tubing, observed on a plain radiograph, indicates distal shunt obstruction.

When shunt dysfunction is suspected, a CT scan of the brain is compared with previous studies (see Figure 31.7). Ventricular enlargement compared with previously small ventricles indicates an obstructed system under high pressure. Markedly enlarged ventricles often indicate shunt malfunction. The CT scan is especially helpful in locating a proximally obstructed catheter that has migrated

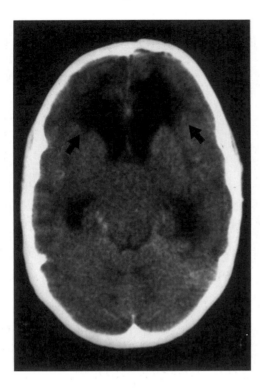

Figure 31.8. CT signs of shunt obstruction with elevated ICP. The periventricular transependymal migration of CSF outside of the lateral ventricular anterior horns (arrows) is observed. The sulci and gyri are flattened against the skull. The perimesencephalic cistern remains visible between the enlarged lateral ventricular temporal horns.

outside the ventricle. The appearance of well-defined sulci and gyri, especially when surrounded by expansive subarachnoid fluid, is in sharp contrast to that of brain parenchyma flattened against the cranial vault as a result of high ICP (Figure 31.7). Absence of the perimesencephalic cistern on CT imaging is especially ominous. Periventricular hypodensity, especially around the anterior horns of the lateral ventricles, indicates transependymal flow of CSF from the ventricles into the parenchyma (Figure 31.8). This extravasation of CSF can be confirmed by magnetic resonance imaging (MRI). If radionuclide studies are unavailable, MRI can assist in diagnosing an obstructed shunt system.

The combination of a shunt tap and radionuclide clearance shuntogram is the most reliable test for investigating shunt obstruction. The technetium phase of this combination allows visualization of the entire tract, assesses flow and reveals sites of degradation and separation of the components of the shunt system (Figure 31.5). A shunt tap is performed through the reservoir whenever possible. When no separate reservoir is present, the pumping chamber of the valve apparatus is accessed. The scalp site is cleaned with an iodine preparation. A 23-gauge "butterfly" needle is inserted percutaneously into the reservoir or the pumping chamber. An accurate pressure measurement is obtained only when the patient is calm. Opening pressure is recorded, and CSF drip frequency or free flow is assessed. CSF is collected, closing pressure is measured, and technetium is injected.

In a normally functioning shunt system, the opening pressure is within the normal range for the valve in place and is always lower than 20 cm CSF. A spontaneous drip rate of at least one drop per 20 seconds is an excellent predictor of proximal patency. The drip test is performed with the butterfly tubing held 5 cm below the ventricles and is accurate 95% of the time. Technetium clearance is measured from the time of injection and the count should diminish by 50% within 5 minutes, unless there is reflux into the ventricle. In this case, 20 minutes are allowed before concluding the test. Technetium diffuses freely throughout the space where the distal tubing terminates. When the shunt system is accessed, CSF is collected for culture, Gram stain, and cell count.

Distal Shunt Malfunction (Distal Catheter Obstruction)

Causes of distal obstruction include disconnection of the catheter, fibrosis or catheter plugging with cellular debris, kinking, catheter migration, and loculations of CSF. Plain radiographs may show a disconnection. On manual evaluation of the system, the pumping chamber refills promptly. Pressure within the shunt system is elevated when measured by a "shunt tap" and flow out of the reservoir is good. Wide changes in the ICP amplitude with each heartbeat imply a stiff, noncompliant brain. The technetium study reveals delayed or absent clearance and may show loculation distally.

Proximal Shunt Malfunction (Proximal Catheter Obstruction)

Proximal obstruction of the ventricular catheter of the CSF shunt system occurs from cellular debris, fibrosis, infection, envelopment by the choroid plexus, and catheter migration. Absent or delayed refill of the pumping chamber can be present. Catheter tip migration outside the ventricular system is obvious on CT imaging. Poor flow through the butterfly tubing and difficulty aspirating CSF can be seen with proximal obstruction. A low CSF drip rate is present 95% of the time when the shunt is "tapped." ICP that does not fall with inspiration suggests proximal obstruction. Combined with low or normal shunt pressure, a technetium study showing delayed or absent clearance confirms the diagnosis of proximal obstruction.

Management

Emergent medical therapy to lower increased ICP includes osmotic agents such as glycerol (1 g/kg given intravenously every 6 hours), mannitol (0.25–1 g/kg given intravenously every 6 hours) and isosorbide (2 g/kg given intravenously every 6 hours). Osmotic agents are effective primarily by extracting water from brain parenchyma but are relatively ineffective when there is little cortical mantle from which to extract fluid. The potential dangers of the use of osmotic agents are (1) osmotic diuresis exacerbates dehydration in a child who may be vomiting and may have had poor oral intake because of increased ICP; (2) when surgical intervention does not take place within 24 hours, and osmotic agents are stopped, rebound intracranial hypertension can occur; and (3) water is drawn from the interstitial space of the entire body in the 10–15 minutes immediately following administration of an osmotic agent. This results in a markedly higher cardiac output and transiently elevated cerebral blood flow and blood volume. When osmotic agents are given, therefore, an already elevated ICP can increase further before it begins to decrease.

Furosemide (1 mg/kg per day) with or without Mannitol is also used to lower elevated ICP. Parenteral diuretic such as furosemide (Lasix) is known to decrease

CSF production by 50–60%. ICP begins to fall within 30 minutes and reaches it nadir at 90 minutes; with duration of effect of up to 2.5 hours after parenteral administration of furosemide. Exacerbation of dehydration is a concern. The routine use of acetazolamide is avoided because it can cause an immediate increase in ICP due to drug-induced cerebral acidosis. The acidosis causes vasodilation and an increase in cerebral blood volume. With this increased intracranial volume, the ICP can increase to 75–150% above baseline. Therefore, acetazolamide is only used in less critical situations or after the intracranial space has been mechanically decompressed. In cases of life-threatening distal obstruction, mechanical decompression is performed by slowly removing manometric amounts of CSF from the ventricular compartment until ICP reaches 10–15 cm CSF. If the ICP is lowered too rapidly, subdural hemorrhage, subarachnoid hemorrhage, and pneumocranium can result.

An emergent neurosurgical consult for ventricular puncture may be required when the ventricular catheter is blocked (proximal obstruction) and the intracranial space cannot be mechanically decompressed through the reservoir or the pumping chamber. The intracranial space is entered through the coronal suture approximately 1 cm lateral to the midline or at the farthest lateral (coronal) margin of an open anterior fontanel. The needle is directed straight to the base of the skull on a plane parallel to the falx. After the dural "pop" is felt, the needle is redirected toward the base of the skull in line with the inner canthus of the ipsilateral eye. Enough CSF is drained (slowly) to achieve ICP of 10–15 cm of CSF.

In addition to the shunt malfunction, the two commonly encountered complications of long-term CSF shunt systems are (1) slit ventricle syndrome and (2) ventriculitis.

Slit Ventricle Syndrome

Small ventricles (slit-like) develop in at least 50% of patients who receive shunts in the first year of life. The term *slit ventricle syndrome* (frequency: 0.9–3.3%) refers to a small subset of shunt-dependent children with slit-like ventricles, who develop disabling chronic or recurring headaches associated with signs and symptoms of increased ICP. In the majority of the cases, these symptoms resolve spontaneously and do not require any intervention. However, the symptoms such as headaches, vomiting, and drowsiness can confound the diagnosis of slit ventricle syndrome because these symptoms also resemble those of shunt malformation.

Slit ventricle syndrome is not considered to be a single pathological entity, but rather a symptom complex with multiple etiologies. Pathophysiological conditions associated with this syndrome include overdrainage of CSF (causing low ICP), intermittent proximal catheter occlusion secondary to periventricular fibrosis, and decreased intracranial compliance. Sudden postural change or exercise can result in intracranial hypotension. Persistent cold sweats appear to be characteristic of intracranial hypotension. Sudden upward traction on the brainstem from significant intracranial hypotension causing sudden respiratory arrest, syncope, bradycardia, opisthotonus, or cranial nerve findings demand prompt attention. Placing the child in a Trendelenburg position at 15–30 degrees helps to alleviate the symptoms.

Ventriculitis

Shunt infection causing ventriculitis is suspected in febrile or ill-appearing children with CSF shunts without any other apparent source of infection. Of all shunts, 2–5% become infected. Almost 50% of shunt infections are caused by *Staphylococcus epidermidis*. Two-thirds of all shunt infections occur within one month of shunt surgery. Shunt infection typically results in only mildly elevated CSF white blood cell counts (50–200 cells/ml), which may not be distinguished from CSF cellularity induced by the presence of the shunt itself. CSF eosinophilia is a sign of ventricular infection. CSF cultures are positive in 96% of shunt system infections causing ventriculitis.

When CSF cannot be aspirated from the shunt system, lumbar puncture is performed cautiously if signs of elevated ICP are not present on CT scan prior to the lumbar puncture. Lumbar CSF is not contiguous with CSF in the lateral ventricles and routinely has elevated protein levels and monocytosis because of decreased CSF circulation. This presentation can lead to an incorrect diagnosis of infection.

PEARLS AND PITFALLS

- Nonspecific complaints of fever, nausea, and vomiting are more likely to be due to common non-shunt-related illness than to shunt malfunction. However, delaying investigations of possible shunt malfunction can have fatal consequences.

- Pumping the shunt is not an adequate shunt evaluation. "Normal pumping" and refill is accurate only 80% of the time. Further investigations to assess possible shunt malfunction are necessary.

- Life-threatening events from shunt malfunction can occur without evidence of ventricular enlargement on CT imaging.

- Altered sensorium, cranial nerve findings, and autonomic instability (especially breathing pattern) can indicate impending brain herniation.

- A child with a CSF shunt who presents with periodic breathing, declining Glasgow Coma Scale score, hypertension for age, or a low-normal or low heart rate for age cannot wait for neurosurgery to assume care. Immediate measures are undertaken in the emergency department to reduce increased ICP. Depending on the clinical condition, ventricular puncture may be needed when CSF cannot be drained from the shunt reservoir.

- In cases of distal shunt obstruction, decompression of the CSF shunt system is easily accomplished and can be life-saving.

SELECTED BIBLIOGRAPHY

Bell WE, McCormick WF. Hydrocephalus. In: Bell WE, McCormick WF, eds. *Raised Intracranial Pressure in Children: Diagnosis and Treatment.* Philadelphia, Pa: WB Saunders; 1978.

Epstein F, Lapras C, Wisoff JF. Slit-ventricle syndrome: etiology and treatment. *Pediatr Neurosci.* 1988;14:5.

Gilmore HE. Medical treatment of hydrocephalus. In: Scott RM, ed. *Concepts in Neurosurgery*. Baltimore, Md: Williams & Wilkins, 1990;3.

Guertin SR. Cerebrospinal fluid shunts; evaluation, complications, and crisis management. *Pediatr Clin North Am*. 1987;34:203.

Jordan KT. Cerebrospinal fluid shunts. *Emerg Med Clin North Am*. 1994;12:779.

Key CG, Rothrock SG, Falk JL. Cerebrospinal fluid shunt complications: an emergency medicine perspective. *Pediatr Emerg Care*. 1995;11:265.

Kiekens R, Mortier W, Pathmann R, et al. The slit-ventricle syndrome after shunting in hydrocephalic children. *Neuropediatrics*. 1982;13:190.

Madsen MA. Emergency department management of ventriculoperitoneal cerebrospinal fluid shunts. *Ann Emerg Med*. 1986;15:1330.

Post EM. Currently available shunt systems: a review. *Neurosurgery*. 1985;16:257.

Shapiro K, Fried A. Pressure-volume relationships in shunt-dependent childhood hydrocephalus. *J Neurosurg*. 1986;64:390.

Sood S, Kim S, Ham SD, et al. Useful components of the shunt tap test for evaluation of shunt malfunction. *Childs Nerv System*. 1993;9:157.

Venus JL. Infections of CSF shunt and intracranial pressure monitoring devices. *Infect Dis Clin North Am*. 1989;3:289.

Wolpert SM. Radiological investigation of pediatric hydrocephalus. In: Scott RM, ed. *Concepts in Neurosurgery*. Baltimore, Md: Williams & Wilkins; 1990;3.

32 Pediatric Infections of the Central Nervous System

Anthony Briningstool and Jane Turner

INTRODUCTION

In infants and young children the signs and symptoms of central nervous system (CNS) infections are frequently nonspecific. Timely recognition of symptoms and early intervention are critical if complications from CNS infections in children are to be avoided. Treatment often is initiated presumptively while definitive diagnostic information is processed. The emergency physician faces special dignostic challenges when a child who has previously been taking antibiotics presents with symptoms consistent with a CNS infection.

Meningitis is the most common CNS infection and is primarily a pediatric disease. In the United States, 75% of all cases occur in individuals under 18 years of age; 60% are under 5 years of age. Most cases of meningitis are aseptic (viral), with seasonal enteroviruses being responsible for more than 75% of all cases. With the advent of *Haemophilus infl uenza* type B vaccine (HiB) there has been a dramatic decline in invasive *H. infl uenza* disease. Use of HiB has resulted in an overall decline in the number of cases of meningitis in children under 5 years of age. However, there has been little decline in the overall prevalence of meningitis due to other pathogens.

Infants Under 2 Months of Age

Meningitis must be considered in the differential diagnosis of any ill infant. Presenting symptoms can be vague and nonspecific (e.g., poor feeding, increased somnolence, irritability, and inconsolable crying). Fevers may be absent. Hypothermia is common in children with meningitis. Organisms associated with meningitis in the newborn typically belong to the maternal flora with Group B streptococci, Gram negative bacilli, and *Listeria monocytogenes* being the most common pathogens affecting the very young infant. Ocassionally, *Haemophilus influenza* type B is responsible for meningitis in this age group, but the rate of associated infection increases with age.

Many infants with herpes simplex (HSV) encephalitis do not have characteristic mucocutaneous vesicles, and approximately 33% of infants with HSV

325

Table 32.1. Cerebrospinal Fluid Analysis

	Normal			Bacterial	Viral
	Preterm	**Term**	**>6 mo**	**Bacterial**	**Viral**
Cell count (WBC/mm^3)					
Mean	9	8	0	>500	<500
Range	0–25	0–22	0–4		
Predominant cell type	Lymph	Lymph	Lymph	80% PMN leukocyte	PMN leukocyte initially, lymphocyte later
Glucose (mg/dl)					
Mean	50	52	>40	<40	>40
Range	24–63	34–119			
Protein (mg/dl)					
Mean	115	90	<40	>100	<100
Range	65–150	20–170			
CSF/blood glucose (%)					
Mean	74	81	50	<40	>40
Range	55–150	44–248	40–60		
Gram stain	Negative	Negative	Negative	Positive	Negative
Bacterial culture	Negative	Negative	Negative	Positive	Negative

Note: CSF, cerobrospinal fluid; PMN, polymorphonuclear neutrophils; WBC, white blood cells.

infection have encephalitis without disseminated disease. Typically, these infants present during the second or third week of life because of poor feeding and failure to thrive. Other clinical findings include seizures, apnea, bradycardia, or cranial nerve abnormalities. There may be no associated history of HSV infection in the mother at delivery. Cerebrospinal fluid (CSF) findings are variable, typically, pleocytosis and increased protein levels are found. CSF cultures with PCR antibody studies for HSV can confirm the diagnosis. When HSV infection of the CNS is suspected clinically Acyclovir (20 mg/kg given intravenously every 8 hours) is recommended.

Evaluation of a child less than 2 months of age presenting with lethargy, poor feeding, somnolence, irritability, or fever begins with a thorough history and physical examination. Specific findings on physical examination such as a bulging fontanel or mucocutaneous vesicles can help, however CNS infections can still exist when these findings are absent. Likewise, an acute illness such as otitis media does not eliminate the possibility of a concurrent CNS infection. Lumbar puncture for CSF analysis is performed in an any infant suspected of having a CNS infection. A catheterized urine specimen is obtained for microscopic analysis and culture and bacterial antigen studies to rule out other diagnoses. The diagnosis of CNS infection is made primarily on the basis of the CSF analysis. Age-specific values of CSF examination are listed in Table 32.1.

Infants 2–24 Months of Age

The presenting symptoms of CNS infections in children 2–24 months of age typically is nonspecific. Fever, seizures, poor feeding, and irritablity are the most common symptoms. The level of responsiveness and interaction with family often provides the best insight into the severity of the child's illness. The child who smiles spontaneously and interacts playfully is unlikely to have a serious infection.

In infants over 2 months of age, the bacteria responsible for meningitis are largely upper respiratory tract flora. These include *Haemophilus influenza* type B, *Streptococcus pneumoniae*, and *Neisseria meningitidis*. Meningitis caused by *Pseudomonas aeruginosa*, *Staphylococcus epidermidis*, *Salmonella*, or *Listeria monocytogenes* is uncommon. The likelihood of identifying an uncommon pathogen is increased in children with immune deficits or anatomical defects. *Mycobacterium tuberculosis*, although uncommon, can cause meningitis in all age groups. Enteroviruses, especially Echovirus and Coxsackievirus, are responsible for most cases of viral meningitis or meningoencephalitis. Other viral agents that cause meningoencephalitis include mumps, Herpes simplex, California equine, St. Louis equine, and western equine viruses. *Mycoplasma pneumoniae* has been implicated in encephalitis and meningoencephalitis in a number of children.

Physical examination findings are often nonspecific as well. A bulging fontanel suggests CNS infection, but a flat or nonpalpable fontanel does not exclude it. Nuchal rigidity can be present in older infants but is not found consistently in children younger than 2 years of age who have meningitis. The level of consciousness, responsiveness to surroundings, and willingness to interact with the care provider or examiner are the most critical components of the physical examination of a child. As with younger infants, a localizing sign that can account for fever does not eliminate the possibility of CNS infection. Otitis media often is present in infants with meningitis. CNS infection is suspected in any febrile infant or toddler who appears toxic or has an altered mental status.

Children 24 Months and Older

In children 2 years of age and older, symptoms and the physical findings are more specific indicating CNS infection. Headache, fever, lethargy, and stiff neck are likely to be present. Physical examination reveals meningismus in most cases, and fever is virtually always present. Examination of the CSF is the definitive diagnostic study to determine the presence of CNS infection. Computerized tomography (CT) of the brain is performed prior to lumbar puncture (LP) when increased ICP or a mass lesion such as tumor or hematoma is suspected. Prompt administration of antibiotics is important when bacterial infection is suspected.

Patients with viral meningitis can also present with fever, headache, and stiff neck. In contrast to children with bacterial meningitis, children with viral CNS infection rarely appear toxic. CSF results usually confirm the diagnosis.

Management and Disposition

Clinical stabilization is followed by administration of antibiotics and occasionally corticosteroids when bacterial meningitis is suspected. Ideally, antibiotics are administered within 30 minutes of arrival. All children suspected of having bacterial meningitis are hospitalized for close observation and treatment.

The standard therapy for newborns with early-onset disease (i.e., under 7 days old) is Ampicillin plus an aminoglycoside, usually Gentamicin or Tobramycin.

Infants over 7 days old can be treated with a third-generation cephalosporin (Cefotaxime or Ceftriaxone) plus Ampicillin. The weight-appropriate dosing for Ampicillin is 100 mg/kg. For the aminoglycocides (Gentamicin or Tobramycin), the weight-appropriate dosing is 2.5 mg/kg. The initial dose for Cefotaxime or Ceftriaxone is 50–75 mg/kg. The total daily dose per kilogram is adjusted according to the gestational age and weight of the infant. Adjustments are made by altering the dosing interval; the initial dose in the emergency department is unchanged.

The recent emergence of penicillin-resistant strains of *Streptococcus pneumoniae* is cause for considerable concern. The incidence of resistance strains varies from community to community, but the problem is growing nationwide. Some experts recommend empirical therapy with Cefotaxime and Vancomycin for all children with meningitis because of emerging resistance to cephalosporins and to penicillin. Others recommend the addition of Vancomycin only when gram-positive diplococci are found in the CSF or when there is strong suspicion of pneumococcal disease clinically. Antibiotic susceptibility testing is critical in guiding therapeutic decisions later in the course of the illness. A repeat LP for another evaluation of CSF at 24–48 hours is recommended in children infected by strains with reduced susceptibility to penicillin.

The use of Dexamethasone has been found to improve the outcome from bacterial meningitis in children in some studies. Neurological sequelae, specifically hearing impairment, occurred less often in children who received Dexamethasone early on. These studies were done at a time when *H. influenza* was the most common pathogen in meningitis in children. It is not known whether steroid treatment is as effective when other pathogens are involved. The recommended dose of Dexamethasone is 0.15 mg/kg given intravenously every 6 hours for 4 days, with the first dose given prior to the first dose of antibiotic.

Supportive treatment in the emergency department includes careful fluid management. Hydration is necessary when the child is dehydrated or hypovolemic on arrival. normovolemia is established, fluids are restricted to 50–66% maintenance to avoid complications of the syndrome of inappropriate antidiuretic hormone (SIADH) secretion.

Seizures occur commonly in children with meningitis. Intravenous administration of Diazepam or Lorazepam is recommended for immediate seizure control. Phenytoin can be administered to reduce the risk of recurrence while avoiding CNS depression.

Special Circumstances

Children currently taking antibiotics at the time of presentation to the emergency department pose a unique challenge. Children with partially treated meningitis present differently and are more likely to have a history of vomiting with prolonged symptoms. They are less likely to show signs of altered mental status or have a temperature over 38.3°C. They are also more likely to have findings of an ear, nose, or throat infection. The threshold for performing an LP is lower for children taking antibiotics who present with apparently minor illnesses. CSF parameters are also altered by partial treatment with antibiotics, making it difficult to distinguish between patients with viral meningitis and those with a partially treated bacterial disease.

Another challenge commonly faced by emergency physicians is the blood-contaminated CSF from a traumatic LP. The difficulty occurs in the interpretation of the white blood cell (WBC) counts in the blood-contaminated cerebrospinal fluid. CSF WBC counts are expected to be proportional to the peripheral blood WBC counts when all the cells are introduced from blood. When this occurs, the existence of a CSF pleocytosis is considered to be unlikely. However, it has been demonstrated that CSF WBC counts can be significantly lower than expected from this assumption, and a clinically significant CSF leukocytosis can be missed when this formula is applied. Interpretation remains problematic. Close clinical monitoring is advised when meningitis is suspected and the LP is traumatic regardless of the WBC count of the specimen.

PEARLS AND PITFALLS

- The younger the child is, the less specific the symptoms and signs of meningitis are.
- Children on an oral antibiotic with meningitis present differently from children who have not been on an antibiotic.
- There is no reliable way to interpret the cell count of a traumatic LP.
- Seizures often accompany meningitis but are rarely or never the only symptom.
- As soon as hypovolemia has been corrected, fluids are restricted to avoid fluid overload due to the potential of development of SIADH.
- Recommendations for antibiotics to treat meningitis may change in the near future as a result of the emergence of resistant organisms.

SELECTED BIBLIOGRAPHY

Al-Eissa YA. Lumbar puncture in the clinical evaluation of children with seizures associated with fever. *Pediatr Emerg Care*. 1995;11:347–50.

Annunziato PW, Gershon A. Herpes simplex virus infections. *Pediatr Rev*. 1996;17:415–23.

Barkin RM, Rosen P, eds. *Emergency Pediatrics*. St. Louis, Mo: Mosby – Year Book; 1994.

Bradley JS, Kaplan SL, Klugman KP, Leggiadro JJ. Consensus: management of infections in children caused by *Streptococcus pneumoniae* with decreased susceptibility to penicillin. *Pediatr Infect Dis*. 1995;14:1037–41.

Guerina NG. Viral infections in the newborn. In: Cloherty JP, Starkf AR, eds. *Manual of Neonatal Care*, 3rd ed. Boston, Mass: Little, Brown and Co.; 1991:114–46.

Prober CG. Infections of the central nervous system. In: Behrman RE, Kliegman RM, Nelson WE, eds. Nelson: *Textbook of Pediatrics*. Philadelphia, Pa: WB Saunders; 1996:707–16.

Report of the Committee on Infectious Diseases of the American Academy of Pediatrics. *Dexamethasone Therapy for Bacterial Meningitis in Infants and Children*, 23rd ed. Elk Grove Village, Ill: American Academy of Pediatrics; 1991:558–9.

Walsh-Kelly C, Nelson DB, Smith DS, Losek JD, Melzer-Lange M, Hennes HM, et al. Clinical predictors of bacterial versus aseptic meningitis in childhood. *Ann Emerg Med*. 1992;21:910–14.

Pediatric Cerebrovascular Disorders

Liza A. Squires and Imad Jarjour

INTRODUCTION

Childhood stroke is being recognized earlier due to increased medical awareness and modern neuroimaging technology. The incidence of ischemic stroke exceeds 3.3 in 100,000 children per year. Risk factors for stroke in children are numerous, differ from risks of stroke in adults, and can be recognized in more than 75% of children with stroke (Table 33.1). The prognosis for children with ischemic infarction is encouraging with 57% achieving a full recovery or having only mild dysfunction, 26% having moderate dysfunction, and only 16% having severe disability. Children with sickle cell disease have a 10% per year risk of stroke. The stroke prevention and sickle cell disease (STOP) trial demonstrated a nearly 90% decrease in incidence when the children were treated with chronic transfusion programs. Recent advances in the adult stroke population such as thrombolytic therapy (tPA) may prove to be safe and effective in children. Development of neuronal protective agents also holds promise in the pediatric population, but further research in this area is needed.

Presentations of Childhood Stroke

Strokes are classified by mechanism as either hemorrhagic or ischemic.

Hemorrhagic infarctions are either subarachnoid or intraparenchymal. No historical feature distinguishes ischemic from hemorrhagic stroke. However, nausea, vomiting, headache, and a depressed level of consciousness are more common in hemorrhagic strokes. Subarachnoid hemorrhage (SAH) generally presents with a sudden onset of severe headache, nausea, vomiting, meningismus, and photophobia. A loss of consciousness or seizure may occur around the onset of hemorrhage. In infants, CNS depression and full fontanel may be the only signs. SAH can be secondary to vascular malformation, Sickle cell disease, rupture of an aneurysm, and accidental or nonaccidental trauma. Secondary vasospasm leads to ischemic cerebral infarction 1–5 days after the hemorrhage. Intraparenchymal hemorrhage presents with a sudden onset of headache and vomiting and with a progressive decrease in the level of consciousness and focal neurological deficits. Etiologies include cavernous hemangiomas, arterial venous malformations,

Table 33.1. Risk Factors for
Pediatric Cerebrovascular Disorders

Congenital heart disease
  Complex congenital defects
  Ventricular septal defect
  Atrial septal defect
  Patent ductus arteriosus
  Aortic stenosis
  Mitral stenosis
  Coarctation of the aorta
  Cardiac rhabdomyoma
  Mitral valve prolapse
Acquired heart disease
  Rheumatic heart disease
  Prosthetic heart valve
  Bacterial endocarditis
  Cardiomyopathy
  Myocardial infarction
  Myocarditis
  Atrial myxoma
  Arrhythmia
Systemic vascular disease
  Systemic hypertension
  Volume depletion
  Systemic hypotension
  Hypernatremia
  Superior vena cava syndrome
  Diabetes
  Atherosclerosis
  Progeria
Vasculitis
  Acquired immunodeficiency syndrome
  Behcet syndrome
  Kawasaki disease
  Meningitis
  Systemic infection
  Polyarteritis nodosa
  Granulomatous angiitis
  Takayasu arteritis
  Rheumatoid arthritis
  Dermatomyositis
  Mixed connective tissue disease
  Varicella
  Inflammatory disease
  Drug abuse (cocaine, amphetamine)
  Primary cerebral angiitis
  Sneddon syndrome
Vasculopathies
  Ehlers-Danlos syndrome
  Moyamoya syndrome
  Fabry disease
  Malignant atrophic papulosis
  Pseudoxanthoma elasticum
  Neurofibromatosis
  Systemic lupus erythematosis

(continued)

Table 33.1. *(continued)*

Metabolic disorders
  Homocystinuria
  Isovaleric acidemia
  MELAS
  NADH-CoQ reductase deficiency
  Methylmalonic acidemia
  Propionic acidemia
  Ornithine transcarbamylase deficiency
Vasospastic disorders
  Alternating migraine hemiplegia
  Primary cerebroretinal vasospasm due to
    subarachnoid hemorrhage
  Migrainous stroke
  Ergot overdose
Hematologic disorders and coagulopathies
  Hemoglobinopathies (Sickle cell disease)
  Immune thrombocytopenic purpura
  Hemolytic uremic syndrome
  Thrombocytopenic purpura
  Thrombocytosis
  Polycythemia
  Congenital coagulation defects
  Disseminated intravascular coagulation
    (DIC)
  Leukemia and other neoplasms
    (neuroblastoma)
  Oral contraceptives
  Twin-twin transfusion
  Pregnancy and postpartum period
  Antithrombin III deficiency
  Vitamin K deficiency
  Protein C deficiency
  Protein S deficiency
  Lupus anticoagulant
  Anticardiolipin antibody
  Antiphospholipid antibody
  Paroxysmal nocturnal hemoglobinuria
  Nephrotic syndrome
Congenital cerebrovascular anomalies
  Arterial fibromuscular dysplasia
  Agenesis/hypoplastic vessels
  Arteriovenous malformation
  Hereditary hemorrhagic telangectasia
  Sturge-Weber syndrome
  Cavernous angioma
  Intracranial aneurysm
Trauma
  Child abuse
  Congenital bony anomalies
  Fat or air embolism
  Fibrocartilaginous embolism
  Foreign body embolism
  Posttraumatic arterial dissection
  Blunt cervical arterial trauma

Intraoral trauma
Penetrating intercranial trauma
Posttraumatic carotid cavernous fistula
Coagulation defect with minor trauma
Iatrogenic
   Anticoagulation arteriography
   Bone marrow transplant
   Carotid ligation (e.g., ECMO)
   Cardiac surgery
   Chemotherapy with thrombocytopenia
   Chiropractic manipulation
   L-Asparaginase
   Maternal anticonvulsants
   Post-irradiation
   Temporal artery catheterization
   Umbilical artery catheterization

Source: Modified from Roach ES, Riela AP. *Pediatric Cerebrovascular Disorders*, 2nd ed. Armonk, NY: Futura; 1995.

hemorrhage into tumor, and secondary hemorrhage into the site of an embolic/thrombotic stroke. Patients receiving cancer treatments may present with radiation vasculopathy or radiation necrosis as an etiology for intraparenchymal hemorrhage.

Ischemic infarctions are thrombotic (arterial or venous) or embolic (arterial). Seizures are a presenting symptom of ischemic stroke in approximately 20% of patients. Subcortical infarction often presents with acute hemiparesis. Cortical infarction may present with hemiparesis with or without other deficits. Cerebral embolism may present with a sudden loss of function followed by subtle improvement upon reperfusion. Embolism may also present with a stuttering course of recurrent deficits followed by improvement. Reperfusion can lead to secondary hemorrhage. Embolic sources include endocarditis in children with congenital heart disease, valvular vegetations, and right-to-left shunts in which the peripheral emboli bypass the lungs. Hypoxemia in children with right-to-left shunts leads to polycythemia and thrombosis. Spontaneous emboli are also known to occur. Fat emboli occur in children with long bone fractures.

Dissections of the carotid artery or less commonly vertebral artery occur after penetrating injuries, sports injuries, child abuse, or inappropriate chiropractic manipulation. Thrombosis of intracranial vessels from arteritis due to bacterial meningitis, chronic tonsillitis, dental infection, cat scratch disease, and mycoplasma pneumonia can also occur. Vasculopathy may cause stroke as a complication of polyarteritis nodosa, systemic lupuserythematosus, and varicella infection.

Cerebral venous thrombosis is more common in children than adults and often presents with altered mental status, seizures, and increased intracranial pressure (headache, vomiting, papilledema). Children with congenital heart disease, malignancy, or hemoglobinopathy are at risk for cerebral venous thrombosis if they develop dehydration, fever, polycythemia, or hypoxemia.

Conditions That Mimic Stroke

The sudden development of focal neurological deficits, headache, seizure, and altered consciousness are typical manifestations of childhood stroke. Other childhood conditions, which have a similar presentation, include migraine, epilepsy, hypoglycemia, and rarely other neurological conditions such as alternating hemiplegia of childhood.

Migraine presents with unilateral neurological symptoms such as numbness, weakness, or aphasia. These symptoms occur before or during the complaint of headache. Hemiplegic migraine can present with loss of consciousness and weakness, with or without paresthesia. Often, as the weakness improves, a vascular headache that is diffuse or contralateral to the weakness develops. Stroke is more likely if weakness persists beyond 24 hours. Young adult females with a history of migraine with aura and the antiphospholipid antibody can present with transient focal deficits and are at higher risk for stroke. Trauma-triggered migraine is an often underrecognized syndrome of dramatic encephalopathy, with or without focal features after a minor head injury. Minutes to hours after a seemingly trivial head injury, the child becomes confused, agitated, and may develop hemiparesis or hemiparesthesia. Blindness and loss of consciousness have also been reported. A family history of migraine and prior complaints of vascular headaches are common.

Epileptic seizures followed with Todd's paralysis mimic stroke. Generally the paralysis lasts only a few hours, but deficits can last up to 48 hours. Children with a history of focal seizures, unilateral headache, and a new focal neurologic deficit warrant brain imaging. Hemiparetic seizures with preserved mental state are a rare form of partial epilepsy.

Alternating hemiplegia is a rare condition of undetermined etiology. The first attack of hemiplegia typically occurs before 18 months of age and may last minutes to days. Dysautonomia, ocular motor dysfunction, and extrapyramidal symptoms have also been reported.

Hypoglycemia may present with acute hemiplegia and is often preceded by dizziness, tremor, confusion, and altered mental status. Transient hemiplegia is known to occur in children with diabetes mellitus during upper respiratory infections.

Intracranial infection rarely presents with focal neurological deficits. Herpes encephalitis, tuberculosis, and neurocysticercosis are examples. Children with congenital heart disease and right-to-left cardiac shunt present with a progressive hemiplegia due to intracerebral abscess.

Intracranial neoplasms typically cause slowly progressive hemiplegia; however, acute hemorrhage into the tumor presents suddenly with seizure or hemiplegia. Traumatic brain injury with resultant epidural or subdural hemorrhage, cerebral contusion, and shear injuries are also known to cause hemiplegia.

Evaluation

Selected historical information helps to determine the etiology of stroke. A recent febrile illness or systemic infection supports a thrombotic or vasculitic etiology. Histories of trauma, chiropractic manipulation, or intraoral trauma suggest an arterial dissection. The presence of congenital heart disease or heart murmur suggests an embolic etiology. It is important to inquire about recurrent headaches and seizures, as well as the use of oral contraceptives, alcohol, and drugs, and family history of stroke, thrombosis, spontaneous abortion, or premature myocardial infarction.

The physical survey includes evaluation of cardiac rhythm and rate, blood pressure, and mental status. Patients with diminished consciousness are evaluated for their ability to protect their airway. Patients with subarachnoid hemorrhage have mild to moderate increases in blood pressure. Blood pressure also becomes labile as intracranial pressure rises. A funduscopic examination may reveal retinal hemorrhages from trauma, subarachnoid hemorrhage, or arterial hypertension. The oral pharynx and neck is evaluated for evidence of injury and inflammation. An abnormality in cardiac rhythm, murmur, or gallop sounds is suggestive of heart failure. The abdomen is palpated for enlarged kidneys, a sign of polycystic kidney disease. Diminished femoral pulses suggest coarctation of the aorta. A careful skin survey shows signs of herpes, varicella, neurocutaneous disorders, or bruising from trauma.

The neurologic examination is tailored to the patient's level of consciousness and developmental stage. Assessment includes level of consciousness, cranial nerves, and motor, sensory, and cerebellar function, including gait and deep tendon reflexes.

Oculomotor nerve palsy with or without ipsilateral mydriasis can be seen with posterior communicating artery aneurysms. Occlusions of the anterior cerebral artery primarily affect frontal lobe function and manifest as altered mental status, contralateral lower extremity weakness, and gait apraxia. Middle cerebral artery occlusions can cause contralateral hemiparesis, hypesthesia, and ipsilateral hemianopsia with gaze preference toward the side of the lesion. Posterior cerebral artery occlusion causes homonymous hemianopsia, visual agnosia, altered mental status, and impaired memory. Vertebral basilar artery occlusion is difficult to detect, as it may present with vertigo, nystagmus, diplopia, visual field defects, dysphasia, dysarthria, facial hypesthesia, syncope, ataxia, and visual hallucinations.

Diagnostic Studies

An emergent head computerized tomography (CT) scan may help to determine whether the stroke is hemorrhagic or ischemic and to guide further diagnostic evaluations. Children with new neurologic deficits are at risk for alteration of mental status and brain herniation and are accompanied by a physician to the radiology department for the required studies. Brain magnetic resonance imaging (MRI) is needed when a CT scan is either normal or inconclusive. MRI is the study of choice if a lesion in the brainstem or cerebellum is suspected. Carotid duplex, transcranial Doppler, and cerebral angiography are done as warranted.

When embolism is suspected, cardiac investigations include electrocardiogram (EKG), transesophageal echocardiography with bubble contrast study, and Holter monitoring.

Laboratory studies include a complete blood count (CBC) with erythrocyte sedimentation rate, chemistry profile including glucose, toxicology, sickle cell prep, pregnancy test when applicable, coagulation studies, platelet count, and blood cultures. Hypercoagulable screening tests include protein C, proteins, antithrombin 3, factor 5 Leiden, and antiphospholipid antibody. Homocystine levels may be obtained, when applicable.

Cerebral spinal fluid analysis is warranted if infection is suspected.

Management

Emergent stabilization and documentation of initial neurological deficits are critically important. Children with suspected infections receive appropriate antibiotics and antiviral agents. Increased intracranial pressure is treated aggressively (see Chapter 23, "Increased Intracranial Pressure and Herniation Syndromes"). Seizures are treated with a nonsedative agent, such as phenytoin. Prophylactic anticonvulsants are usually unnecessary but are often considered in the presence of SAH.

Benefits and risks of using anticoagulant agents in children are based on the likelihood of either extension of the infarct or development of a second infarction when embolism is suspected versus the risk of hemorrhage. Aspirin is used especially in children who are at risk of developing recurrent stroke. Anticoagulation with warfarin is also used in selected patients but is generally avoided in children because of the risk of trauma-related hemorrhage. Children with neurological deficits are observed in the hospital, typically in an intensive care unit.

PEARLS AND PITFALLS

- Stroke in children occurs from fetal life to adolescence.
- The etiologies and manifestations of stroke are different in children compared to adults.
- Congenital heart disease is a common underlying cause of stroke in children.
- Stroke occurs in approximately 6% of patients with sickle cell disease.
- Migraine, epilepsy, hypoglycemia, and alternating hemiplegia of childhood can mimic stroke.
- Consider substance abuse and physical abuse in children as a possible cause of stroke.
- Thrombolytic therapy has not yet been approved to treat stroke in children.

SELECTED BIBLIOGRAPHY

Adams RJ, Brambilla DJ, McKie VC, et al. Prevention of a first stroke by transfusions in children with Sickle cell anemia and abnormal results on transcranial Doppler ultrasonography. *N Engl J Med.* 1998;339:5–11.

Broderick J, Talbott GT, Prenger ES, Leach A, Brott T. Stroke in children within a major metropolitan area: the surprising importance of intra-cerebral hemorrhage. *J Child Neurol.* 1993;8:250–5.

DeVeber GA, McGregor D, Curtis R, Mayank S. Neurologic outcome in survivors of childhood arterial ischemic stroke and sinovenous thrombosis. *J Child Neurol.* 2000; 15:316–24.

Dusser A, Goutieres F, Aicardi J. Ischemic stroke in children. *J Child Neurol.* 1986; 1:131.

Roach ES, Riela AR. *Pediatric Cerebrovascular Disorders*, 2nd ed. Armonk, NY: Futura; 1995.

34 Pediatric Seizures

Mont R. Roberts and Rae R. Hanson

INTRODUCTION

The incidence of seizures and epilepsy is increased at the extremes of age – infants and elderly. The prevalence of epilepsy is similar in children and adults; however, the etiology and therapy of seizures differs. Parental concerns are important; sequelae, prognosis, medication side effects, and social stigmata may need to be discussed.

When a previously normal child has a seizure and recovers to a normal baseline, a focused evaluation is indicated. A more extensive evaluation in the emergency department is based on factors other than the occurrence of the seizure. Management of status epilepticus requires aggressive treatment that adheres to a timetable based on a clear understanding of the pharmacokinetics of the antiepileptic drugs used.

Status Epilepticus

Status epilepticus (SE) is defined as a condition characterized by an epileptic seizure that is sufficiently prolonged or repeated at sufficiently brief intervals to produce an unvarying and enduring epileptic condition. In clinical practice, SE is any seizure that lasts 30 minutes or more, or occurs so frequently that the patient does not return to normal mental status between seizures.

Differential Diagnosis

An episode of SE may be the first or only seizure in 50% of children (when febrile seizures are included). The average age of childhood SE is under 3 years old. Causes of SE include prior central nervous system (CNS) injury (13%), progressive encephalopathy (5%), and a roughly even division of the remaining 82% between febrile, idiopathic, and acute symptomatic causes (CNS infection, anoxia, stroke, hemorrhage, trauma, antiepileptic drug [AED] withdrawal, intoxication, and metabolic abnormalities). The outcome of SE is related to the etiology of the convulsion. Morbidity is 9–28% and is more common in younger children, and less likely in previously healthy children with idiopathic or remote causes of SE

337

Table 34.1. Classification of Status Epilepticus

Generalized	Partial
Convulsive	Simple (consciousness preserved)
Tonic–clonic	
Clonic	
Tonic	
Myoclonic	
Nonconvulsive	Complex (clouding of consciousness or unconscious)
Absence	
Partial absence	
Atonic	

when they are rapidly treated. Mortality is 3–11%. See Table 34.1 for a seizure classification scheme. It can be difficult to clinically discriminate a generalized seizure from a partial seizure with secondary generalization.

Evaluation and Management

See Tables 34.2 and 34.3.

Generalized Convulsive SE

The acute management requires a planned treatment schedule and a specific time line. The duration of SE is the greatest risk to the patient – the longer SE lasts, the more difficult it is to treat. There are three goals of treatment: (1) control seizures, (2) preserve vital functions, and (3) diagnose the underlying pathology.

Patients who are going to respond to the first dose of benzodiazepine will usually do so within 60 seconds. Lorazepam is less sedating and longer acting than diazepam, making it the preferred drug. Midazolam is increasing in popularity, and may prove to be the drug of choice. Phenytoin takes nearly 20 minutes to reach peak brain levels with intravenous infusion, although clinically most patients respond earlier. Fosphenytoin, the prodrug of phenytoin, can be infused two to three times as rapidly as phenytoin and can be administered intramuscularly. Phenobarbital can alternatively be administered as intermittent boluses in the management of SE, rather than a single large bolus, to minimize respiratory depression.

Nonconvulsive SE

Absence SE, partial absence SE, or complex partial SE may present as nonconvulsive SE. Typical symptoms include waxing and waning levels of consciousness and motor activity that varies from multifocal twitching to frank automatisms. Complex partial SE is treated like generalized convulsive SE. Absence SE and atypical absence SE are treated most effectively with benzodiazepines. When needed, valproic acid can be given.

Neonatal SE

Neonatal seizures occur in patients under 29 days old, and they are usually related to significant neurological disease. These are rarely idiopathic. (See Table 34.4.) The investigation is directed toward identifying an underlying etiology. If the

Table 34.2. Evaluation and Management of Status Epilepticus in Children

Time 0–5 minutes
Maintain open airway, apply oxygen, obtain vital signs, apply cardiac monitor and pulse oximeter
Obtain IV access, draw blood for lab tests as indicated (CBC, lytes, BUN, glucose, Ca^+, Mg^+, ABGs, drug levels, tox screen, ammonia level, blood cultures)
Perform history (past med history, prior seizures, meds, compliance, recent illness, trauma, drug abuse)
Examine patient

Time 5–10 minutes
Antidotes to Consider
dextrose 2–4 cc/kg as D50W (D25W if <2 yr, D10W if neonate) if glucose <60
pyridoxine 100 mg IV for children under 18 months with new onset seizures
calcium gluconate 10% solution 2 cc/kg IV
magnesium sulfate 50% 0.2 cc/kg IM
thiamine 100 mg IV if malnourished or alcoholism
naloxone 0.1 mg/kg IV up to 2 mg/dose if suspicion of drug exposure
Anticonvulsants
lorazepam 0.05–0.1 mg/kg IV (max dose 4 mg); can be repeated in 5–10 minutes
OR
midazolam 0.05–0.3 mg/kg IV (0.3–0.8 mg/kg IM if no IV access)
OR
diazepam 0.2–0.5 mg/kg IV, at 1.0 mg per minute (max 10 mg), or 0.5–1.0 mg/kg rectal (max 10–30 mg)
AND
fosphenytoin 20 mg/kg (as phenytoin equivalents) at 150 mg per minute (or 3 mg/kg per minute if <50 kg) IVP or in normal saline infusion, or IM
OR
phenytoin 20 mg/kg at 50 mg per minute (or 1 mg/kg per minute if less than 50 kg) IVP or in normal saline infusion; must have cardiac monitor
OR
phenobarbital 20 mg/kg at 1 mg/kg per minute IVP; repeat 5–10 mg/kg boluses (max 1 g); usually used as the initial drug in neonatal seizures

Time 20–30 minutes
Use a loading dose of fosphenytoin (or phenytoin) or phenobarbital in doses above, whichever was not used as initial first-line therapy
OR
midazolam continuous infusion – bolus as above, then 0.05–0.4 mg/kg per hour
OR
valproate 15–30 mg/kg (3–6 mg/kg per minute) IV

Time 45–60 minutes – refractory SE
Endotracheal intubation if not already done; hemodynamic support as needed
AND
midazolam continuous infusion as recommended above
OR
continued phenobarbital loading as recommended above
OR
thiopental 1.0–4.0 mg/kg IVP, then 3–5 mg/kg per hour infusion
OR
pentobarbital 5–12 mg/kg IV, then 1.0—3.0 mg/kg per hour infusion
OR
general anesthesia

Table 34.3. AEDs Used in the Treatment of Pediatric Status Epilepticus

Drug	Dosage Range (mg/kg)	Route	Rate of infusion	Recommended Dose (mg/kg)	Maximum Dose (mg)
Lorazepam	0.05–0.1	IV		0.1	4
	Same	Rectal		0.1	4
Midazolam	0.05–0.3	IV	Bolus may be followed by infusion at 0.05–0.40 mg/kg per hour		
	0.3–0.8	IM			
Diazepam	0.2–0.5	IV	1–2 mg per minute	0.3	20
	0.5–1.0	Rectal		0.5	10–30
Phenytoin	20–30	IV	50 mg per minute or 1–2 mg/kg per minute	20	
Fosphenytoin	20–30 phenytoin equivalents	IV	150 mg per minute or 3 mg/kg per minute if <50 kg; IVP or in normal saline if infusion	20 phenytoin equivalents	
		IM			
Phenobarbital	20 mg/kg	IV	1–2 mg/kg per minute; May repeat additional 5–10 mg/kg boluses	20	1000
Valproic acid	15–30 mg/kg	IV	3–6 mg/kg per minute	15	
		Rectal		30	

Table 34.4. Neonatal Seizures

	Causes	Onset		
		Day 1–2	Day 3–7	Day 7–10
More common	Hypoxic-ischemic encephalopathy	X		
↓	Intracranial hemorrhage	X	X	
	Hypoglycemia	X		
	Intracranial infection		X	
	Cerebral dysgenesis	X	X	X
	Hypocalcemia	X		X
	Drug withdrawal		X	
	Inborn errors of metabolism		X	
Less common	Neonatal epilepsy		X	X

Source: Adapted from Hill A. Neonatal seizures. *Pediatr Rev*. 2000;21(4):117–21.

basic laboratory evaluation fails to identify a cause, other studies to consider include measurement of serum amino acids, lactate, and urine organic acids and testing for congenital viral infections and chromosome karyotype. Clinical manifestations may be subtle with oral-buccal, ocular, or swimming and pedaling movements, as well as tonic, clonic, or myoclonic movements of the extremities.

Initial drug therapies to consider include: calcium, magnesium, and pyridoxine. Next, the use of phenobarbital as the initial AED is recommended. One protocol begins with phenobarbital, 20 mg/kg given intravenously, followed by repeated boluses of 5–10 mg/kg until the seizures stop or a level of 40 μg/ml is achieved. In another protocol, phenobarbital 30 mg/kg is given intravenously over 15 minutes. If these measures fail, the infant is loaded with phenytoin, 20 mg/kg given intravenously, and the algorithm for convulsive SE is used.

Childhood Epileptic Syndromes

Epilepsy is defined as two or more unprovoked seizures. Pediatric patients are unique in that several characteristic epileptic syndromes have an age-dependent appearance, one or more characteristic seizure types, a natural history, and a prognosis. Some major syndromes include febrile seizures, infantile spasms, Lennox-Gastaut syndrome, and benign rolandic epilepsy (BRE). Of this group, febrile seizures are the most commonly encountered in the emergency department (ED).

Febrile Seizures

A febrile seizure is a seizure occurring with high fever in a child between 3 months and 5 years of age, with no cause identified other than the fever itself. "High fever" commonly refers to a temperature greater than 102°F. Etiology is typically a viral illness. Children who present with seizures and meningitis virtually always have other abnormal findings that do not mimic those in children with uncomplicated febrile seizures. Febrile seizures are typically described as simple or complex. Simple febrile seizures are generalized, brief (less than 15 minutes), do not repeat within 24 hours, and generally do not repeat during the same illness.

Evaluation and Management

See Figure 34.1.

Parent Counseling

Parents need to be reassured that the febrile seizure itself is benign whether it is simple, focal, prolonged, or presenting as SE. The probability of recurrence is based on risk factors and the presence of an underlying neurological condition. Risk factors for additional febrile seizures include a lower temperature, a shorter duration of fever (especially less than 1 hour), a family history of febrile seizures, and age less than 18 months. A family history of epilepsy and complex febrile seizures does not correlate with an increased risk for recurrent febrile seizures. Overall, approximately 30% of children will have a recurrent febrile seizure with a risk of 13–50%; 50% of these experience a third seizure. Frequently occurring simple febrile seizures slightly increase the risk for the development of nonfebrile

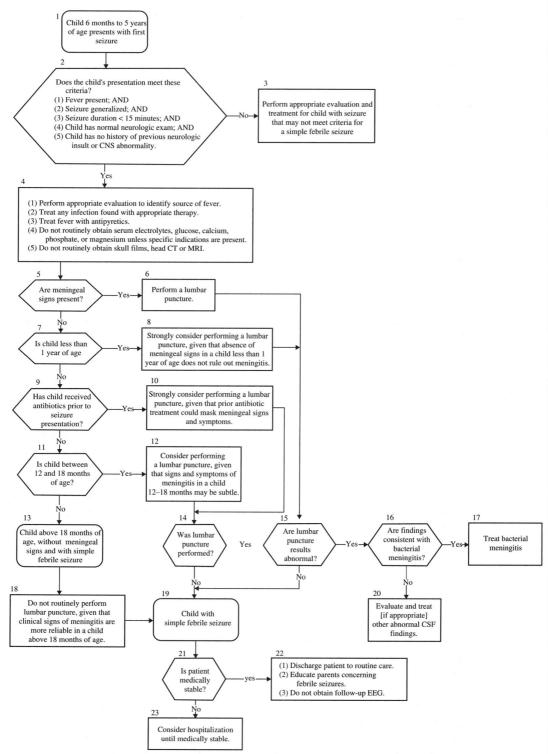

Figure 34.1. Algorithm: The Neurodiagnostic Evaluation of the Child with a First Simple Febrile Seizure.

seizures. Complex febrile seizures raise this risk by 10%. Regardless of the risk, no treatment for febrile seizures has decreased the risk of subsequent epilepsy. Parents can be advised that the decision to treat or monitor for further febrile seizures should be discussed in detail with the child's primary physician.

The Child with a First Nonfebrile Seizure

See Figure 34.2 and Table 34.5.

Evaluation

A history is obtained. When no cause is immediately apparent, prior unrecognized seizures, neurological problems such as developmental delay, or remote events that can predispose to subsequent seizures and epilepsy are investigated. A family history of genetic, metabolic or neurological disease can be helpful. A detailed description of the seizure is important in order to determine if it was partial or generalized from the outset. A parent who witnesses a seizure may need help in considering the sequence of seizure activity, which side of the body it started on, the duration, changes in the level of consciousness, and the presence of a postictal state. The neurological examination is directed toward any focal or lateralizing findings that may suggest a focal onset of seizures, or the possibility of a focal structural lesion.

Prognosis

The risk of seizure recurrence after a first nonfebrile seizure is 23–71%. Factors found to correlate with risk of recurrence are etiology, electroencephalogram (EEG) findings, and type of seizure; patients with partial seizures, nocturnal seizures, or an abnormal EEG have an increased risk of recurrent seizure. Recurrence rates are highest immediately after the first seizure and rapidly decrease thereafter, with 80–90% of second seizures occurring in the first year. Patients with a second seizure have a 80–90% probability of having a third seizure. Treatment with AEDs does not appear to affect the chance of a second seizure, despite the clear efficacy of AEDs in patients with epilepsy.

Treatment

Most pediatric neurologists do not treat the patient until criteria are met for the diagnosis of epilepsy: two or more unprovoked nonfebrile seizures. For BRE including repeated seizures, treatment usually is not prescribed, unless they are very frequent or unacceptably disturbing to the patient or the family. Phenobarbital, primidone, phenytoin, and carbamazepine are used to treat complex partial or generalized tonic–clonic seizures. Carbamazepine is the drug of choice for children older than 1 year. It can be used in children younger than 1 year in certain instances. For children older than 1 year, phenytoin is the second choice, and barbiturates are the third. For children younger than 1 year, barbiturates are the accepted first-line medication. Phenytoin is not recommended in this age group because of difficulty obtaining and maintaining adequate blood levels. Recently marketed AEDs such as gabapentin, lamotrigine, topirimate, and tiagabine have

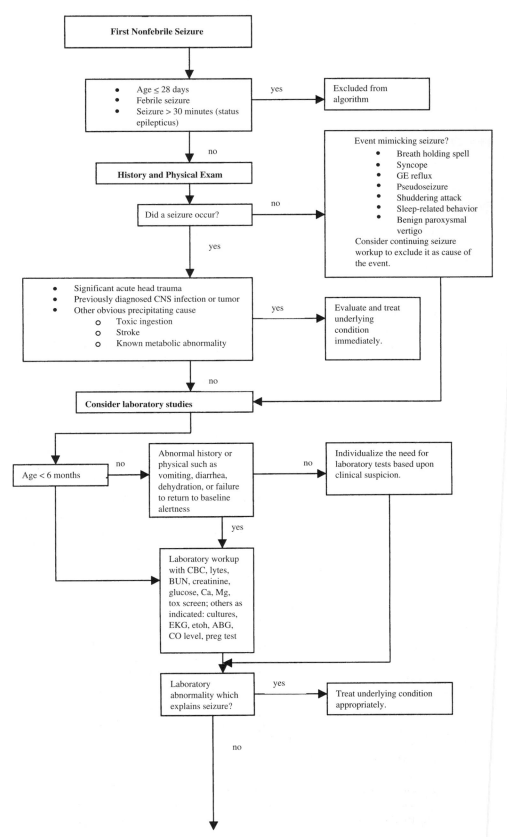

Figure 34.2. Evaluation of a First Nonfebrile Seizure in Children.

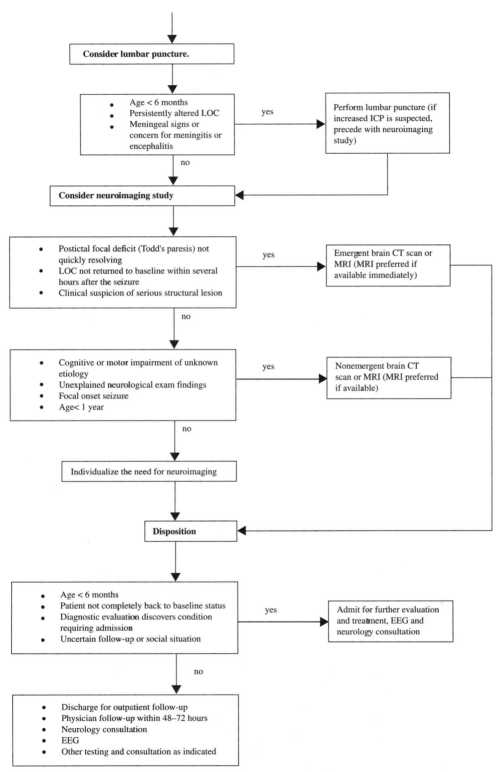

Figure 34.2. *(continued)*

Table 34.5. Common AEDs for Initial Treatment of Seizures in Children

Medication	Formulation (mg)	Starting Dose[a] (mg/kg per day)	Maintenance Dose[a] (mg/kg per day)	Schedule	Significant Drug Interactions
Carbamazepine (CBZ)	Liquid, 100 mg/5 ml Chewable tab, 100 mg Tablet, 200 mg	3 × 5 days, 6 × 5 days, 10 per day final	10–20	tid–qid bid bid	Erythromycin increases levels dangerously VPA increases 10, 11-epoxide
Phenytoin (PHT)	Liquid, 125 mg/5 ml Chewable tab, 50 mg Capsule, 30, 100 mg	5	4–7	tid bid bid	VPA increases free fraction
Phenobarbital (PB)	Liquid, 20 mg/5 ml Tablet, 15, 30, 45 mg	5	2 mo–1 yr: 4–11 1–3 yr: 3–7 3+: 3–5	qd	VPA increases levels
Valproic acid (VPA)	Liquid, 250 mg/5 ml Sprinkles, 125 mg 125, 250, 500 mg	5 × 5 days, 10 × 5 days, 15 per day final	15–30	tid–qid bid bid	PB decreases levels

[a] Doses recommended are for children on initial monotherapy who are not taking other medications.

Source: American Academy of Pediatrics. Provisional Committee on Quality Improvement, Subcommittee on Febrile Seizures. Practice parameter: the neurodiagnostic evaluation of the child with a first simple febrile seizure. *Pediatrics.* 1996;97(5):769–72; discussion 773–5.

Table 34.6. Causes of Recurrent Seizures

- Underlying medical problem
  - Progression of preexisting neurological problem
  - New metabolic or structural CNS disorder
  - Acute illness
- Medication related
  - Inadequate AED levels
    - Drug interactions causing increased protein binding or increased metabolism
    - AED Noncompliance
  - AED toxicity
  - Lowered seizure threshold secondary to medications

---

better kinetics and less toxicity and may replace the older AEDs in the future. They have not been adequately studied for use as monotherapy in children and should not be used in the ED. Pediatric formulations and doses of first-line medications for generalized tonic–clonic and complex partial seizures are given in Table 34.7.

Recurrent Seizures

See Tables 34.6 and 34.7.

AED Toxicity

AED toxicity can occur because of increased blood levels of the parent drug, decreased protein binding in highly bound drugs such as phenytoin, increased metabolites, or a consequence of polypharmacy with decreased tolerance for high, but still therapeutic, serum levels of individual AEDs. It is important to remember that therapeutic ranges of serum AED levels are only guidelines for treatment. Patients can be toxic in the therapeutic range of an AED or tolerate serum levels well above the published maximums. Valproic acid increases the level of unbound phenytoin, which can cause toxicity with total phenytoin levels within the therapeutic range. Valproic acid can cause a 50% or more increase in carbamazepine metabolites when they are coadministered. Valproic acid significantly decreases the clearance of phenobarbital and the newer AED, lamotrigine, leading to increased serum levels of these AEDs. Valproic acid is associated with many more

---

Table 34.7. Treatment of Subtherapeutic AED Levels

Loading dose = Weight $\times$ V_d $\times$ (Desired level − Actual level)

Loading dose = Bolus in milligrams
Weight = Weight of patient in kilograms
V_d = Volume of distribution of the AED in liters/kg
- Phenytoin – 0.75
- Carbamazepine – 1.0
- Phenobarbital – 0.6–0.7 (pediatric only)
- Valproic acid – 0.25–0.35

Table 34.8. Events Mimicking Seizures

- Breath holding spell
- Syncope
- Gastroesophageal reflux (Sandifer's syndrome)
- Shuddering attack
- Sleep-related behavior
- Benign paroxysmal vertigo
- Pseudoseizure

serious side effects in children age 2 years or younger. It is toxic at normal levels in those with carnitine deficiency.

Events Mimicking Seizures

Events that mimic seizures are listed in Table 34.8.

PEARLS AND PITFALLS

- Treatment of status epilepticus requires a treatment strategy and timetable.
- Healthy children who present with status epilepticus as their first seizure do not need to be started on antiepileptic medication in the emergency department.
- Febrile seizures are usually benign; many children will require no workup other than the evaluation and treatment of their fever.
- Febrile seizures do not require treatment with chronic antiepileptic medication.
- Children presenting to the emergency department with new-onset seizures who recover to a normal baseline require a focused evaluation.
- The disposition in patients stable for discharge home must be arranged in conjunction with the patient's primary physician or a neurologist.
- Not everything that looks or sounds like a seizure is a seizure.

SELECTED BIBLIOGRAPHY

American Academy of Pediatrics, Provisional Committee on Quality Improvement, Subcommittee on Febrile Seizures. Practice parameter: the neurodiagnostic evaluation of the child with a first simple febrile seizure. *Pediatrics.* 1996;97(5):769–72; 773–5.

Bradford JC. Evaluation of the patient with seizures: an evidence based approach. *Emerg Med Clin North Am.* 1999;17(1): 203–20, ix–x.

Dunn DW. Status epilepticus in infancy and childhood. *Neurol Clin.* 1990;8:647–57.

Fountain NB. Midazolam treatment of acute and refractory status epilepticus. *Clin Neuropharmacol.* 1999;22(5):261–7.

Hauser WA, Hesdorffer DC. *Epilepsy: Frequency, Causes and Consequences.* New York, NY: Demos Publications; 1990.

Hauser WA. Status epilepticus: epidemiologic considerations. *Neurology.* 1990;40(suppl 12):9–13.

Hauser WA. Status epilepticus: frequency, etiology, and neurologic sequelae. *Adv Neurol*. 1983;34:3–14.

Hill A. Neonatal seizures. *Pediatr Rev*. 2000;21(4):117–21.

Hirtz D. Practice parameter: evaluating a first nonfebrile seizure in children: report of the quality standards subcommittee of the American Academy of Neurology, The Child Neurology Society, and The American Epilepsy Society. *Neurology*. 2000; 55(5):616–23.

Painter MJ, Gaus LM. Phenobarbital: clinical use. In: Levy RH, Mattson RH, Meldrum BS, eds. *Antiepileptic Drugs*. New York, NY: Raven Press; 1995.

Roberts MR, Eng-Borquin J. Status epilepticus in children. *Emerg Med Clin North Am*. 1995;13(2):489–507.

Sabo-Graham T. Management of status epilepticus in children. *Pediatr Rev*. 1998; 19(9):306–9.

35 Hypotonic Infant

Marsha D. Rappley and Sid M. Shah

INTRODUCTION

It is important to clarify the terminology used in describing hypotonia and muscle weakness in infants. Hypotonia refers to decreased muscle tone. This is the least resistance that a quiet, alert infant offers when the examiner passively moves the extremities and head. Weakness refers to a decrease in muscle power generated by the infant. Muscle strength can be felt in the active movement of a healthy infant. A weak baby is always hypotonic, but a hypotonic baby may be able to generate muscle strength. A focused history and a careful physical examination will distinguish hypotonia from weakness, essential to diagnosis and treatment.

Evaluation

History

The chief complaint concerning a hypotonic infant includes feeding problems, recurrent respiratory infection, or delay in motor milestones. Infants who present with lethargy or a potential acute life-threatening event require assessment for sepsis, apnea, and trauma. Premature infants are hypotonic compared to full-term infants. Onset of hypotonia at 12–24 hours of age is suggestive of a metabolic disorder related to feedings. Hypotonia that improves and develops over time into hypertonia suggests cerebral palsy.

The family history is particularly important. A maternal history of neurological disease or muscle weakness, which might indicate neonatal myasthenia gravis or a hereditary disorder, is sought. A negative family history does not exclude a neuromuscular disorder because many families have too few known members, and the expression of many disorders is extremely variable.

Physical Examination

Observation of the infant in various stages of arousal is critical. The normal-term infant shows active movement of flexed limbs when placed in a supine position.

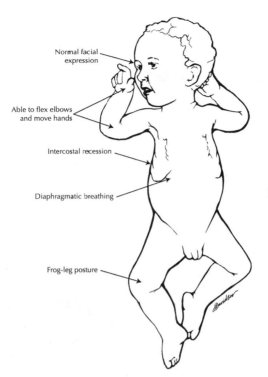

Normal facial
expression

Able to flex elbows
and move hands

Intercostal recession

Diaphragmatic breathing

Frog-leg posture

Figure 35.1. Infant with hypotonia.

A classic presentation of hypotonia is the frogleg position, with abduction of hips and extension of limbs when the infant is supine (Figure 35.1). Observation includes assessment of possible dysmorphic features, abnormalities of the skin, and relative proportion of head, trunk, and limbs. The examination assesses respiratory rate, excursion, diaphragmatic movement, and the use of accessory muscles. Also noted are the condition of the heart, the size of the liver and spleen, status of the genitalia, range of motion of the joints, tendon length or contractures, the quality of muscle mass and subcutaneous fat.

The mental status examination of an infant assesses the level of alertness, nature of the cry, degree of irritability, consolability, and interaction. Primitive reflexes are characteristic of the newborn. Moro's reflex, reflex stepping, and plantar and palmer grasps are examples of primitive reflexes present at birth. These reflexes persist after a few months with central nervous system (CNS) dysfunction. The cranial nerve examination assesses facial symmetry, the ability to suck and swallow, the ability to fixate and follow, eye movements with the oculocephalogyric reflex using gentle rotation of the head, condition of the fundi, and tongue movements or possible fasciculations.

Muscle tone is assessed and hypotonia confirmed by (1) decreased resistance of limbs through passive range of motion; (2) the frogleg posture in supine position; and (3) abnormal axillary suspension when the infant is held under the axillae and slips through the examiner's hands.

Muscle strength is assessed and weakness confirmed by (1) decreased ability of the limbs to resist gravity, which can be demonstrated by holding the infant in horizontal suspension causing the limbs to fall loosely; (2) abnormal ventral suspension with curvature of head, trunk, and limbs when the infant is held prone over the examiner's arm and hand; (3) abnormal head lag when the infant is pulled from a supine to a sitting position; and (4) decreased trunk and head control with these maneuvers, or with sitting position for older infants. Muscle strength is apparent when the infant is able to keep the extremities in a flexed position, pushes against the examiner or parent, and withdraws extremities or moves against gravity.

Distribution of weakness is important to note (see Figure 35.2). Proximal muscle weakness can be associated with muscular dystrophy and progressive spinal atrophy. Distal weakness is characteristic of peripheral neuropathies and myotonic dystrophy. Weakness of the facial muscles may indicate congenital myopathy, myotonic dystrophy, or fascioscapulohumeral muscular dystrophy. Fatigability, characteristic of myasthenia gravis, is demonstrated in an infant who appears hungry and starts feeding with a good suck but tires quickly.

Deep tendon reflexes (DTRs) are most easily elicited in the biceps, knees, and ankles of the normal infant. Increased or absent DTRs can be associated with CNS lesions. Decreased reflexes are associated with weak muscles. Sensory levels can be determined by a withdrawal response of the infant and are used to differentiate transection of the spinal cord from spinal muscular atrophy. Weakness can make evaluation of sensation difficult because of the dependence of the withdrawal response on adequate muscle strength. Rare disorders of infancy resulting in decreased sensation include Charcot-Marie-Tooth and Dejerine-Sottas syndromes.

Differential Diagnosis

The differential diagnosis of infantile hypotonia can be generated by first determining whether hypotonia is associated with weakness (see Figure 35.3). Global CNS disorders are suggested by the loss of developmental milestones or evidence of mental retardation. These disorders can be obscured by severe malnutrition, systemic illness, or weakness that prevents the infant from normal interaction. Isolated connective tissue disorders are suggested by laxity of joint movements; weakness and hypotonia are not prominent features. Examples of CNS disorders that can present with hypotonia but without significant weakness include hypoxic-ischemic encephalopathy and intracranial hemorrhage. Chromosomal disorders associated with hypotonia include Prader-Willi syndrome and Down's syndrome. Osteogenesis imperfecta is an example of a connective tissue disorder that also affects the CNS. It presents with hypotonia, blue sclera, multiple fractures, and retarded development.

The following disorders are associated with significant *weakness and secondary hypotonia*.

➤Spinal muscular atrophy, Werdnig-Hoffmann syndrome, is characterized by profound symmetrical weakness and loss of spontaneous movement. Muscle atrophy can be obscured by subcutaneous fat. The diaphragm is affected late in the disease process. DTRs are reduced or absent. Infants are alert, and there is no loss of cognitive function. In its most severe form, onset of spinal muscular atrophy is noted at birth or within the first month of life. These infants rarely survive to 2nd year of life.

➤Congenital muscular dystrophies are inherited disorders with slow onset in early life. They are characterized by preferential involvement of proximal muscles, loss

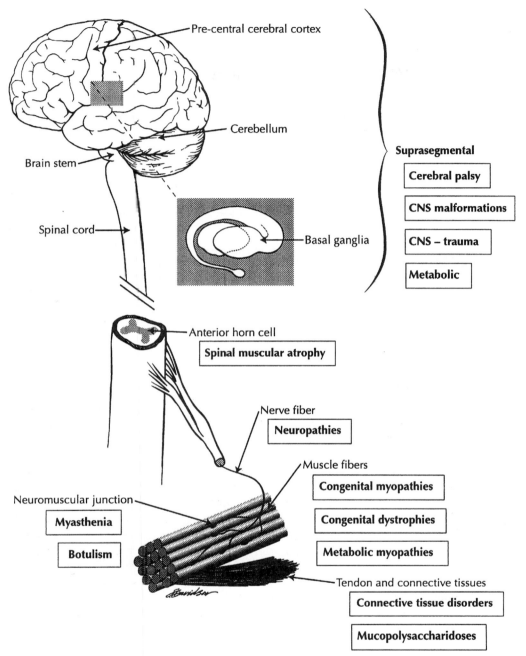

Figure 35.2. Anatomical approach to disorders producing hypotonia.

of DTRs, and pseudohypertrophy of muscle. This form has onset at birth and is commonly associated with contractures. Other types typically present at age 2–5 years or older, depending on the type. There is no effective treatment for the muscular dystrophies.

➤ Myasthenia gravis of infants can be of two types: (1) transient neonatal or (2) congenital type. Transient neonatal disease occurs in approximately one in seven

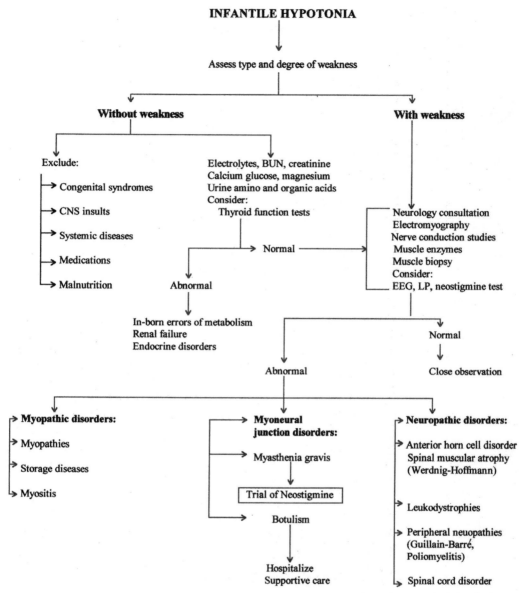

Figure 35.3. Algorithm for infantile hypotonia (adapted from Berman S. Infantile hypotonia. In: Berman S, ed. *Pediatric Decision Making*. Philadelphia, Pa: BC Decker and CV Mosby; 1985:137.

infants born to mothers with myasthenia gravis. There are elevated antibodies against the acetylcholine receptors in mother and baby. Symptoms appear at from 1 to 3 days of life. There is a weak cry and difficulty in swallowing. The duration of transient neonatal myasthenia gravis is commonly less than 5 weeks, but symptoms can be severe. With early hospital discharge, close observation must be maintained for infants born to mothers with myasthenia gravis. Congenital myasthenia gravis occurs in infants born to mothers without myasthenia gravis. The symptoms of congenital disease in infancy usually are not as severe

Table 35.1. Diagnosis of 107 Cases of Floppy Infant

Diagnosis	Number of Cases
Infantile muscular atrophy	67
Congenital muscular dystrophy	3
Polymyositis	1
Myasthenia gravis	1
Scurvy	2
Cerebral disease (atonic cerebral palsy)	14
"Benign congenital hypotonia"	17

Source: Menkes JH. Diseases of the motor unit. In: *Textbook of Child Neurology*. Baltimore, Md: Williams & Wilkins, 1995;819.

as those of the transient neonatal type, but they persist and are typically refractory to therapy. The hallmark of the history is fatigability. Diagnosis is confirmed by transient improvement in muscle strength with edrophonium or neostigmine. Treatment of infants usually is symptomatic.

➤Congenital myotonic dystrophy can present with choking, difficulty sucking and swallowing, respiratory problems, arthrogryposis, skeletal deformities, facial diplegia, diminished or absent DTRs, mental retardation, abdominal distension, and ileus. These abnormalities are the result of failure of voluntary muscle to relax after contraction. Many genetic and biochemical defects are associated with the various forms of myotonic dystrophy. The congenital form is commonly associated with an affected mother. The clinical course is one of gradual deterioration.

➤Guillain-Barré syndrome is uncommon but described in infants ranging from 1 to 16 months of age. Presentation is typically that of remarkable respiratory infection with profound hypotonia. Characteristic elevation of the protein level of the cerebrospinal fluid is found.

➤Toxic causes of hypotonia include *Clostridium botulinum*, *C. tetani*, and venom of the cobra and of the black widow spider, all of which affect the neuromuscular junction. Infantile botulism presents in 95% of cases between 3 weeks and 6 months of age with poor suck and swallow, weak cry, drooling, or obstructive apnea. These symptoms relate to bulbar palsies. A classic presentation of infantile botulism includes internal and external ophthalmoplegia.

A list of diagnoses resulting in hypotonia of infancy is listed in Table 35.1.

Diagnostic Studies

Results of blood chemistry analysis are age-referenced. Creatine phosphokinase (CPK), for example, can be increased tenfold in the first week of life. However, elevations associated with muscular dystrophies range in the thousands. Evaluation of chemistries should include CPK, lactate dehydrogenase (LDH), alanine aminotransferase (ALT), aspartate aminotransferase (AST), calcium, and electrolytes. Thyroid function tests are obtained because neonatal screens of thyroid disease do not examine all levels of the hypothalamic-pituitary-thyroid axis. When the history suggests a metabolic disorder, glucose level, venous pH, ammonia, serum amino acids, and complete blood count with differential, serum and urine organic acids are considered. Chromosomal analysis with a specific request for karyotyping of suspected Prader-Willi syndrome or Down's syndrome may be indicated. Lumbar puncture is indicated for consideration of an infectious etiology or possible Guillain-Barré syndrome. Neuroimaging can be useful for detecting disorders of the CNS suggested by hypotonia without weakness.

Hypotonia with weakness requires the use of electrophysiology and biopsy studies, interpreted in the context of the infant's age. Electromyography, nerve conduction studies, and biopsies of muscle and nerve have normal developmental expressions in the neonate and young infant that can mimic pathological findings in an older infant or child. These studies can be useful in differentiating specific disorders or localizing lesions, but they require expertise. Ultrasound imaging of muscle can be useful in identifying the characteristic muscle patterns of Werdnig-Hoffmann disease or Duchenne's muscular dystrophy.

Management and Disposition

Hospitalization is commonly required to observe a hypotonic infant and to continue with diagnostic evaluation (e.g., when a metabolic disorder is suspected and feedings are withheld). Typically, acute management is directed at problems secondary to the hypotonia and weakness such as respiratory compromise, feeding difficulties, and aspiration. A pediatric neurologist is consulted to determine the need for further diagnostic procedures or to initiate treatment of an underlying neurological disorder.

PEARLS AND PITFALLS

- Decreased muscle tone (hypotonia) is distinct from decreased muscle power (weakness).
- Hypotonia is considered in an infant who has feeding problems with poor suck and swallow, recurrent respiratory infections, or a delay in developmental milestones.
- Hypotonia might not be apparent until 8–12 weeks of age.
- Proximal muscle weakness can be associated with muscular dystrophy and progressive spinal atrophy.
- Distal muscle weakness is characteristic of peripheral neuropathies and myotonic dystrophy.
- Diagnostic evaluation of hypotonia with weakness requires electrophysiological studies and a muscle biopsy.
- Transient neonatal myasthenia gravis is considered in an infant born to a mother with myasthenia gravis; this might be associated with severe symptoms.
- In infantile botulism, 95% of cases present between 3 weeks and 6 months of age with poor suck, swallow, weak cry, drooling, or obstructive sleep apnea.
- An infant with hypotonia is hospitalized for observation and evaluation when symptoms or diagnostic procedures place the child at risk for complications secondary to the hypotonia.

SELECTED BIBLIOGRAPHY

Berman S. Infantile hypotonia. In Berman S, ed. *Pediatric Decision Making*. Philadelphia, Pa: BC Decker and CV Mosby; 1985:137.

Dubowitz V. *The Floppy Infant*. Philadelphia, Pa: JB Lippincott; 1980.

Fanaroff AA, Martin RJ, eds. *Neonatal-Perinatal Medicine, Diseases of the Fetus and Infant*, 7th ed. St. Louis, Mo: CV Mosby; 2002.

Gay CT, Bodensteiner JB. The floppy infant: recent advances in understanding of disorders affecting the neuromuscular junction. *Neurol Clin North Am*. 1990;8:715–25.

Menkes JH, Sarnat HB. *Child Neurology*, 6th ed. Baltimore, Md: Lippincott, Williams & Wilkins; 2000.

Miller G. Hypotonia and neuromuscular disease. In: Fanaroff AA, Martin RJ, eds. *Neonatal-Perinatal Medicine, Diseases of the Fetus and Infant*. 6th Ed. St Louis, Mo: CV Mosby; 1997; 1.

Spiro AJ. Hypotonia. In: Hoekelman RA, Adam HM, Nelson NM, Weitzman ML, Wilson MH, eds. *Primary Pediatric Care*, 4th ed. St. Louis, Mo: CV Mosby; 2001.

36 Neurological Emergencies of Pregnancy

Mary Hughes and Page Pennell

INTRODUCTION

The challenging spectrum of neurological disorders in pregnancy extends from life-threatening eclamptic seizures to self-limiting meralgia paresthetica. Eclampsia, a disorder specifically related to the pregnant or newly delivered patient, carries a significant morbidity and mortality to the mother and the fetus. The pregnant patient is likely to present to the emergency department (ED) with not only the conditions resulting directly from pregnancy but also preexisting conditions changed by the gravid state of the patient. Certain types of neuropathies and movement disorders occur specifically during pregnancy or result from the gravid state.

Eclampsia

Eclampsia is the occurrence of seizures (not caused by other neurologic disease such as epilepsy) in a woman whose condition also meets the criteria for preeclampsia. Eclampsia can occur during pregnancy, during labor, or within 1–2 weeks of delivery. It is a condition with an obscure cause which primarily affects young primigravidas and those over 35 years of age. Other risk factors include nulliparity, plural gestation, low socioeconomic class, poor nutrition, and molar pregnancies.

Preeclampsia is pregnancy-induced hypertension (PIH), proteinuria, and/or edema of marked degree. Proteinuria is defined as 300 mg or greater of urine protein per 24 hours, or 100 mg/dL or greater on at least two random urine samples done at least 6 hours apart. Increasing proteinuria is a marker of a worsening clinical condition. Hypertension is the sine qua non of preeclampsia. Once the blood pressure exceeds 140/90, or a rise of at least 30/15 occurs, PIH is considered to be present.

Evaluation and Differential Diagnosis

When convulsions and altered sensorium occur in the pregnant patient past 20 weeks gestation or in the first 2 weeks postpartum, eclampsia is the prime

> **Table 36.1.** Medications for Seizure Management in Eclampsia
>
> **Magnesium Sulfate Dosage Schedule**
> 1. Give 4 g of magnesium sulfate ($MgSo_4 \cdot 7H_2O$, USP) as a 20% solution intravenously at a rate not to exceed 1 g per minute.
> 2. Follow with 10 g of 50% magnesium sulfate solution, one half (5 g) injected deep in each buttock. (Addition of 1.0 mL of 2% lidocaine may be used to decrease discomfort.)
>   a. If convulsions persist after 15 minutes, give up to 2 g more intravenously as a 20% solution at a rate not to exceed 1 g per minute. If the woman is large, up to 4 g may be given slowly.
> 3. Every 4 hours thereafter give 5 g of a 50% solution of magnesium sulfate injected deep into alternate buttocks, if:
>   a. the patellar reflex is present.
>   b. respirations are not depressed.
>   c. urine output the previous 4 hours exceeded 100 mL.
> 4. Magnesium sulfate is discontinued 24 hours after delivery.

suspect. Unrelenting headache, visual disturbances, and occasionally right upper quadrant abdominal pain in the preeclamptic patient frequently can precede convulsions. Coma can be caused from a sudden rise in blood pressure resulting in the inability of the brain to autoregulate cerebral flow, causing overt cerebral edema. Another cause of coma in these patients is intracranial hemorrhage, including subarachnoid, cortical, and deep intracerebral hemorrhages.

Seizures can occur any time before, during, or after labor. Seizures may be focal or generalized tonic–clonic (grand mal). The incidence of seizures increases as the patient approaches term. Approximately 25% of eclampsia develops postpartum and can be encountered up to 10–14 days postpartum, and rarely up to 26 days postpartum. Seizures can even occur as the first sign of eclampsia.

Epigastric or right upper quadrant abdominal pain is thought to result from hepatocellular necrosis and edema that stretches the liver capsule. This is accompanied by elevated serum liver enzymes secondary to periportal hemorrhagic necrosis. Most often these enzyme elevations are accompanied by thrombocytopenia. This constellation of findings is known as the HELLP syndrome (hemolysis, elevated liver enzymes, low platelets). Bleeding may rarely cause hepatic rupture resulting in free fluid in the abdomen or may be contained as in subcapsular hematoma. Thrombocytopenia increases the risk of maternal intracranial hemorrhage and excessive bleeding during parturition.

Laboratory findings are inconsistent in eclampsia, and none are pathognomonic. Delivery of the fetus and placenta is the definitive treatment of eclampsia. Delivery is generally delayed until seizures and hypertension are controlled, and hypoxia and acidosis have been corrected.

Management of Eclamptic Seizures

Since 1955, Parkland Hospital (Dallas, Texas) has popularized a regimen that incorporates the use of magnesium sulfate in the management of eclamptic seizures, and that has been accepted as the preferred therapy by the American College of Obstetrics and Gynecology (Table 36.1). Although controversy surrounded this treatment for several decades, two large trials of preeclamptic and eclamptic patients published in 1995 established that magnesium sulfate is the medication of choice for control of eclamptic seizures. Diuretics and hyperosmotic agents are avoided and intravenous fluids are limited unless fluid loss is excessive. Prompt delivery of the fetus is necessary. Early symptoms and signs of magnesium toxicity include nausea, a sensation of warmth and flushing, somnolence, diplopia, dysarthria, and weakness.

Magnesium Toxicity (magnesium level: usual symptoms or signs)

4–8 mg/dL: usually controls seizures

8–12 mg/dL: lose patellar reflexes

15–17 mg/dL: respiratory compromise, muscular paralysis

30–35 mg/dL: cardiopulmonary arrest

At the first signs of toxicity, 1 g calcium gluconate should be given intravenously and infusion of magnesium sulfate should be discontinued. Magnesium is contraindicated in the patient with myasthenia gravis. Benzodiazepines such as diazepam and lorazepam can be used as adjunctive agents for acute seizures and can be given rapidly but should be used with caution as large doses are known to suppress fetal activity and respirations and cause maternal hypoventilation.

Phenytoin can be used to control seizures that are resistant to magnesium. Phenytoin is also a good choice if a woman is identified as high risk for eclamptic seizures and needs treatment for a prolonged period of time. Phenytoin has little effect on the respiratory drive, gastric emptying time or the level of consciousness. Phenytoin is free of tocolytic activity, and neonatal effects are nonexistent. Contraindications to the use of phenytoin include allergy to phenytoin, or marked bradycardia, especially if associated with atrial flutter or fibrillation. To prevent bleeding associated with phenytoin-induced coagulopathy, the mother should receive 10 mg. of vitamin K daily by mouth during the last month of gestation. If this has not been done the mother may receieve parenteral 10 mg of vitamin K at the time of the delivery. A single 1 mg dose of vitamin K intramuscularly should be given to neonates born of mothers on phenytoin at the time of delivery.

Management of Hypertension

Adequate control of hypertension is essential for prevention of centeral nervous system (CNS) complications in these patients. The Parkland formula uses hydralazine intravenously whenever the diastolic blood pressure is greater than 110 mm Hg. The usual initial dose is 5 mg, titrated in 5- to 10-mg doses at 15- to 20-minute intervals until the patient achieves a diastolic blood pressure of 90–100 mm Hg. Lower blood pressure or precipitous decline of blood pressure is generally not desired as it may compromise placental perfusion. Parenteral labetalol is also effective for the treatment of acute hypertension during pregnancy and is often used as a second-line drug. Oral nifedipine is third line but should be used cautiously in association with magnesium sulfate. It has also been reported to cause maternal hypotension with fetal distress, precipitating the need for caesarean delivery. In rare cases, sodium nitroprusside can be used if the former three agents fail to adequately control the blood pressure.

Antihypertensive medicines that are avoided in the pregnant patient include diazoxide, angitensin-converting enzyme (ACE) inhibitors, diuretics, trimethaphan, reserpine, and hyperosmotic agents. ACE inhibitors are contraindicated during pregnancy because of associations with fetal growth restrictions, toxic effects on the fetal kidneys, and neonatal death.

Fluid therapy is aimed at replacing physiological losses unless excessive fluid loss from diaphoresis, nausea, vomiting, diarrhea, or blood loss from delivery are encountered.

Disposition

All patients with eclampsia and many with preeclampsia need hospitalization. Patients with preeclampsia or eclampsia should also be evaluated for HELLP syndrome. It is often misdiagnosed as hepatitis, pyelonephritis, cholelithiasis, or other gastrointestinal diagnoses.

Seizures in Pregnancy

Seizures are one of the most frequent neurological disorders encountered in pregnancy and carry an increased risk to the fetus from trauma, hypoxia, and metabolic acidosis. Rarely, seizures have been reported to cause fetal intracranial hemorrhage and stillbirth. Even a single brief convulsive seizure has been shown to cause depression of the fetal heart rate for greater than 20 minutes. Status epilepticus is especially risky with a high maternal and fetal mortality rate.

Immediate ED management of the convulsing pregnant patient is similar to that of the nonpregnant patient. For details see Chapter 9, "Seizures." Benzodiazepines can be used initially to abort a cluster of seizures or status epilepticus. Fetal monitoring is suggested because of the potential prolonged effects of a brief seizure on fetal heart rate. Use of a longer-acting antiepileptic drug (AED) is often indicated in addition to initial benzodiazepines. Basic knowledge of the risks of the major AEDs during pregnancy should be considered and eventually discussed with the patient or family members. ED management of the pregnant patient in the postictal state is similar to that of the nonpregnant patient. It is important to position the patient in the left lateral Sims position placing a pillow under the right hip.

Hyperemesis gravidarum, medication noncompliance, and pregnancy itself can lower AED levels and precipitate seizures. Sleep deprivation is another common cause of a lower seizure threshold.

A coagulopathy related to the maternal use of anticonvulsants can occur in the fetus. The mother should receive oral vitamin K_1 10 mg daily for the last month of pregnancy. If this has not been given, then 10 mg intramuscularly 4 hours before delivery should be given. Vitamin K 1 mg intramusculary should always be given to the baby at the time of delivery. Internal hemorrhage resulting from the coagulopathy may occur in the fetus or neonate, and fresh frozen plasma may be necessary. This coagulopathy may also lead to stillbirth.

Headache

Quite common during pregnancy, headache is generally benign, but it can occasionally herald serious pathology. Headache with new onset in the pregnant patient should alert the emergency physician to serious disorders such as preeclampsia, eclampsia, uncontrolled hypertension, pheochromocytoma, vasculitis, arteriovenous malformation, stroke, subarachnoid hemorrhage, cerebral venous thrombosis, pituitary tumor, choriocarcinoma, pseudotumor cerebri, a rapidly expanding tumor, and infectious etiologies such as encephalitis and meningitis. Some of these disorders are more common during pregnancy. If intracranial pathology is suspected, the appropriate radiographic tests and/or lumbar puncture should not be avoided due to pregnancy.

A high proportion of women with migraines experience significant improvement of their headaches during pregnancy, usually beginning in the third or fourth month. Medication use should be limited especially during the first trimester, but it is not absolutely contraindicated during pregnancy. The risk to the fetus of medications could be less than the headache syndrome itself if the headaches are associated with nausea, vomiting, and possible dehydration. First-line medications for headache during pregnancy include acetaminophen, nonsteroidal anti-inflammatory drugs (NSAIDs), except perhaps indomethacin; and codeine or other narcotics. Most NSAIDs can be used safely during the first trimester, but their use should be avoided during later pregnancy as they may constrict or close the fetal ductus arteriosus. Medications that should be limited in their use for headache include aspirin, barbiturates, benzodiazepines, the ergot alkaloids, and triptans. The associated symptom of nausea can be treated with metoclopramide, Emetrol, doxylamine succinate, and vitamin B_6. More severe nausea may require injections or suppositories of trimethobenzamide, chlorpromazine, prochlorperazine, and promethazine. Prednisone (in preference to dexamethasone, which crosses the placenta more readily) can be used occasionally. Intravenous narcotics can supplement these treatments, especially in status migrainosus.

Preventive treatment with use of daily medication is the last resort during pregnancy. Propranolol has been used during pregnancy, but it is known to cause fetal bradycardia and occasionally intrauterine growth retardation.

Movement Disorders

Chorea gravidarum (CG) is chorea occurring during pregnancy. Chorea gravidarum is generally a diagnosis of exclusion. Inherited and other identifiable causes of choreiform movements are excluded before making the diagnosis of CG. In developing nations, the vast majority of chorea gravidarum cases are associated with rheumatic heart disease, whereas in industrialized nations the etiology is usually autoimmune and most frequently associated with systemic lupus erythematosus. Rarely, chorea gravidarum can be due to medications. Psychiatric symptoms may precede the chorea and be as subtle as emotional lability or as flagrant as frank psychosis.

Chorea gravidarum may resolve spontaneously in a few months when associated with rheumatic disease, or after parturition. See Chapter 13, "Movement Disorders." For symptomatic treatment of the chorea in the first trimester, phenothiazines are often used. Haloperidol can be used after the first trimester but not before, as it has been associated with limb deformities.

Restless legs syndrome has an incidence of 11–19% during pregnancy and can be confused with chorea gravidarum. It is characterized by crawling dysesthesias,

Table 36.2. Common Drug-Induced Movement Disorders

Movement Disorder Syndrome	Drugs
Akathisic movements	DDA, DRA, cinnarizine, ethosuximide, flunarizine, levodopa, reserpine, tetrabenazine
Ataxia	Alcohol, lithium carbonate
Chorea	AC, amphetamines, cocaine, DDA, DRA, estrogen (birth control pill and vaginal cream) levodopa, lithium, methylphenidate, TCA, theophylline
Dystonia	DDA, DRA, levodopa
Myoclonus	AC, DRA, levodopa, TCA
Restless legs	None
Rigidity (neuroleptic malignant syndrome)	DRA, withdrawal of antiparkinsonian medication in Parkinson's disease
Tics	Carbamazepine, DDA, DRA, IDA, levodopa
Tremors (postural)	Adrenocorticosteroids, aminophylline, amiodarone, cyclosporin A, DRA, epinephrine, levodopa, levothyroxine, lithium carbonate, oxytocin, terbutaline, valproic acid, withdrawal state (alcohol, sedatives)
Symptomatic parkinsonism	Alpha-methyldopa, DRA, lithium carbonate, reserpine, tetrabenazine, toxins (carbon monoxide, carbon disulfide, cyanide, disulfiram, manganese, methanol)

Notes: AC, anticonvulsants; DRA, dopamine receptor antagonists; DDA, direct dopamine agonists (apomorphine, bromocriptine, lisuride, pergolide); IDA, indirect dopamine agonists (amantadine and others); TCA, tricyclic antidepressants.
Source: Rogers JD, Fahn S. Movement disorders and pregnancy. In: Devinsky O, Feldman E, Hainline B, eds. *Neurological Complications of Pregnancy.* New York, NY: Raven Press; 1994: 163–78.

primarily involving the legs, that is most common at night when the patient is relaxed, resulting in an urge to move about. The neurological examination is normal, and symptoms usually resolve after delivery. The treatment is supportive but if symptoms are severe treatment with carbidopa/levodopa, pergolide, or opiates may be useful. Table 36.2 lists common drugs associated with a variety of movement disorders.

Peripheral Nerve Disorders

See Chapter 14, "Peripheral Nervous System and Neuromuscular Disorders."

Carpal Tunnel Syndrome

Carpal tunnel syndrome (CTS) is the most common nerve entrapment syndrome associated with pregnancy. It is usually self-limited and generally resolves postpartum. Supportive treatment in the form of nocturnal wrist splints, occasional local steroid injections, supplemental oral Vitamin B_6, or diuretics usually suffice. In severe cases with disabling pain, surgery can be performed under local anesthesia with little risk to the fetus.

Bell's Palsy

The incidence of Bell's palsy is increased in pregnancy to 3.3 times that of age-matched nonpregnant women, with 85% of cases occurring in the third trimester or within 2 weeks postpartum. Most cases resolve spontaneously and completely. The provision of artificial tears and systemic corticosteroids, particularly if the patient presents early in the course of the disease are considered.

Lateral Femoral Cutaneous Neuropathy/Meralgia Paresthetica

Meralgia paresthetica is a self-limiting sensory syndrome in which the lateral femoral cutaneous nerve is trapped under the inguinal ligament medial to the anterior superior iliac spine or retroperitoneally where the nerve angulates over the sacroiliac joint. It is manifested by pain, paresthesias, or dysesthesias in the middle one-third of the lateral thigh and may be bilateral. The onset is often the 30th week of gestation and is thought to be secondary to increased weight gain and exaggeration of the lumbar lordosis during pregnancy. Meralgia paresthetica is exaggerated by standing in hip extension and relieved by rest. Management includes reassuring the patient of the transient nature of the syndrome.

Traumatic Neuropathies

The passage of a large fetal head through the birth canal, use of forceps, improper leg position in the stirrups, or trauma with hematoma secondary to Cesarean section can cause certain peripheral nerves of the mother to be injured during labor and delivery. The most common injury is postpartum foot drop secondary to compression of the lumbosacral plexus by the fetus' head or a mid-forceps rotation. It may also result from poorly positioned stirrups that cause compression of the common peroneal nerve as it crosses the fibular head laterally. The second most common injury is a femoral neuropathy, which may occur secondary to compression of the femoral nerve during vaginal delivery or Cesarean section. It manifests as difficulty climbing steps and anterior thigh paresthesias. Occasionally the obturator nerve is compressed causing weakness in hip adduction and rotation with decreased sensation to the upper medial thigh.

Myasthenia Gravis

See Chapter 16, "Myasthenia Gravis."

Myasthenia gravis (MG) worsens in 40% of women with pregnancy, usually in the puerperium. Exacerbations tend to be most sudden and dangerous in the postpartum period, often with respiratory failure. Patients with MG have been reported to have an increased incidence of spontaneous abortion, a slightly increased risk of premature delivery, and up to a 10% maternal mortality. Many medications have adverse side effects to the patient with MG, and each medication should be evaluated prior to use in the pregnant patient. (See Table 36.3.) Anticholinesterase medication (pyridostigmine) should be continued during

Table 36.3. Drugs Potentially Harmful in Myasthenia Gravis

Antibiotics	Neuromuscular blocking agents	Cardiovascular	Antirheumatic	Anticonvulsants	Others	Psychotropics
Aminoglycoside	Curare	Lidocaine	Chloroquine	Phenytoin	Magnesium sulfate	Lithium carbonate
Neomycin	Pancuronium	Quinidine	D-Penicillamine	Trimethadione	Corticosteroids	Chlorpromazine
Streptomycin	Succinylcholine	Quinine			Thyroid replacement	Phenelzine
Kanamycin		Procainamide			ACTH	Promazine
Gentamicin		Beta-blockers			Anticholinesterases	
Tobramycin		Ca^{++}				
Amikacin		channel blockers				
Polymyxin A		Trimethaphan				
Polymyxin B						
Colistin						
Lincomycin						
Clindamycin						
Tetracyclines						

Source: Gilchrist JM. Muscle disease in the pregnant woman. In: *Neurological Complications of Pregnancy.* New York, NY: Raven Press; 1994:199.

pregnancy. Principles of management of myasthenic crises are similar to that of a nonpregnant patient. See Chapter 16, "Myasthenia Gravis," for details.

Neonatal myasthenia gravis (NMG) occurs in 12–19% of live born infants of myasthenic mothers. The onset may be within hours of birth to 14 days postpartum and may last 10 days to 15 weeks. Symptoms include feeding difficulties (87%), generalized weakness (69%), respiratory difficulty (65%), feeble cry (60%), and facial weakness (54%). Treatment includes anticholinesterase drugs and supportive care. (See Chapter 16, "Myasthenia Gravis.")

Magnesium is contraindicated in the pregnant patient with MG because it increases muscle weakness by decreasing acetylcholine release and by decreasing the excitability of the postsynaptic membrane. Alternative therapy for preeclampsia/eclampsia is diazepam, phenobarbital, or phenytoin.

Cerebrovascular Disease

For years it was thought that during pregnancy the risk of stroke was substantially increased, but data to convincingly support this belief are lacking. A large population-based study revealed that ischemic stroke occurs in 11 per 100,000 deliveries with a relative risk during pregnancy of only 0.7. However, the relative risk during the postpartum period is 9.7. Intracerebral hemorrhage (exclusive of subarachnoid hemorrhage) occurs in 9 per 100,000 deliveries with a relative risk during pregnancy of 2.5 and during the postpartum period of 28.3. Subarachnoid hemorrhage (SAH) occurs in 1 in 2,000–10,000 pregnancies.

The causes of stroke in pregnancy are the same as for any young stroke patient and include atherothrombotic, cardioembolic, and hematologic disorders; substance abuse; migraine; and other vasculopathies. During pregnancy and the postpartum period, there is an overall increase in hypercoagulable state, and several conditions unique to pregnancy can present as stroke, including eclampsia, postpartum cerebral angiopathy, peripartum cardiomyopathy, choriocarcinoma, and amniotic fluid embolism. Eclampsia should not be the assumed cause, as only 24% of the ischemic infarcts and 14% of the intracerebral hemorrhages in Kittner's series had eclampsia. The blood volume and hormonal changes postpartum are likely to contribute to postpartum ischemic stroke, and pregnancy itself may increase the risk in patients with underlying hematologic diseases such as sickle cell anemia, antiphospholipid antibody syndrome, and hypercoagulopathy. Additionally, TTP has an increased incidence in pregnancy.

Cerebral venous thrombosis is more common in the postpartum period, when hemoconcentration and hypercoagulopathy are likely to be at their peak. The clinical syndrome of venous thrombosis generally presents with progressive headache, associated with nausea, vomiting, visual disturbances, and altered mentation secondary to increased intracranial pressure. Focal and generalized seizures may occur. Focal stroke-like signs such as monoparesis or hemisensory loss are more likely to represent secondary infarctions, which are often hemorrhagic. Hemorrhagic stroke can be classified as either subarachnoid or intracerebral. SAH has been reported to be the third most common nonobstetrical cause of maternal death. Aneurysmal SAH tends to occur during the second or third trimesters, labor, and the postpartum period with a mortality rate of

35%. Intracerebral hemorrhage (ICH) can complicate eclampsia. Other causes of ICH are poorly controlled hypertension not related to eclampsia, ruptured vascular malformations, intracranial venous thrombosis, vasculitis, and choriocarcinoma. It is important to differentiate eclampsia with intracerebral hemorrhage from a ruptured aneurysm or arterio-venous malformation (AVM) because definitive treatment differs. Previous studies are divided as to whether there is an increased risk of bleeding due to an AVM during pregnancy. Many of the previously reported high rates may be due to an artifact of case ascertainment. One series of women referred for AVM radiosurgery reported a more modest risk with a rate of hemorrhage during the "pregnancy years" of 9.3% compared to 4.5% when not pregnant. One group reported that for ICH associated with pregnancy, 77% were due to aneurysms and 23% were due to AVMs.

Management of Cerebrovascular Events

The ED management of the pregnant patient with an acute cerebrovascular event should focus on prompt evaluation and identification of any underlying cause(s). Appropriate radiographic studies are utilized with shielding of the abdomen to limit fetal exposure. Magnetic resonance imaging appears to be safe, but computerized tomography (CT) or magnetic resonance contrast agents should be avoided if possible. Surgery is known to reduce mortality in patients with a ruptured aneurysm and should not be withheld in the pregnant patient. Endovascular treatments can also be considered as a treatment option. Dias and Sekhar could not define a significant reduction in maternal or fetal mortality with surgical treatment of an AVM, although there may be a significant increased short-term maternal risk in pregnancy-associated AVM hemorrhages, with maternal mortality as high as 23–32%.

Pseudotumor Cerebri

Pseudotumor cerebri (PC) is defined as prolonged elevation of intracranial pressure, with normal CSF, and without focal neurological deficits or intracranial pathology. PC is an uncommon condition generally presenting in young, obese females and is associated with headache and visual disturbances including diplopia, an enlarged blind spot, blurred vision, and papilledema. It is seen most often in the first half of gestation but can occur at any time. If PC is suspected, a CT scan of the brain should be followed by lumbar puncture. If the opening pressure of lumbar puncture is 25 cm H_2O (250 mm H_2O) or higher in a relaxed patient, then ICP is considered to be elevated.

Management of PC to prevent visual loss may include carbonic anhydrase inhibitors to decrease cerebrospinal fluid (CSF) production. Diuretics should be used cautiously in pregnant patients due to decreased placental blood flow from decreased circulating blood volume. Monitoring the amniotic fluid levels with ultrasound is suggested if carbonic anhydrase inhibitors or diuretics are used. If these measures are unsuccessful, repeated lumbar puncture for CSF evacuation can be used. A lumboperitoneal shunt may be needed in refractory cases. Occasionally optic nerve decompression can improve the vision.

Permanent visual damage is a known complication. Visual fields must be monitored closely. The recurrence risk in patients during a subsequent pregnancy is 10–30%, which necessitates close follow-up.

Brain Tumors

The effects of brain tumors may mimic common complaints in pregnancy such as headache and nausea/vomiting. A constant daily headache should never be attributed to pregnancy alone, especially in the patient with no prior history of headache. Hyperemesis gravidarum is generally maximal in the first trimester and improves thereafter. The nausea and vomiting of brain tumors can occur at any time and persists. Magnetic resonance imaging (MRI) or CT scan of the brain should be obtained to assess for intracranial pathology in patients in whom symptoms are persistent or progressive. New-onset seizures, especially if focal, can be the initial presenting sign of a brain tumor. However, an evaluation for eclampsia is also essential. Any of the different types of brain tumors can present during pregnancy. Pituitary adenomas and meningiomas in particular may grow more rapidly during pregnancy. Choriocarcinomas can metastasize to the brain and have a tendency to hemorrhage spontaneously with rapid neurologic deterioration. The type of brain tumor and the clinical course determine the management. If corticosteroids and/or anticonvulsants are indicated, they need to be used in the context that they both carry some risk to the fetus.

PEARLS AND **PITFALLS**

- Preeclampsia may progress rapidly to eclampsia and status epilepticus.
- In eclampsia, the mainstays of therapy are controlling seizure, controlling blood pressure, and limiting fluid intake unless there is documented fluid loss. Use of central nervous system depressants, diuretics, and osmotic agents may worsen maternal, and thus fetal, outcome.
- In eclampsia, delivery is the ultimate goal of therapy. When possible, delivery is delayed until the mother is stable.
- Each patient has her own autoregulatory control of cerebral blood flow and blood pressure. Abnormally high blood pressure may begin at 140/90 in a teenager or at 180/110 in a patient with previous hypertension, resulting in a wide range of blood pressures at the onset of eclampsia. Therefore, there is no absolute blood pressure value above which the diagnosis of eclampsia is certain or below which eclampsia can be excluded.
- Management of seizures may include use of diazepam in small doses; it also involves the use of magnesium sulfate or phenytoin when the etiology is eclampsia.
- In the evaluation of the pregnant patient with upper abdominal pain, a diagnosis of the HELLP syndrome is always considered because imminent delivery is indicated regardless of the fetal gestational age.
- Differentiation of generalized convulsive seizures due to epilepsy from those due to eclampsia is important because delivery is part of the definitive treatment in the latter.
- Magnesium is contraindicated in the eclamptic patient with MG.

SELECTED BIBLIOGRAPHY

Aminoff MJ. Pregnancy and disorders of the nervous system. In: Aminoff MJ, ed. *Neurology and General Medicine*, 2nd ed. New York, NY: Churchill Livingstone; 1995: 567–83.

Cohen BS, Felsenthal G, Peripheral nervous system disorders and pregnancy. In: Goldstein PJ, ed. *Neurological Disorders of Pregnancy*. Mount Kisco, NY: Futura; 1986: 153–96.

Dias MS, Sekhar LN. Intracranial hemorrhage from aneurysms and arteriovenous malformations during pregnancy and the puerperium. *Neurosurgery*. 1990;27:855–65.

Donaldson JO. Neuropathy. In: Donaldson JO, ed. *Neurology of Pregnancy*, 2nd ed. Philadelphia, Pa: WB Saunders; 1989: 23–59.

Cunningham FG, MacDonald PC, Grant NF, et al. Common complications of pregnancy. *Williams Obstetrics*, 19th ed. Norwalk, Conn: Appleton & Lange; 1993:763–803.

Dias MS, Sekhar LN. Intracranial hemorrhage from aneurysms and arteriovenous malformations during pregnancy and the puerperium. *Neurosurgery*. 1990;27:855–65.

Gilchrist JM. Muscle disease in the pregnant woman. In: Devinsky O, Feldmann E, Hainline B, eds. *Neurological Complications of Pregnancy*. New York: Raven Press; 1994:193–208.

Gilmore J, Pennell PB, Stern BJ. Medication use during pregnancy for neurologic conditions: iatrogenic disorders. *Neurol Clin*. W. B. Saunders: 1998;16:189–206.

Johnson CJ, Jangula JC. Cerebrovascular disease in women. In: Kaplan PW, ed. *Neurologic Disease in Women*. New York, NY: Demos Medical Publishing; 1998:219–28.

Kaplan PW. Eclampsia. In: Kaplan PW, ed. *Neurologic Disease in Women*. New York, NY: Demos Medical Publishing; 1998:173–87.

Khurana RK. Migraine. In: Kaplan PW, ed. *Neurologic Disease in Women*. New York, NY: Demos Medical Publishing; 1998:173–87.

Kittner SJ, Stern BJ, Feeser BR, et al. Pregnancy and the risk of stroke. *NEJM*. 1996;335:768–774.

Koren G, Pastuszak A, Ito S. Drugs in pregnancy. *N Engl J Med*. 1998;338:1128–37.

Pritchard JA, Cunningham FG, Pritchard SA. The Parkland Memorial Hospital protocol for treatment of eclampsia: evaluation of 245 Cases. *Am J Obstet Gynecol*. 1984; 148(7):951–63.

Repke JT, Klein VR. Myasthenia gravis in pregnancy. In: Goldstein PJ, ed. *Neurological Disorders of Pregnancy*. Mount Kisco, NY: Futura; 1986:213–34.

Report of the Quality Standards Subcommittee of the American Academy of Neurology. Practice parameter: management issues for women with epilepsy (summary statement). *Neurol*. 1998;51(4):944–8.

Rogers JD, Fahn S. Movement Disorders and Pregnancy. In: Devinsky O, Feldman E, Hainline B, eds. *Neurological Complications of Pregnancy*. New York, NY: Raven Press; 1994: 163–78.

Silberstein SD. Migraine and pregnancy. *Neurol Clin*. 1997;15:209–31.

Yerby MS, Collins SD. Pregnancy and the mother. In: Engel J, Pedley TA, eds. *Epilepsy, A Comprehensive Textbook*. Philadelphia, Pa: Lippincott-Raven; 1997:2035–7.

37 Neurotoxicology

Fred Harchelroad, Mary Beth Hines, Janet Eng,
David Overton, and David Rossi

INTRODUCTION

Neurological signs of central or peripheral origin are common to many emergency medicine patients, whether they are poisoned by pharmaceutical agents, drugs of abuse, occupational exposures, or environmental hazards. The key to successful treatment is not only the correct diagnosis but also good supportive care. Specific antidotes may not be available for most poisoned patients. Yet knowledge of the pharmacology of the toxin and physiology of the disease process will allow more appropriate interventions and better patient outcomes. Many poisonous substances produce their primary toxic effects by affecting neurotransmission. The nervous system's vulnerability to chemical attack depends heavily on its developmental state and its postdevelopmental organization and functional specialization. Neuromodulators and neurotransmitters of special concern include acetylcholine, adenosine, gamma-aminobutyric acid, dopamine, epinephrine, glutamate, gamma-hydroxybutyrate, norepinephrine, and serotonin.

General Approach to the Patient with Altered Mental Status

In the emergency department (ED), vital signs, as well as airway, breathing, and circulation are assessed and stabilized before further treatment is instituted or history obtained. External warming or cooling measures are initiated to correct abnormal core body temperatures. The unconscious patient requires determination of blood glucose level at the bedside, and levels of less than 80 mg/dL are treated with 50 mL of 50% dextrose in the adult, 4 mL/kg of 25% dextrose in children, and 5 mL/kg of 10% dextrose in neonates. Thiamine, 100 mg, is given intravenously in adults. The use of naloxone is indicated for patients in coma, with respiratory depression, and pinpoint pupils, or circumstantial evidence of opioid overdose. The initial dose is 2 mg given intravenously in adults and children (0.01 mg/kg in neonates). Flumazenil is used in the stuporous patient if there is clinical evidence of sedative-hypnotic ingestion and no contraindication such as concomitant ingestion of a proconvulsant compound. The initial dose of 0.2 mg intravenously may be titrated to 1 mg depending on response.

Table 37.1. Common Drugs that Induce Delirium

Amphetamines
Anticholinergics
Cocaine
Ethanol/sedative-hypnotic withdrawal
Hallucinogens
Phencyclidine

A comprehensive history and physical examination follows. Family members, friends, or EMS personnel can provide pertinent information for those patients who are unable or unwilling to provide a history. The time, type, and route of exposure and all substances to which the patient had access are determined. A list of all nonprescription medications, vitamins, herbal preparations, and household chemicals is helpful. Treatments rendered at home are required. A medical, psychiatric, and alcohol or substance abuse history is sought. A social history including occupation and hobbies can be helpful. A thorough physical and neurological examination are required, especially when the diagnosis is unclear. A careful examination can reveal a clinical pattern consistent with one of the classic toxidromes. See Table 37.1 for drug-induced delirium.

Laboratory evaluation may include analysis of arterial blood gas and serum electrolyte levels to determine the presence of acidosis. The presence of a high anion-gap acidosis requires determination of the osmolal gap. A pregnancy test in women of childbearing age is done when applicable. An electrocardiographic tracing helps to determine the presence of drugs such as cyclic antidepressants. Alcohol and acetaminophen levels should be obtained. Toxicological screening tests may detect the presence of unexpected substances but rarely alter decisions regarding clinical management. Specific drug levels (lithium, aspirin, theophylline, etc.) are obtained when specific ingestion is suspected, and the quantitative level may define further therapy.

Decontamination is performed for every patient with suspected poisoning, whether it is inhalational, dermal, or gastrointestinal. Care is taken to prevent the ED staff from additional exposure. Activated charcoal can absorb many orally ingested compounds by virtue of its large surface area and thus help prevent the absorption of compounds from the gastrointestinal (GI) tract. Activated charcoal can be self-administered by cooperative patients, or it can be placed through a small-bore nasogastric tube. Charcoal is administered orally in a dose of 1 g/kg to patients who have ingested a substance in a potentially toxic dose. Drugs not absorbed significantly by charcoal are listed in Table 37.2.

Recognition of several known toxidromes may narrow the diagnostic focus and aid in management. These include:

➤ Cholinergic syndrome
➤ Anticholinergic syndrome
➤ Adrenergic syndrome
➤ Sedative hypnotic syndrome
➤ Opioid syndrome
➤ Withdrawal syndromes

Table 37.2. Substances Not Absorbed Significantly by Activated Charcoal

Borates
Bromide
Ethyl alcohol
Ethylene glycol
Iron
Lithium
Methyl alcohol
Mineral acids/alkalis
Potassium

Cholinergic Syndrome

The neurotransmitter acetylcholine is found throughout the nervous system and binds to receptors in the sympathetic and parasympathetic nervous systems and the neuromuscular junction. Its effects are terminated by the enzyme acetylcholinesterase (AChE). Inhibition of AChE by compounds such as organophosphates and carbamate insecticides leads to the accumulation of acetylcholine and overstimulation of its receptors, causing a characteristic set of symptoms and signs commonly known as the cholinergic syndrome.

Organophosphate and carbamate insecticides are readily absorbed by dermal, inhalation, and oral routes. The military agents Sarin (GB), sorman (GD), GF, and VX are more potent organophosphate agents. The characteristic findings of excessive muscarinic activity are summarized by the mnemonic SLUDGE (salivation, lacrimation, urination, defecation, gastric emptying) or DUMBELS (defecation, urination, miosis, bronchorrhea, emesis, lacrimation, salivation). Because AChE is not restricted to the parasympathetic nervous system, other findings can be present. Increased sympathetic tone can cause tachycardia or mydriasis, and stimulation of nicotinic receptors can cause fasciculations, weakness, and eventually paralysis.

Bronchospasm and increased secretions pose an immediate threat to the airway. Endotracheal intubation is performed when appropriate. Atropine is a competitive inhibitor of muscarinic receptors and is used to control excess parasympathetic findings. Patients receive atropine until bronchospasm is resolved and oral secretions are controlled. The dosage is higher than usually used (2–5 mg of atropine sulfate, given by intravenous push every 2–3 minutes for adults, and 0.05 mg/kg given by intravenous push every 2–3 minutes in children). Atropine has no effect on nicotinic cholinergic receptors and does not reverse weakness or paralysis.

Pralidoxime (2-PAM) is an antidote for organophosphate poisoning. 2-PAM is most effective when administered early in the course of therapy. The dose for adults is 1–2 g given intravenously over 10–15 minutes followed by an infusion of 250–500 mg per hour; for children, there is a loading dose of 25 mg/kg and an infusion of 10–20 mg/kg per hour. The rise or fall of red blood cell (RBC) and plasma cholinesterase values is used to direct therapy, not initiate treatment. Most patients with a significant exposure require hospitalization for at least 3 days. Patients who recover from severe acute toxicity can exhibit confusion, depression, fatigue, and behavioral changes. Organophosphate-induced delayed neurotoxicity (OPIDN) is characterized by lower extremity weakness, paresthesias, and pain. The "intermediate syndrome" (IMS) is the third neurologic syndrome associated with organophosphorous compounds. IMS occurs about 48–96 hr after resolution of acute severe cholinergic crisis, with bulbar weakness and respiratory paralysis.

Anticholinergic Syndrome

Many medications have anticholinergic properties (Table 37.3). These drugs exert their effects by blocking muscarinic cholinergic receptors throughout the nervous system. Central manifestations include sedation, confusion, delirium, agitation, and hallucinations. Patients exhibit a characteristic mumbling speech or repetitive picking at bedsheets and clothing. When exposure is severe, coma and seizures can result. Peripheral effects include fever, flushing, dry skin, anhydrosis (particularly of the axilla), tachycardia, diminished gastrointestinal motility, mydriasis, and urinary retention. Patients can exhibit these findings during varying times after the poisoning.

Management of an anticholinergic syndrome includes adequate hydration and sedation. Though intravenous benzodiazepines are given frequently as a first-line agent, the use of physostigmine (1–2 mg intravenously) in patients with pure anticholinergic toxicity will reverse the central nervous system (CNS) delirium. Smaller doses should be used in patients with underlying bronchospastic disease. Physostigmine should not be used in patients with cyclic antidepressant overdoses. In expectation of urinary retention, a Foley catheter should be placed in the bladder. Agitation can contribute to fever and lead to rhabdomyolysis and is controlled with intravenous benzodiazepines when physostigmine was not successful. Seizures are treated with benzodiazepines or barbiturates.

Adrenergic Syndrome

Both pharmaceutical and illicit compounds can exert adrenergic effects (Table 37.4). Symptoms caused by excess catecholamines include tachycardia, hypertension, agitation, seizures, tremulousness, mydriasis, hyperreflexia, and metabolic acidosis. These findings are best treated with benzodiazepines intravenously. Patients with an adrenergic syndrome may appear very similar to those with an anticholinergic syndrome.

Sedative Hypnotic Syndrome

A variety of drugs are classified as sedative hypnotics because of their ability both to reduce anxiety and to induce sleep (see Table 37.5). The classic example is ethyl alcohol. Clinical effects of sedative hypnotic toxicity include ataxia, nystagmus, hypotonia, coma, apnea, bradycardia, hypotension, and hypothermia. Prolonged and cyclical coma is characteristic of glutethimide and meprobamate. Coma produced by ethchlorvynol has been reported to last almost 2 weeks. Many of the ultrashort acting sedative-hypnotics are used as "date rape" drugs (e.g., gamma hydroxybutyric acid, flunitrazepam) and are difficult to identify in the laboratory.

Treatment consists of aggressive airway management and supportive measures. Beacuse of its unique pharmacokinetics, the elimination of phenobarbital

Table 37.3. Substances with Anticholinergic Effects

Antiarrhythmic agents
  Disopyramide
  Quinidine
  Procainamide
Antipsychotic agents
  Acetophenazine
  Chlorprothixene
  Chlorpromazine
  Clozapine
  Fluphenazine
  Loxapine
  Fluphenazine
  Mesoridazine
  Molindone
  Perphbenazine
  Promazine
  Thioridazine
  Thiothixene
  Trifluoperazine
Plants
  Amanita muscaria
  Amanita pantherine
  Aropa belladonna
  Datura stramonium
  Mandragora officinarum
Antihistamines
  Astemizole
  Brompheniramine
  Carbinoxamine
  Clemastine
  Chlorpheniramine
  Cyclizine
  Cyporheptadine
  Diphenhydramine
  Hydroxyzine
  Loratadine
  Methscopolamine
  Phenyltoloxamine
  Pyrilamine
  Terfenadine
  Tripelennamine
  Trimeprazine
  Tripolindine
Antispasmodic agents
  Cinnamedrine
  Clidinium
  Dicyclomine
  Flavoxate
  Hycosamine
  Methantheline
  Oxybutynin
  Propantheline
  Tridihexethyl

(continued)

Table 37.3. *(continued)*

Skeletal muscle relaxants
    Cyclobenzaprine
    Orphenadrine
Antinausea drugs/motion sickness agents
    Dimenhydrinate
    Meclizine
    Prochlorperazine
    Promethazine
    Scopolamine
    Trimethobenzamide
Cyclic antidepressants
    Amitriptyline
    Amoxapine
    Clomipramine
    Desipramine
    Doxepin
    Imipramine
    Maprotiline
    Nortriptyline
    Protriptyline
    Trimipramine
Sleep aids
    Diphenhydramine
    Doxylamine
Anti-Parkinsonian agents
    Amantadine
    Benztropine
    Biperiden
    Ethopropazine
    Procyclidine
    Trihexyphenidyl
Ophthalmic agents
    Cyclopentolate
    Homatropine
    Tropicamide
Miscellaneous
    Atropine
    Bupropion
    Carbamazepine
    Glutethimide
    Glycopyrolate
    Meperidine
    Quinine

is enhanced by alkalinizing the urine. A bolus of 1 mEq/kg of sodium bicarbonate is administered intravenously. A maintenance infusion is prepared by adding 100 mEq sodium bicarbonate and 40 mEq KCl to 1 liter of D5W and administered to attain a urine pH of 7.5–8.0. Flumazenil (Romazicon) is a competitive inhibitor specific to the benzodiazepine binding site of the GABA$_A$ receptor and does not reverse the effects of barbiturates or other non-benzodiazepine sedatives. Its use is not recommended in those suspected of having an ingestion that may predispose to seizures.

Table 37.4. Substances Causing Adrenergic Syndrome

Albuterol
Amphetamines and derivatives
Caffeine
Cocaine
Dopamine
Dobutamine
Ephendrine/pseudoephedrine
Epinephrine/norepinephrine
Isoproterenol
Methylphenidate
Phenylephrine
Phenylpropanolamine
Theophylline

Opioid Syndrome

Opioids act on the various receptors to mediate the body's natural response to pain. The classic presentation of opioid overdose is coma, respiratory depression, and pinpoint pupils. Meperidine (Demerol) and diphenoxylate (Lomotil) in particular may present with mydriasis. Propoxyphene (Darvon) shares the sodium channel–blocking properties commonly associated with the cyclic antidepressants and may prolong ventricular conduction or cause seizures.

Naloxone is the opioid receptor antagonist used for both the diagnosis and the treatment of opioid intoxication. It can be administered orally, endotracheally, intramuscularly, intravenously, or sublingually. Some compounds are relatively resistant to the effects of naloxone (propoxyphene, methadone, etc.), thus requiring doses of up to 10 mg. Because the half-life of naloxone is shorter than many opioids, repeat doses may be used. Nalmefene is a longer acting, intravenously available opioid antagonist. It may be given in doses from 200 μg to 1 mg.

Table 37.5. Sedative-Hypnotic Agents

Barbiturates
Benzodiazepines
Bromides
Buspirone
Chloral hydrate
Ethanol
Ethchlorvynol (Placidyl)
Gamma hydroxybutropic acid
Glutethimide (Doriden)
Isopropanol
Meprobamate (Miltown, Equanil)
Methylqualone
Zolpidem (Ambien)

Table 37.6. Drugs Causing Respiratory
Depression

Antipsychotics
Chlorinated hydrocarbon solvents
Clonidine
Cyclic antidepressants
Botulism toxin
Cobra envenomation
Neuromuscular blocking agents
Nicotine
Organophosphate
Insecticides
Strychnine
Tetrodotoxin
Opioids
Sedative-hypnotics

Withdrawal Syndromes

Opioid withdrawal is characterized by intact cognition. No neurologic deficits should be associated with a pure opioid withdrawal state. Piloerection is objective evidence consistent with opioid withdrawal. Treatment is supportive. Clonidine will help alleviate most of the symptoms of opioid withdrawal except diarrhea.

Sedative-hypnotic withdrawal occurs in a time course consistent with the half-life of that particular agent. Clinical manifestations are indistinguishable from the numerous sedative-hypnotic agents. Agitation, tachycardia, tachypnea, hypertension, hyperthermia, hallucinations, and seizures all contribute to the high morbidity and mortality associated with this withdrawal syndrome.

Specific Neurotoxins

Coma and Respiratory Depression

Although many drugs depress the level of consciousness and respiratory drive, the agents most frequently responsible for these effects include opioids or sedative/hypnotics. The toxicity from any of these agents can cause hypotension, hypothermia, pulmonary edema, and hyporeflexia. Naloxone will reverse the opioid effects. Flumazenil will reverse any benzodiazepine effect. Other drugs causing respiratory depression are listed in Table 37.6.

Seizures

A variety of substances (Table 37.7) cause seizures by lowering seizure threshold, or secondarily from respiratory depression and hypoxia. Poisoning from a select few compounds presents with seizure as the initial manifestation of the toxicity. Both anticholinergies and adrenergies may produce seizures. The most effective way to control seizure activity caused by poisoning is by increased gamma-aminobutyric acid (GABA) inhibition of the CNS. Both benzodiazepines and barbiturates enhance the activity of GABA and are used in controlling

Table 37.7. Drug- or Toxin-Induced Seizures

Analgesics and nonprescription (OTC) preparations
    Antihistamines
    Caffeine
    Mefenamic acid
    Phenylbutazone
    Salicylates
Prescription medications
    Antihistamines
    Carbamazepine
    Chlorambucil
    Chloroquine
    Clonidine
    Digoxin
    Ergotamines
    Fenfluramine
    Isoniazid
    Lidocaine
    Methotrexate
    Phenytoin
    Procarbazine
    Quinine (cinchonism)
    Sulfonylureas
    Theophylline
Psychopharmacologic Medications
    Antiemetics
    Cyclic antidepressants
    Lithium
    Methylphenidate
    Monoamine oxidase inhibitors (esp. w/food or drug reaction)
    Neuroleptics
    Opioids (propoxyphene, meperidine)
    Pemoline
    Sedative-hypnotics (W)
Psychopharmacologic medications
    Barbiturates
        Benzodiazepines
        Other nonbarbiturate sedative-hypnotics
Alcohols and drugs of abuse
    Amphetamines
    Cocaine
    Disulfiram reaction
    Ethanol (W)
    Ethylene glycol
    MDMA (methylenedioxymethamphetamine)
    Methanol
    Phencyclidine
Botanicals
    Ackee fruit
    Coprinus spp. (disulfiram-like reaction w/alcohol)
    Daphne
    Herbal preparations (lobelia, jimson weed, gaiega, pokeweed,
        mandrake, passion flower, periwinkle, wormwood)
    Mistletoe

(continued)

Table 37.7. *(continued)*

  Nicotine
  Rhododendron
Heavy metals
  Arsenic
  Copper
  Lead
  Manganese
  Nickel
Household toxins
  Benzalkonium chloride
  Boric acid (chronic)
  Camphor
  Fluoride
  Hexachlorophene
  Phenol
Pesticides
  Diquat
  Organochlorines (lindane)
  Organophosphates
  Paraquat
  Pyrethrins
  Rodenticides (thallium, sodium monofluoroacetate, strychnine, zinc
    phosphide, arsenic)
Occupational and environmental toxins
  Carbon disulfide
  Carbon monoxide
  Chlorphenoxy herbicides
  Cyanide
  Hydrocarbons
  Simple asphyxiants (methane, ethane, propane, butane, natural gas)
  High volatility (benzene, toluene, gasoline, naphtha, mineral spirits, light
    gas oil)
  Halogenated (carbon tetrachloride, trichloroethane)
  Hydrogen sulfide
  Methyl bromide
  Toxic inhalants (simple asphyxiants producing hypoxia – helium, nitrogen)
  Triazine
Toxic envenomation and marine animal ingestion
  Marine animals (gymnothorax, saxitoxin [shellfish])
  Pit viper
  Scorpion
  Tick bite (*Rickettsia rickettsii*)

poison-induced seizures. The use of phenytoin to control seizures is not recommended when the etiology of seizure is suspected to be poisoning. Several compounds require special attention.

Theophylline and other methylxanthines exert their effect by competitive inhibition of adenosine receptors. The CNS symptoms of theophylline toxicity are agitation, tremulousness, and seizures. Similarly, effects of theophylline on the peripheral adrenergic nervous system include tachycardia, cardiac arrhythmias, metabolic acidosis, and rhabdomyolysis. Because seizures are the main cause of mortality in theophylline toxicity, prophylactic use of

Table 37.8. Anion Gap Metabolic Acidosis

Acetylene
Benzyl alcohol
β-Adrenergics
Boric acid
Caffeine
Carbon monoxide
Epinephrine
Ethanol
Ethylene glycol
Formaldehyde
Hydrogen sulfide
Ibuprofen
Iron
Isoniazid
Methanol
Methylphenidate
Salicylates
Theophylline

phenobarbital or a benzodiazepine is recommended in severely poisoned patients. Hemoperfusion is recommended in treating patients with severe theophylline toxicity.

The most significant properties of cyclic antidepressants are the anticholinergic effects and the inhibition of sodium channels. The latter phenomenon accounts for the prolongation of the QRS interval of the electrocardiogram. Prolongation of the QRS interval of greater than 110 ms results in an increased probability of developing cardiac arrhythmias, but a QRS interval greater than 160 ms is associated with increased risk of seizures. Sodium bicarbonate is given as the first-line treatment of both ventricular arrhythmias and seizures in the patient poisoned with a cyclic antidepressant.

Isoniazid (INH) is a competitive inhibitor of the enzyme pyridoxine kinase, which is necessary for the synthesis of GABA. Signs of toxicity include vomiting, abdominal pain, coma, metabolic acidosis, and seizures. Seizures are refractory to standard treatment because potentiation of GABA receptor-mediated inhibition by benzodiazepine or barbiturates may not be sufficient when GABA levels are depleted. Administration of pyridoxine (vitamin B_6) restores this deficiency. For every gram of INH ingested, 1 gm of pyroxidine is given intravenously; 5 gm are given initially when the amount of ingested INH is unknown.

Lithium has a narrow therapeutic index. Symptoms of chronic toxicity occur despite "therapeutic" serum levels. Clinical findings of toxicity include nausea, bradycardia, muscle rigidity, mental status changes, agitation, hyperreflexia, coma, and seizures. Adequate hydration enhances the renal excretion of lithium. Hemodialysis is recommended for symptomatic patients.

Coma and Metabolic Acidosis

An overdose of many compounds can cause metabolic acidosis (Table 37.8) and subsequent mental status changes. Overdose of these drugs should be considered in the differential diagnosis of delirium/coma if a high anion gap metabolic acidosis is noted.

A significant overdose of salicylate can result in initial symptoms of vomiting, tinnitus, confusion, and respiratory alkalosis and can progress rapidly to metabolic acidosis, coma, and seizures. Glucose levels in cerebrospinal fluid may be low despite normal serum levels. Management of salicylate toxicity includes alkalinization of the urine, which enhances renal elimination. Bicarbonate therapy helps maintain a blood pH of 7.45–7.5 and urine pH of greater than 7.5. The Done nomogram has many limitations, and a decision to initiate hemodialysis is best made on clinical data. The most common presentation of chronic salicylate toxicity is confusion. Salicylate levels may be within therapeutic range. Treatment is similar to that of acute salicylate toxicity.

Methanol and ethylene glycol are alcohols found in numerous industrial and household products. Methanol is used as a gasoline antiknock additive and windshield wiper fluid. Ethylene glycol is used in antifreeze, deicing agents, fire extinguishers, and refrigerator coolants. The toxic alcohols methanol and ethylene glycol are both metabolized through the alcohol dehydrogenase system as ethyl alcohol. Methanol is initially metabolized to formaldehyde and subsequently converted to formic acid, leading to metabolic acidosis. Ethylene glycol is metabolized initially to glycolaldehyde and eventually oxalic acid.

Symptoms of methanol poisoning typically take 12–24 hours to develop after ingestion, secondary to the slow metabolism of methanol to formic acid. Symptoms are very similar to ethyl alcohol intoxication except for visual problems and dilated pupils. Physical examination reveals impaired visual acuity, dilated pupils with a poor pupillary light reflex, and papilledema. Severe metabolic acidosis is noted by this stage. Residual permanent symptoms are similar to those of Parkinson's disease, with predominant findings of dystonias and hypokinesis. Although improvement in motor impairment is observed in some patients when given levodopa, others have little response. It is unknown why the basal ganglia and, specifically, the putamen are preferentially affected in methanol poisoning.

Ethylene glycol poisoning is divided into three clinical stages. Stage 1 develops within 30 minutes of ingestion and lasts for approximately 12 hours. Patients appear inebriated. Progressive CNS depression can lead to coma. Stage 2 occurs 12–24 hours postingestion. Findings in this stage are secondary to the development of a severe metabolic acidosis and include tachypnea, acute respiratory distress syndrome, and cardiovascular collapse. Stage 3 is characterized by acute renal tubular necrosis with anuria, oliguria, and flank pain. This stage develops between 48 and 72 hours after ingestion. Cranial nerve VII is consistently affected by ethylene glycol poisoning, which can result in facial diplegia. Dysarthria, dysphagia, and hearing loss can also occur. The effects can be permanent despite aggressive treatment of this poisoning.

Confirmation of ethylene glycol or methanol poisoning is obtained through specific measurement of these alcohols in blood. Because alcohol levels may not be readily available in the ED, and treatment delay can lead to serious sequelae, calculations of anion and osmolar gaps aid in the early diagnosis of poisoning.

If an anion gap acidosis is present, measurement of serum osmolality helps make the diagnosis of toxic alcohol poisoning. Serum osmolality is calculated by the following formula and expressed as mOsm/kg H_2O:

$$2(Na^+) + Glucose/18 + Blood\ urea\ nitrogen/2.8 + Ethanol\ (mg/dL)/4.5$$

Low-molecular-weight alcohols such as ethylene glycol and methanol are osmotically active and increase serum osmolality. An osmolar gap is determined by subtracting the calculated serum osmolality (derived from the preceding formula) from the serum osmolality as measured by freezing point depression. A normal osmolar gap is considered less than 10 mOsm/kg. Therefore, the presence of an osmolar gap may support the diagnosis of toxic alcohol poisoning, but its absence does not exclude this possibility. Urine calcium oxalate crystals and hypocalcemia can be observed with ethylene glycol poisoning.

Initial treatment of these toxic alcohol ingestions is correcting the acidosis and preventing further metabolism of them.

Ethanol has a much higher affinity for alcohol dehydrogenase than does methanol or ethylene glycol. Administration of ethanol, by either oral or intravenous routes, successfully blocks further metabolism of these toxic alcohols. Ethanol may be given empirically when poisoning with a toxic alcohol is suspected, even before laboratory confirmation. Oral loading doses of 700 mg ETOH/kg followed by 150 mg/kg given intravenously every hour infusions are initiated until hemodialysis (HD) may be started. When HD is initiated, the maintenance infusion of ethyl alcohol (ETOH) must be increased to 300 mg/kg per hour. Alternative treatment is with 4-methyl pyrazole (15 mg/kg) given intravenously. Unlike treatment with ETOH, 4-methylpyrazole (fomepizole) does not cause the CNS effects noted with ETOH treatment. Nevertheless, HD may still be needed to remove the toxic metabolites of methanol and ethylene glycol, so repeat treatment with formepizole may be needed because it is also removed by hemodialysis.

Adjunctive therapy includes administration of sodium bicarbonate and vitamins. Folic acid, a cofactor in the metabolism of formic acid, is given intravenously, 50 mg every 4 hours, in methanol poisoning. Thiamine and pyridoxine are cofactors in the metabolism of glyoxilic acid. Thiamine, 100 mg, and pyridoxine, 50 mg, are given intravenously every 6 hours. As poisoning with these agents is infrequent, consultation with a medical toxicologist should be considered.

Altered Mental Status, Rigidity, and Hyperthermia

Neuroleptic malignant syndrome (NMS) is a disorder associated with dopamine blockade or depletion in the CNS. Symptoms can develop 1–7 days after the initiation of the offending agent, typically a neuroleptic, and can occur regardless of the duration of its use. Patients who appear to be ill present with mental status changes, elevated temperature, and autonomic instability. Rigidity can lead to respiratory compromise and rhabdomyolysis. Treatment consists of supportive measures and institution of rapid cooling measures. Dantrolene (0.8–3.0 mg/kg given intravenously every 6 hours) and bromocriptine (5 mg given orally followed by 2.5–10 mg given orally every 8 hours) are commonly used for muscle relaxation and dopamine receptor agonism, respectively. Neuromuscular blocking agents can be used when rhabdomyolysis is severe.

Table 37.9. Drug- and Toxin-Induced Parkinsonism

Neuroleptics	Other Drugs	Toxins
Chlorpromazine	Alpha-methyldopa	Alcohol withdrawal
Chlorprothixene	Calcium-channel blockers	Carbon disulfide
Clozapine	Captopril	Carbon monoxide
Droperidol	Lithium	Cyanide
Fluphenazine	Metoclopramide	Manganese
Haloperidol	Phenytoin	Methanol
Loxapine	Prochlorperazine	
Mesoridazine	Reserpine	
Molindone	Tetrabenazine	
Perphenazine		
Pimozide		
Thioridazine		
Thiothixene		
Treifluoperazine		

Serotonin Syndrome

Serotonin syndrome is caused by an excess stimulation of serotonin receptors that results from a combination of drugs affecting serotonin receptors, not from an overdose of a single drug. Serotonin syndrome is known to occur with discontinuation of one drug and the initiation of another before the therapeutic effects of the initial drug have dissipated. A common example is the patient who stops taking monoamine oxidase inhibitor (MAOI) medication and is immediately started on a selective serotonin reuptake inhibitor (SSRI) medication. Symptoms such as head turning, shivering, and leg rigidity can distinguish this syndrome from NMS. The patient's medication list may provide important clues. Treatment includes discontinuation of the offending agent(s) and supportive measures. Cyproheptadine, an antihistamine with nonspecific serotonin antagonist properties, has been used with success in some cases.

Movement Disorders

Virtually all the abnormal movements caused by primary neurologic disease can be induced by a drug/toxin. It is imperative to review a patient's medications and obtain an appropriate exposure history in those patients who present with an acute movement disorder. Tables 37.8 through 37.15 list those drugs that have been implicated.

Peripheral Neuropathies

A common, and difficult-to-diagnose, complaint of patients presenting to the ED is that of extremity weakness or paresthesias. Although the classifications of these neuropathies vary, the importance of investigating the exposure to the selected toxins that may cause these neuropathies is of paramount importance. (See Table 37.16.) Transverse myelitis is a neurological complication of heroin use. This can occur with intravenous use of heroin following several months of drug abstinence. Heroin also causes a variety of peripheral nerve lesions. Brachial and

Table 37.10. Causes of Drug- and Toxin-Induced
Postural Tremor

Drugs
  Amiodarone
  Amphetamines
  Beta-adrenergic agonists
  Caffeine
  Cocaine
  Corticosteroids
  Cyclic antidepressants
  Ergotamine
  Levodopa
  Lithium
  MAOIs (toxic interaction with food or drug)
  Monosodium glutamate
  Neuroleptic agents
  Phenytoin
  Theophylline
  Valproic acid
Toxins
  Arsenic
  Bismuth
  Carbon disulfide
  Carbon monoxide
  Lead
  Mercury
  Methylbromide
  Phencyclidine
Withdrawal
  Ethanol
  Sedative-hypnotics

Table 37.11. Causes of Drug- and Toxin-Induced
Kinetic Tremor

Alcoholic cerebellar degeneration
Amiodarone
Barbiturates
Benzodiazepines
Carbamazepine
Chloral hydrate
Colistin
Ethanol
Ethchlorvynol
Glutethimide
Lithium
Methaqualine
Methyl mercury
Phenytoin
Piperazine
Valproic acid

Table 37.12. Causes of Drug- and Toxin-Induced Chorea

Drugs
  Anticholinergics
    Antihistamines
    Benztropine
    Cyclic antidepressants
  Anticonvulsants
    Carbamazepine
    Phenobarbital
    Phenytoin
  Anti-Parkinsonians
    Amantadine
    Bromocriptine
    Levodopa
    Pergolide
  Corticosteroids
  Lithium
  Metoclopramide
  Neuroleptics
    Butyrophenones
    Phenothiazines
  Oral contraceptives
  Sympathomimetics
    Amphetamines
    Caffeine
    Cocaine
    Methylphenidate
    Theophylline
Toxins
  Carbon monoxide
  Ethanol
  Manganese
  Thallium
  Toluene

Table 37.13. Drugs Associated with Induction of Acute and/or Tardive Dystonia/Dyskinesia

Drug	Dystonia	Dyskinesia
Anticonvulsants		
Carbamazepine, phenytoin	X	
Antidepressants		
Fluvoxamine	X	X
Calcium-channel blockers		
Flunarizine, cinnarizine		X
Dopamine agonists		
Levodopa	X	
Neuroleptic agents		X
Orthopramides and substituted benzamides		
Metoclopramide	X	X
Clebopride		X
Sulpride		X
Veralipride		X

Table 37.14. Drugs Associated with Induction of Akathisia

Neuroleptic drugs
Metoclopramide, prochlorperazine
Dopamine storage and transport inhibitors
    α-Methytyrosine, reserpine, tetrabenazine
Levodopa and dopamine agonists
Antidepressants
    Selective serotinin-reuptake inhibitors
    Tricyclic antidepressants
    Phenelzine
Calcium-channel blockers
    Flunarizine, cinnarizine

lumbosacral plexitis are not associated with needle trauma and are characterized by intense neuritic pain, weakness, and sensory deficits. Mononeuropathy can occur as painless weakness of an extremity hours after intravenous injection of heroin. The mononeuropathy is also known to occur at a remote location from the site of injection. Acute and subacute polyneuropathies that resemble Guillain-Barré syndrome can occur with the use of heroin. Heroin use can affect muscle, resulting in acute rhabdomyolysis with myoglobinuria, localized myopathy at recurrent injection sites, and localized crush syndromes.

Myopathies

Myopathies may be focal or diffuse, but all present with weakness. Drugs and toxins may act through a variety of mechanisms causing injury to skeletal muscle. (See Table 37.17.)

Headaches

Most headaches associated with toxic-metabolic disorders are poorly understood, yet the emergency physician should investigate the numerous drug causes

Table 37.15. Toxic Causes of Asterixis and Multifocal Myoclonus

Anticholinergics
Anticonvulsants
Benzodiazepines
Bismuth
Crotalid venom
Cyclic antidepressants
DDT
Ethanol
Lead
Levodopa
Mercury
Methylbromide
Sedative-hypnotics

Table 37.16. Classification of Selected Toxin- or Drug-Induced Peripheral Neuropathies

Neuropathy	Axonopathy	Myelinopathy	Transmission Neuropathy
Acute Toxic Neuropathies			
Pyridoxine (S)	Hexacarbons (SMA)	Arsenic (SM)	Black widow spider
	Thallium (SM)	Diphtheria (SM)	Botulism
	Triorthocresylphosphate (SM)		Ciguatoxin
	Vacor (MA)		
			Elapid and crotalid venoms
			Gymnothoratoxin
			Saxitoxin
			Scorpion venom
			Tetradotoxin
			Tick paralysis
Subacute/Chronic Toxic Neuropathies			
None convincingly demonstrated	Acrykanude (SM)	Amiodarone (SM)	
	Allyl chloride (SM)	Buckthorn	
	Arsenic (SM)	Diphtheria (SM)	
	Buckthorn (SM)	Gold (SM)	
	Carbon disulfide (SM)	Trichlorethylene (SM)	
	Colchicine (S)		
	Disulfiram (SM)		
	Dapsone (M)		
	2',3'-dideoxycytidine (ddC), ddl		
	Ethanol (M)		
	Ethambutol (S)		
	Ethionamide (S)		
	Ethylene oxide (SM)		
	Glutethimide (S)		
	Gold (SM)		
	Hexacarbons (SM)		
	Hydralazine (SM)		
	Isoniazid (SM)		
	Methyl bromide (SM)		
	Mercury (M)		
	Metronidazole (SM)		
	Misonidazole (SM)		
	Nitrofurantoin (SM)		
	Platinum (S)		
	Podophylin (SM)		
	Taxol (S)		
	Thallium (SM)		
	Vincristine (SM)		
	Nitrous oxide (S)		
	Nucleosides (S)		
	Organophosphorous esters (SM)		
	Polychlorinated biphenyls (SM)		
	Phenytoin (SM)		

Table 37.17. Myopathies Caused by Drugs and Toxins

Diffuse toxic myopathies
  Necrotizing myopathy
  Aminocaproic acid
  Clofibrate
  Heroin
  Ipecac
  Lovastatin and other HMG-CoA reductase inhibitors
  Phencyclidine
  Vincristine
  Zidovidine
  Autophagic myopathy
    Amiodarone
    Chloroquine
  Corticosteroids
  Ethanol
  Hypokalemia caused by
    Barium salts
    Cathartic abuse
    Emetic abuse
    Glycrrhizic acid
  Inflammatory myopathy (myositis)
    D-Penicillamine
    Eosinophilia-myalgia syndrome (L-tryptophan)
  Other Drugs
    Beta-adrenergic antagonists
    Cimetidine
    Cyclosporine
    Doxylamine
    Ethchlorvynol
    Penicillin
    Propylthiouracil
    Rifampin
    Sulfonamides
  Envenomation (species indigenous to North America)
    Snakes
      Copperhead
      Rattlesnake
      Water moccasin
    Spiders
      Brown recluse spider
    Insects
      Hornets
      Wasps
    Microbial myotoxins
      Clostridium perfringens
Focal toxic myopathies
  Needle myopathy
  Opioids

Table 37.18. Chemicals, Drugs, and Toxins Associated with Headache

Analgesics and nonprescription (over the counter – OTC) preparations
  Alpha-adrenergic agonists (e.g., pseudoephedrine)
  Butyl nitrite
  Caffeine withdrawal (in many OTC medications)
  Indomethacin
  Isobutyl nitrite
  Vitamin A
Prescription medications
  Amyl nitrite
  Anesthetics (halothane, ketamine, enflurane, *d*-tubocurare)
  Antibiotics (nalidixic acid, tetracycline, minocycline, nitrofurantoin,
    metronidazole, sulfamethoxazole, griseofulvin)
  Antihypertensives (hydralazine, nifedipine, proazosin, reserpine)
  Corticosteroids and steroid withdrawal
  Danocrine (Danazol)
  Ergotamines
  Hypoglycemic agents
  Isoamyl nitrite
  Isosorbide dinitrate
  Nitroglycerin (oral, transdermal)
  Oral contraceptives
  Quinine (cinchonism)
  Theophylline
Psychopharmacologic agents
  Monoamine oxidase inhibitors when ingested with
    Tyramine-containing foods (red wine, aged cheese, bananas)
    Medication (phenylephrine, ephedrine)
  Phenothiazines
Alcohol and drugs of abuse
  Amphetamines
  Cocaine
  Disulfiram (when mixed with ethanol)
  Ethanol withdrawal ("hangover")
  Ethylene glycol
  Methanol
  Phencyclidine
Food and drink
  Aged cheese (cheddar, mozzarella, Gruyere, Stilton, brie, Camembert)
  Caffeine
  Chocolate
  Ethanol
  Fermented or pickled foods (herring, sour cream, yogurt, vinegar,
    marinated meats, smoked fish)
  Fruits (bananas, plantain, avocado, figs, passion fruit, raisins, pineapple,
    oranges, citrus fruits)
  Monosodium glutamate
  Nitrite-containing meat (hot dogs, bologna, pepperoni, salami, pastrami,
    bacon, sausages, corned beef)
  Sugar substitutes (diet drinks)
  Sulfites (salad bars, shrimp, soft drinks, some wines)
  Vegetables (onions, pods of broad beans [lima, navy], nuts)
  Yeast products (yeast extract, fresh bread, doughnuts)

Botanicals
  Coprinus spp. (disulfiram-like reaction if ingested with ethanol)
  Herbal preparation (Lobelia, Galega)
  Nicotine
  Various plants
Heavy metals
  Lead, especially tetraethyl lead
  Metal fume fever (caused by welding or smelting of brass, cadmium,
    chromium, cobalt, copper, iron, magnesium, manganese, nickel, tin, zinc)
Pesticides
  Carbamates
  Organophosphates
Occupational and environmental
  Carbon monoxide
  Cyanide
  Hydrocarbons
  Hydrogen sulfide
  Methemoglobin inducers
  Toxic inhalants (and simple asphyxiants)
Toxic envenomation and marine animal ingestion
  Arthropods (bite: *Rickettsia rickettsii*)
  Lyme disease
  Marine animals (Ciguatoxin [vertebrate fish], Scombroid [mahimahi fish],
    Gymnothorax poisoning [eels], Tetrodon [puffer fish])

when obtaining the history of a patient with this common complaint. (See Table 37.18.)

Environmental Neurotoxins

Electrical, Lightning, and Thermal Injuries

Electrical injuries can result in numerous immediate and delayed neurological complications. Electrical injuries kill approximately 1,200 individuals annually in the United States. The most common cause of death by either alternating current or direct current (lightning strike) is cardiorespiratory arrest. The most common cause of death in persons with significant thermal injury is multiple organ failure and its complications.

Alternating current typically induces ventricular fibrillation; lightning strike (direct current) commonly causes asystole. Permanent neurological sequelae can now be anticipated in the patient who appears healthy but has underlying serious pathophysiology caused by electrical injury.

According to Ohm's law of physics, amperage (A), voltage (V), and resistance (R) are related according to the following formula:

$$A = V/R$$

Tissue factors interact to produce electrical injury of varying severity and distribution. Although voltage can be determined from the patient's history, other factors such as amperage, resistance, and susceptibility of tissues may be unknown. The neurological effects of electrical injury can be classified as immediate (often transient) and delayed (often permanent).

A recent study using postmortem examinations of 139 burn patients over a 21-year period demonstrated a 50% incidence of CNS complications. Peripheral nerve abnormalities following major burn injuries are estimated to occur in 15–29% of patients. Approximately 10–50% of post–burn injury patients have long-term psychological morbidity.

An unusual prehospital aspect of lightning injury is the often-distorted appearance of the injured individuals. The blast energy can hurl the individual several yards, resulting in further trauma. Sudden depolarization of the myocardium causes asystole.

Disaster triage protocols for care of multiple patients are altered in cases of electrical and lightning injury. Because cardiorespiratory arrest is the leading cause of death in individuals who have sustained electrical injuries, immediate attention is focused on individuals who appear pulseless and unconscious. When standard triage protocols are used in this setting, victims with a moderate chance of survival can be inappropriately considered expired at the scene. Basic and advanced life support protocols are initiated and do not need to be altered in patients with electrical injuries. Fluid resuscitation is begun early because fluid requirements for electrical burn patients exceed those of standard burn protocols. This is most likely due to undetected deep tissue burn injuries.

A careful physical examination and frequent repeat examinations can help differentiate injury due to alternating versus direct current. Alternating current tends to produce entrance and exit wounds of approximately the same size; direct current produces a small entrance wound and a much larger exit wound. A feather or "ferning" pattern has been described in association with skin surface burns caused by lightning strike. The CNS is the most commonly affected organ system in electrical injuries, with 33–100% of patients developing neurological deficits.

The two mechanisms of neuropathological change resulting from electrical injury are (1) direct injury caused by the effect of the blast (in lightning injury) or mechanical trauma and (2) thermal injury caused by tissue exposure to current. This type of thermal injury can injure brain tissue and vascular endothelium, resulting in thrombotic or hemorrhagic infarction. Thermal injury of peripheral nerves can result in irreversible loss of function.

Histological and electrophysiological changes in peripheral nervous tissue have been implicated in transient peripheral nerve injury. The pathological findings are summarized as cavitation, chromatolysis of anterior horn cells, fragmentations of axons, myelin degeneration, petechial hemorrhages, reactive gliosis, and swelling and softening of the spinal cord.

Following initial stabilization, the electrically injured patient is assessed for spinal injury. Continuous cardiac monitoring is established. Other early complications of thermal injury include fluctuations in serum electrolytes, especially sodium, magnesium, and calcium. Tetanus immunization status is assessed. The electroencephalogram (EEG) may demonstrate the absence of alpha rhythms and a predominance of low-amplitude slow waves. Baseline hearing and visual acuity measurements are performed. Early referral to a neurologist, neurosurgeon, or burn specialist is considered.

Most patients injured by a high-voltage electrical source require hospital admission with cardiac monitoring. In patients with very mild electrocution, the prognosis is good, and a period of monitoring in the ED may be adequate to allow discharge. Estimates of long-term psychological morbidity are as high as 50% in burn patients.

Dysbarism

Each year in the United States, 500–600 diving-related injuries occur, with 75–100 fatalities occurring. *Dysbarism* is a term used to describe three main clinical syndromes resulting from SCUBA (self-contained underwater breathing apparatus) diving: barotrauma, dysbaric air embolism (or arterial gas embolism – AGE), and decompression sickness.

Type I decompression sickness is a mild form, from which the term *the bends* originated. Shoulder and elbow periarticular joint pain is the most common symptom of type I decompression sickness. However, descriptions have included more unusual presentations such as temporomandibular joint pain. All joint spaces can develop periarticular pain secondary to the effects of decompression sickness. Type I decompression sickness syndrome is characterized by skin, lymphatic, and musculoskeletal system involvement and typically results in very low morbidity when treated appropriately.

Type II decompression illness is more severe than type I and may involve the CNS, peripheral nervous system (PNS), and inner ears. Hence, the term *neurological decompression sickness* is often used interchangeably with *type II decompression sickness*. Treatment of patients with type II (neurological) decompression sickness involves prolonged and repeated hyperbaric oxygen therapy. Despite treatment, long-term neurological deficits or death can occur.

Decompression sickness occurs when there is a sufficient volume of gas (usually nitrogen) dissolved in tissue, which under decreased pressure comes out of solution and forms bubbles within vascular and tissue spaces. The mechanisms of injury include direct tissue injury, obstruction of blood flow, and foreign body reaction. Clinical manifestations reflect the amount and location of bubble formation. Bubbles that obstruct the paravertebral venous system result in spinal cord symptoms. Bubbles that embolize to the CNS cause cerebral, cerebellar, or other CNS symptoms. Preferential involvement of the lower thoracic, upper lumbar, and lower cervical spinal cord have been described in postmortem studies of divers with decompression sickness who had significant residual impairments following recompression.

Management of patients with neurological decompression sickness in the prehospital environment usually does not involve advanced life-saving measures. Although it is possible that a diver may become unresponsive shortly after a dive, immediate loss of consciousness is more commonly associated with AGE. Most decompression sickness presents as delayed joint pain. Among symptomatic divers, 90% exhibit joint pains and 20–50% exhibit neurological symptoms as a delayed consequence of diving. Approximately 50% of patients with decompression sickness demonstrate symptoms within 30 minutes postdive, 95% within 3 hours, and nearly 100% within 6 hours.

When dysbaric air embolism is suspected, the Trendelenburg and left lateral decubitus positions are maneuvers that may prevent further gas embolism. Additionally, these maneuvers increase venous distension and pressure and facilitate the elimination of air emboli through the venous pulmonary system. One hundred percent oxygen should be administered to increase tissue oxygenation, to help remove excess nitrogen gas dissolved in tissues ("nitrogen washout"), and to prevent further bubble formation. Patients with immediate loss of consciousness and suspected air embolism are transferred to a recompression chamber as soon as possible. A fixed-wing aircraft capable of low-altitude flying with cabin pressures of 1 atm is optimal. Both dehydration and hemoconcentration compound ischemia and should be treated with intravenous fluids.

Immediate assessment in the ED includes evaluation of airway patency, breathing, and circulation. The history is most important in diagnosing decompression sickness. The following questions can elicit useful information: How long and how deep was the dive? What type of equipment was used? Were there repeat dives? What was the water temperature? Where did the dive take place? Was this dive particularly fatiguing? Advanced age, obesity, dehydration, recent alcohol intoxication, and local physical injury have all been related anecdotally to increased risk of developing decompression sickness.

Physical examination precedes recompression therapy because patients can have associated medical problems. In patients with pulmonary barotrauma, chest pain, cough, dyspnea, or tachypnea is usually present. The oropharynx may be deeply red. Skin lesions may also be present. These lesions are typically tender, warm to touch, pruritic, and occur over the chest.

Numerous neurological manifestations of decompression sickness include headache, confusion, delirium, coma, visual loss, blurred vision, vestibular deficits, nausea, equilibrium disorder, paraplegia, quadriplegia, paresis, lower extremity paresthesias, tremor, bladder dysfunction, and death. These reports reinforce the fact that history is usually the best way to differentiate between AGE and decompression sickness. Definitive care includes the earliest possible hyperbaric oxygen treatment, whether the patient exhibits symptoms of AGE or neurological decompression sickness.

Laboratory evaluation of decompression sickness should not delay recompression therapy. Serum creatine kinase levels can reflect the size and severity of AGE.

Neuroimaging and neurophysiological studies may be helpful in evaluating a patient with decompression sickness. Magnetic resonance imaging (MRI) provides a more sensitive technique than conventional CT scanning in localizing spinal cord lesions related to decompression sickness. Intravenous injection with gadolinium (Gd-DTPA) increases the sensitivity of MRI scans in patients with decompression sickness and AGE. Additionally, electronystagmography (ENG) is useful in evaluation of inner ear decompression sickness.

Neurological symptoms can develop due to AGE after decompression in a diver who has an atrial septal defect. Complete recovery from decompression sickness can occur with recompression therapy initiated more than a week after the inciting event.

Conditions that resemble decompression sickness include motion sickness, near drowning, envenomations, carbon monoxide poisoning, nitrogen toxicity, psychological disorders, hypothermia, and cardiac dysfunction. Patients with decompression sickness can present in delayed fashion with headache, nausea, and fatigue and can be misdiagnosed as with a viral illness. Diagnoses that can coexist with diving injuries include pulmonary barotrauma, aural barotrauma, squeeze syndromes, hypoxia, alternobaric vertigo, physical trauma, and exhaustion.

In cases of very mild (type I) decompression sickness, patients commonly have resolution of symptoms with recompression therapy and can be discharged from the ED. When neurological symptoms or signs are present, patients are hospitalized because manifestations of neurological decompression sickness can recur after the first recompression treatment. Some patients never recover full function and experience life-long sequelae.

Accidental Hypothermia

Mild hypothermia is defined as a core temperature of 33-35°C; moderate hypothermia, as 28–32.9°C; and severe hypothermia, as less than 28°C. The lowest recorded temperature for revival after hypothermia was a 23-month-old boy with an initial temperature of 15°C. The rapid detection and correction of core body temperature is the ultimate goal of prehospital care providers and emergency physicians. Permanent neurological abnormalities may not be immediately apparent and may be detected only after complete neurological evaluation. Neurological outcome remains difficult to predict in the acute setting. A hypothermia outcome score has been developed based upon the progressive depression of the CNS by hypothermia. Cerebral metabolism decreases 7% for each 1°C decrease in body temperature. At 19°C, the EEG is flat. As the patient's temperature continues to fall, judgment becomes impaired and hallucinations may develop. By 30°C, patients typically have dilated, sluggish pupils. Patients exhibit loss of muscular reflexes, loss of pain responses, and fixed, dilated pupils by the time core temperature has reached 28°C. The corneal reflex, mediated by CNS pathways, disappears at approximately 25°C.

The management of hypothermic patients focuses on recognition of hypothermia (using a low-reading thermometer), establishment of intravenous catheter(s), administration of supplemental oxygen, cardiac monitoring, and prevention of further heat loss.

Patients are assessed quickly for adequacy of airway, breathing, and circulatory function. Supplemental oxygen is humidified and warmed to 46°C. Severely hypothermic patients can have adequate oxygenation with a respiratory rate as low as 4–6 breaths per minute. Prevention of further heat loss and rewarming are started during the initial resuscitation.

Patients are handled very carefully because of increased risk of cardiac arrhythmias. Because most severely hypothermic patients demonstrate some degree of volume depletion, intravenous fluids are given generously.

A variety of active, external, and core-warming modalities exist, including warmed blankets, radiant heat lamps, aerosol masks, gastric lavage, bladder lavage, peritoneal lavage, thoracic lavage, and cardiopulmonary bypass. The method(s) used depend on the extent of hypothermia and the cardiovascular status of the patient. Cardiopulmonary bypass is rapid, with little afterdrop phenomenon, but is typically not readily available. Unconscious patients receive naloxone, thiamine, and glucose. Patients in whom hypothermia develops gradually are prone to hypoglycemia because prolonged shivering utilizes glycogen stores. However, the inactivation of insulin that occurs with hypothermia can lead to hyperglycemia.

Laboratory evaluation includes arterial blood gases, complete blood count, liver function, coagulation, blood glucose, electrolyte, blood urea nitrogen, serum creatinine, and amylase levels, electrocardiogram, urinalysis, and chest radiograph. Aggressive correction of acidosis is not recommended in hypothermic patients because the acidosis corrects itself with rewarming and alkalosis may precipitate dysrhythmias. Studies have reported a wide range of significant clinical and laboratory factors in hypothermic patients. Poor prognostic signs include prehospital cardiac arrest, low or absent presenting blood pressure, and elevated blood urea nitrogen levels.

Many patients with mild hypothermia can be rewarmed in the ED and discharged once evaluation for associated injuries and illness is complete. Patients with more severe hypothermia are hospitalized for thorough assessment, rewarming, and stabilization. Subtle neurological complications may persist with slow resolution.

Snake Envenomations

Neurotoxicity from snake envenomation in the Unites States is rare. Many snake venoms contain more than one neurotoxin in addition to many different toxins affecting other organ systems. Neurotoxicity from a snake bite is produced by snakes of the family Elapidae, which includes coral snakes, cobras (*Naja*), kraits (*Bungarus*), mambas (*Dendroapsis*), and all terrestrial poisonous snakes of Australia. Other snakes that possess neurotoxins include sea snakes of the family Hydrophiidae, the Mojave rattlesnake, the Brazilian rattlesnake (*Durissus terifficus*), and the Russell's viper (*Vipera russeli*).

Elapids have a distinctive appearance. The bullet-shaped heads of the elapids contrast with the more triangular heads of the crotalids (rattlesnakes). Elapids lack a facial pit and have round pupils. The fangs of the Australian elapids are small and have limited rotation; the coral snake's fangs are fixed to the maxillae and are short. These characteristics of venomous snakes produce a bite that can appear either as fang marks or more often as scratch marks on the skin. The coral snake can be recognized by its characteristic markings. The coral snakes have a black snout, along with red and black bands separated by yellow bands.

Elapid venom has a curare- and myasthenia gravis-like effect. In the past, toxins from the krait and cobra were used to help identify the acetylcholine receptor (AChR) abnormality of myasthenia gravis. The two major sites of action for the neurotoxins are the pre- and postsynaptic AChR. β-Bungarotoxin and γ-bungarotoxin are found in the Formosan krait (*Bungarus multicinictus*). These toxins bind presynaptically to cause depletion of acetylcholine and cannot be reversed by a cholinesterase inhibitor or antivenom globulin. Structurally similar to phospholipase A_2, toxins from *B. multicinictus* are similar in action to botulinum toxin.

The cobra neurotoxin and the α-bungarotoxin from the Formosan krait (*B. multicinictus*) bind hydrophobically to the postsynaptic nicotinic AChR to cause nondepolarizing neuromuscular blockade. This blockade is reversed by cholinesterase inhibitors and antivenom globulin. Clinically, these toxins produce a curare-like neuromuscular blockade and muscle paralysis.

The onset of neurotoxic symptoms is typically delayed. Mild local paresthesias occur within 15 minutes; subsequent weakness progresses to paralysis 12 hours or later. This delayed onset of symptoms is characteristic of the presynaptic neurotoxins and is commonly observed in coral snake and krait envenomations. These bites do not typically present with the marked local reaction that is common with

Table 37.19. Toxicologic Causes of Fasciculations

Amphetamines
Arsenic
Barium salts
Black widow spider envenomation
Brucine
Caffeine
Camphor
Cholinergic agents (including organophosphates and
  carbamates)
Cocaine
Ergotamines
Fluorides
Hypoglycemic agents
Lead
Lithium
Manganese
Mercury
Nicotine
Phencyclidine
Quaternary ammonium compounds (including
  muscarinic mushrooms)
Scorpion envenomation
Shellfish poisoning (saxitoxin)
Strychnine
Tetrodotoxin poisoning (puffer fish)

crotalid bites. The presenting symptoms include headache, nausea, vomiting, and abdominal pain.

Neurotoxic signs manifest as weakness and do not affect the sensorium. The initial signs of toxicity are of the "bulbar type," which includes ptosis, blurred vision, and difficulty swallowing. A sixth cranial nerve palsy or ophthalmoplegia may be followed by progression of paralysis leading to respiratory paralysis. Excessive salivation is common because of an inability to swallow, not from the increase in secretions. Progression of clinical findings can be rapid.

Symptoms of the Mojave rattlesnake envenomation are similar to those of Elapid envenomations. Victims of rattlesnake envenomation develop respiratory distress, muscle fasciculations (Table 37.19), spasm and weakness, ptosis, dysphagia, and paralysis. Victims of the Brazilian rattlesnake bite present with cranial nerve palsies, weakness, and convulsions.

Prehospital treatment for snake envenomations includes rapid patient transport to a health-care facility. In the ED, tetanus prophylaxis and general supportive care including wound care and respiratory support are provided. Prophylactic antibiotics are not recommended.

A snake identification kit available in Australia utilizes an enzyme-linked immunosorbent assay (ELISA). Aspirate from the bite site or venom from skin or clothing can help to identify the species of snake. Because venom is concentrated and excreted in the urine, a severe envenomation is assumed when the venom is identified in the urine.

Different antivenins are available worldwide. A polyvalent antivenin against all venomous species would be ideal but is not yet available. In the United

States, an antivenin that neutralizes venom from the eastern North American and Texas coral snake is available. One vial of coral snake antivenin neutralizes approximately 2 mg of venom. Typically, three to four vials are administered to a patient with no signs of envenomation. In symptomatic patients with severe pain, numbness, or presence of other neurological findings, five to six vials are administered.

Indications for antivenin use in Australia includes neurotoxic paralysis, coagulopathy, myolysis, renal impairment, venom detection in urine, seizures, headache, nausea, vomiting, and abdominal pain.

Hospitalization for observation of patients with suspected coral snakebites is recommended because of the potential for delayed onset of neurotoxicity. Given the rarity of such envenomation in the United States, consultation to a medical toxicologist should be considered.

Scorpion Envenomation

The vast majority of scorpion envenomations in the United States occur in Arizona. Of the eight species of scorpions found in North America, *Centruroides exilicanda* (the bark scorpion) is the most common and the most lethal. *Centruroides* is found in Arizona, parts of California, Texas, Nevada, and New Mexico. *Centruroides* envenomation primarily affects the CNS. The clinical findings of *Centruroides* envenomation include local pain, restlessness, roving eye movements, and cranial nerve dysfunction. Each species of scorpion has a unique combination of toxins that produce varying degrees of cholinergic, adrenergic, and other neurotoxic effects. The size and the age of the victim are also important because the severity of the envenomation is dose-dependent. There is no need for incision and suction of the bite site.

Symptoms generally begin within minutes following scorpion envenomation but can be delayed up to an hour. Pain at the site of the sting is variable. CNS symptoms include paresthesias, irritability, tremor, muscle rigidity, extraocular muscle dysfunction, decreased level of consciousness, coma, and seizures. Scorpion envenomation in young children can result in apneic episodes or centrally mediated respiratory compromise caused by acute hypertensive encephalopathy. Abdominal pain, nausea, and vomiting are common manifestations of scorpion envenomation and can be caused by the development of pancreatitis.

Aggressive symptomatic management is the mainstay of therapy for the victims of scorpion envenomation. A scale grading the severity of symptoms associated with acute *Centruroides* envenomations has been developed (Table 37.20). Rapid onset of neurological symptoms (within 6 hours) associated with grade III and IV envenomations requires aggressive management. Management includes stabilization of the airway and maintenance of hemodynamic stability. Fluid balance is assessed and monitored closely. Hypertension that does not respond to sedation and analgesia is treated with antihypertensive agents. The use of vasodilators and diuretics is recommended when signs of acute left ventricular failure, pulmonary edema, and elevated pulmonary capillary wedge pressure are present. Adequate hydration for optimum renal perfusion is important when signs of rhabdomyolysis are present.

Specific antivenins for scorpion venoms have been developed, but they are not commercially available. A goat-derived antivenin is available for use only

Table 37.20. Grades of Severity of Envenomation by *Centruroides sculpturatus*

Grade	Description
I	Local pain and/or paresthesias at the site of envenomation
II	Local pain and/or paresthesias at the site of envenomation, accompanied by pain or paresthesias remote from the site
III	Either cranial nerve or somatic skeletal neuromuscular dysfunction: 1. Cranial nerve dysfunction such as blurred vision, irregular eye movements, difficulty swallowing, tongue fasciculations, slurred speech, occasional upper airway incoordination 2. Somatic skeletal neuromuscular dysfunction such as jerking of extremities, restlessness, severe involuntary shaking, and jerking that may be mistaken for seizures
IV	Both cranial nerve and somatic skeletal neuromuscular dysfunction

in Arizona. Patients with grade III or IV symptoms require hospitalization and intensive-care management whether or not antivenin is used. Patients with grade I or II symptoms of scorpion envenomation can be discharged from the ED when the symptoms resolve.

Marine Envenomations

There are three classes of marine vertebrates with neurotoxic envenomations: Chondrichthyes, Osteichthyes, and Reptilia. The Chondrichthyes include stingrays, mantas, and rays. Osteichthyes are bony fishes such as scorpionfish and stonefish. Reptilia include sea snakes.

Stingrays reside in moderate to shallow depths of temperate and tropical waters and strike only in self-defense. They vary in size from several inches to 20 feet. Stingray venom is composed of heat-labile, water-soluble proteins including serotonin, 59-nucleotidase, and phosphodiesterase. Exposure to low concentration of the venom produces cardiac conduction disturbances with mild hypotension; larger doses cause vasoconstriction and cardiac ischemia. A centrally mediated neurotoxic effect of the stingray venom is respiratory depression. Seizure activity can also occur.

Stingray envenomations cause immediate pain that increases over the next 1–2 hours and peaks at 2–3 days. The site appears pale and blanched with dusky wound margins. Systemic symptoms and signs include diaphoresis, nausea, vomiting, vertigo, headache, fasciculations and muscle cramps, tachycardia, hypotension, and death.

Treatment begins with wound irrigation with nonscalding hot water (40.5°C) applied for at least 30–90 minutes as tolerated by the patient. The patient can be safely discharged from the ED after 3–4 hours of observation following stingray envenomation in the absence of systemic symptoms.

Species of the family Scorpaenidae, or scorpionfish, have approximately 11 to 17 venom-containing spines that are used primarily for protection. The stonefish, probably the most venomous fish in the world, belongs to the same family as the lionfish. The weeverfish, a member of the Trachinidae family, has dorsal spines containing deadly toxins similar to the stonefish. Stonefish toxin is both antigenic and heat-labile. The venom causes paralysis of cardiac and skeletal muscle by acting on the presynaptic and postsynaptic membranes of the neuromuscular junction, depleting neurotransmitter stores and causing irreversible depolarization. Weeverfish venom also contains a hemotoxin that causes hemolysis.

Envenomation by the scorpionfish or weeverfish is usually nondescript, painful, and not suspected on initial presentation. Radiation of the pain occurs quickly and can be sufficiently severe to cause unconsciousness. Peak intensity of the pain occurs within 60–90 minutes and resolves in 6–12 hours. Swelling, fasciculations, and paralysis can develop rapidly in the involved extremity. Systemic symptoms include anxiety, headache, tremors, nausea, vomiting, diaphoresis, delirium, seizures, abdominal pain, dysrhythmias, and death. Signs of mild heart failure are common. Respiratory compromise can occur because of pulmonary edema or paralysis of the chest muscles. When the victim survives, convalescence can take months. Because of the heat lability of the toxins, immediate irrigation of the wound with nonscalding hot water is initiated and continued for up to 90 minutes.

There are 52 known species of sea snakes distributed in the tropic and temperate Pacific and Indian Oceans. Sea snakes are not found in the Atlantic Ocean, but there are reports of sea snake sightings in Caribbean waters. All are venomous and potentially lethal. Their fangs are short, are easily dislodged, and usually cannot penetrate a wet suit. Most bites do not result in significant toxicity from the small amount of venom injected; however, sea snake venom is considered to be approximately 20 times more toxic than cobra venom. The venom is a mixture of proteins that include cardiotoxins, myotoxins, coagulants, anticoagulants, and hemolytic enzymes.

Victims of sea snake envenomation who remain asymptomatic 8 hours after the bite generally do not develop systemic symptoms. Anxiety and restlessness herald impending toxicity. Rhabdomyolysis with myoglobinuria can develop within 3–4 hours. Muscle fasciculations, trismus, and an ascending paralysis originating from the envenomation site can occur. Respiratory distress, bulbar paralysis, aspiration-related hypoxia, acute renal failure, and coma can complicate sea snake envenomation. Symptoms begin within 1 hour but may not progress for up to 8 hours.

The treatment of sea snake envenomation is rapid administration of antivenin. Polyvalent sea snake antivenin from Commonwealth Serum Laboratories in Melbourne, Australia, is effective against several different species of sea snakes.

Approximately 100 species of Coelenterates (jellyfish) are venomous. Most of these are hydrozoa (Portuguese man-of-war), scyphozoa, (box jellyfish), and anthozoa (anemones), which are found on soft and stony corals. *Chironex fleckeri*, the box jellyfish, is reported to be the most venomous sea creature and can cause death within 30–60 seconds of envenomation. It is found in the waters off the coast of Australia. The box-shaped body can measure 20 cm on a side. Its tentacles are covered with nematocysts (small coiled cystic structures that uncoil, releasing the toxin) and can measure up to 3 m in length.

Three biochemical properties of box jellyfish venom are a hemolytic component, a dermatonecrotic factor that causes rapid skin death, and a lethal component that is cardiotoxic and neurotoxic. Myocardial paralysis occurs during the contraction phase, resulting in cardiac arrest. Envenomation can cause apnea by paralyzing the respiratory muscles. Central respiratory depression can also result in apnea. The overall mortality of a box jellyfish sting is estimated at 15–20%.

To prevent further discharge of venom from nematocysts, the affected region is covered with acetic acid 5% (vinegar). Local application of vinegar helps prevent further envenomation. Health-care providers should wear gloves while removing the tentacles. Rapid administration of box jellyfish antivenin ensures the best possible patient outcome. Analgesics, local anesthetic sprays, or steroid preparations provide relief from local discomfort and pain.

Three of the five main classes of mollusks are hazardous to humans: cephalopods (squid, octopus, and cuddlefish), gastropods (snails and slugs), and pelecypods (oysters, scallops, mussels, and clams). The latter cause hypersensitivity reactions when ingested by people who are allergic to "shellfish." The blue-ringed or Australian ringed octopus, *Hapalochlena lunulata*, is colored yellow-brown with rings on its tentacles, is found in tidal pools and seaweed, and is the most common offending species. Initially, the bite is nondescript and may remain unnoticed. Edema and blister formation develop, followed by localized paresthesias. Maculotoxin interferes with sodium conductance in excitable membranes. Rapid neuromuscular blockade occurs primarily at the phrenic nerve. Oral and facial paresthesias develop within 10–15 minutes. Systemic symptoms include visual disturbances, ptosis, mydriasis, dysphagia, dysphonia, generalized weakness, and difficulty in coordination. These symptoms persist for approximately 4–12 hours; weakness can persist longer. Peripheral and respiratory paralysis are potential complications. Treatment is supportive care.

PEARLS AND **PITFALLS**

General Neurotoxicology

- Poisoning is considered in the differential diagnosis of a patient with a "neurological presentation."
- Coexisting medical illness and occult trauma is considered in a patient with poisoning.
- Patients with anticholinergic syndrome can be misdiagnosed as having psychiatric illness.
- Coingestants are considered in a poisoned patient with a known ingestion.
- Alcohol-intoxicated patients require a comprehensive evaluation. Failure to recognize and treat coexisting medical problems or associated trauma is a major pitfall in caring for such patients.
- Intravenous ethanol therapy is begun in suspected cases of ethylene glycol or methanol poisoning, even before the results of serum levels are available.
- Nontraumatic mononeuropathy is common in intravenous drug abusers.
- Transverse myelitis can occur in heroin abusers who inject the drug after several months of abstinence.

Envenomations

- The mainstay of therapy for snake and scorpion envenomations is rapid patient transport to a health-care facility where aggressive symptomatic care can be delivered.
- Incision and suction at the site of envenomation and routine application of a tourniquet in the field are not recommended. However, when a tourniquet is placed, it should be removed gradually in the ED under controlled conditions.

- The use of antivenin for snake envenomation is considered especially when signs of neurotoxicity are present. The antivenin is administered in an intensive care unit where signs of anaphylaxis can be monitored and treated.
- Specific antivenin is available for the stonefish, box jellyfish, and sea snakes.
- Decompression sickness (parasthesias, abdominal cramping, muscular spasms, and seizures) can mimic symptoms produced by certain neurotoxins. A careful history can help to differentiate the two.
- When patient transport times are prolonged in an area where marine envenomation occurs, access to a first aid kit containing vinegar, latex gloves, oral analgesics, steroids (oral and topical), antihistamines, and bandaging material is crucial.

Electrical, Lightning, and Thermal Injuries

- Cardiopulmonary arrest is the leading cause of death in individuals with electrical injuries.
- Significant head, chest, and abdominal injuries are considered present until proven otherwise in the electrically injured patient.
- Fractures and dislocations are commonly associated with electrocution.
- Alternating current commonly causes ventricular fibrillation and exhibits entry and exit wounds of nearly equal size.
- Direct current commonly causes ventricular asystole and exhibits a larger exit wound.

Decompression Sickness

- The most common form of decompression sickness is type I, "the bends," and nearly 90% of patients exhibit musculoskeletal symptoms only.
- Associated injuries, envenomations, or intoxications are reviewed with suspected decompression sickness.
- The left lateral decubitus or Trendelenburg position is used for patient transport.
- Immediate supplemental oxygen can help to remove excess nitrogen dissolved in tissues.
- The use of positive airway pressure devices is avoided because associated pulmonary barotrauma may be present.

Accidental Hypothermia

- Movement of patients with hypothermia can precipitate cardiac dysrhythmias and is done as gently as possible.
- Nearly all hypothermic patients exhibit some degree of volume depletion.
- Once rewarming has been initiated, it is not discontinued until core temperature has reached a minimum of 30°C.
- Target organs become progressively more unresponsive to pharmacological agents as core temperature drops. This may lead to toxic levels when pharmacological therapy is aggressively pursued prior to rewarming.
- Correction of metabolic acidosis occurs with rewarming and usually is not treated.

SELECTED BIBLIOGRAPHY

Goldfrank LR, Flomenbaum NE, Lewin NA, Weisman RS, Howland MA, Hoffman RS, eds. *Goldfrank's Toxicologic Emergencies,* 6th ed. Stamford, Conn.: Appleton & Lange; 1998.

Greer HD, Massey EW. Neurologic injury from undersea diving. *Neurol Clin.* 1992;10:1032–43.

Pattern BM. Lightning and electrical injuries. *Neurol Clin.* 1992;10:1047–57.

Spencer PS, Schaumburg HH, eds. *Experimental and Clinical Neurotoxicology*, 2nd ed. New York, NY: Oxford University Press; 2000.

38 Brain Death

David K. Zich and Jon Brillman

INTRODUCTION

Brain death criteria have been established to determine the irreversible loss of all functions of the entire brain, including the brainstem. Although these criteria have general acceptance in the medical community, minor variations may exist from institution to institution. Brain death determination is performed infrequently in the emergency department. Ideally, brain death criteria include assessment of the following: (1) normothermia; (2) cause of brain death; (3) unresponsiveness; (4) absence of brainstem reflexes; and (5) apnea.

Evaluation

Normothermia

When a patient is significantly hypothermic, active rewarming measures should be taken to normalize body temperature prior to initiating a brain death evaluation because severe hypothermia can suppress brainstem function. The old adage that no patients are pronounced dead until they are warm and dead pertains to both traditional cardiovascular concepts of death as well as modern brain death criteria.

Cause of Death

In general, the cause of brain death should be sought to prevent overlooking potentially reversible conditions mimicking brain death. These conditions include drug or alcohol overdoses or iatrogenic administration of hypnosedatives and/or paralytics. When the patient has not been under the direct care of the physician conducting the brain death protocol prior to obtundation, the set of criteria should be documented twice, at least 6 hours apart. This allows for the effects of unknown substances to dissipate and for reversible causes to become evident. In some cases, the cause of unresponsiveness may be obtained by history, examination, or supplemental tests. However, this is not always possible, and brain death remains a clinical diagnosis that can be augmented by, but not dependent upon, electroencephalography (EEG) and other advanced forms of neuroimaging.

Unresponsiveness

Unresponsiveness means the lack of response to any applied stimulus (Glasgow Coma Scale of 3). The presence of withdrawal reflexes, typically seen in the lower extremities, do not preclude the diagnosis of brain death given that withdrawal reflexes can be spinally mediated.

Absence of Brainstem Reflexes

Absence of brainstem reflexes includes pupillary responses, eye movements, and lower brainstem reflexes such as response to tracheal stimulation. Because the diagnosis of brain death requires loss of all function of both cerebral hemispheres and brainstem, assessment is made of pupillary reactions, corneal reflexes, cough reflex to deep endotracheal suction, and response to cold calorics. Cold calorics testing is performed by injecting 30 cc of ice water into the external ear canal on both sides while observing for any eye movement.

Apnea

Apnea testing is performed to demonstrate lack of respiratory effort, even in the presence of elevated p_{CO_2} levels. The test is performed by providing adequate oxygenation of the brain while p_{CO_2} levels rise to greater than 60 mm Hg. Initially, an arterial blood gas (ABG) should be obtained to verify that the patients p_{CO_2} level is in the range of 38 to 42 mm Hg. This may require that the ventilator be adjusted and the ABG be rechecked. Once this is achieved, the patient is disconnected from the ventilator. Supplemental oxygen is usually required, usually 10 L/min by a suction catheter near the carina or by a T-tube. After approximately 10 minutes, another ABG is obtained. If the p_{CO_2} is over 60 mm Hg and the patient has not attempted to breathe, this is confirmatory evidence of complete brainstem unresponsiveness. If an arrhythmia occurs or the O_2 saturation drops below 90 mm Hg during the test, the patient must be reconnected to the ventilator and resuscitated; brain death cannot be diagnosed.

Criteria for Death

When no respiratory effort is made during the apnea test and the other criteria have been met, the patient may be pronounced dead. Time of death is usually the time recorded on the ABG that confirms a p_{CO_2} of greater than 60 mm Hg. Support is withdrawn at this time provided that family members do not object and the patient is not considered for organ donation. However, when organ donation is to occur, the patient is maintained on ventilatory support and preparation is made for organ harvesting. This usually includes contacting the appropriate supervising agency, drawing a specific panel of laboratory tests to assess organ viability and compatibility, and gaining central venous access as well as arterial blood pressure monitoring when not already established.

Supplemental investigations may be helpful but are not necessary. These include transcranial Doppler blood flow studies, nuclear angiography, magnetic resonance imaging (MRI), or an EEG to look for electrocerebral silence. The latter investigation is most commonly used; however, all supplemental tests are subject to artifact, which may be misinterpreted as brain activity, and false negatives have been produced by sedative/hypnotic medications. In addition, these tests are often not available in emergent situations or after regular dayshift hours. Therefore, these studies are to be used strictly as adjuncts in special circumstances and do not replace or override a thorough clinical evaluation.

Conducting brain death protocols in the emergency department is impractical in most circumstances for several reasons. The process is time-consuming and most institutions require the criteria to be conducted by physicians only. Completing the entire series of requirements usually takes an hour or more at the patient's bedside and ideally should be repeated in 6 hours to confirm. In addition, it is imperative that proper facilities and support staff be available for the patient's family and friends who await confirmation of their loss.

Finally, the diagnosis of brain death is not without controversy. For instance, thermoregulation is regarded as a brainstem function; therefore, some argue that those patients who maintain their body temperature cannot be declared brain dead. In the future, "near-death" or "imminent death" criteria may be established. Use of current death criteria remains the best, objective clinical practice to indicate the irreversible loss of all brain function and must be performed meticulously and conscientiously by qualified physicians.

PEARLS AND **PITFALLS**

- Brain death means the irreversible loss of all brain function, including that of the brainstem.
- Hypothermia and the effects of some medications can cause or contribute to unresponsiveness and must be evaluated thoroughly.
- Lower extremity withdrawal reflexes may be spinally mediated and do not preclude a diagnosis of brain death.
- Tests supplemental to the bedside brain death evaluation are not necessary for a diagnosis of brain death.

SELECTED BIBLIOGRAPHY

Ball WS Jr. Neuroimaging in brain death. *Ajnr: American Journal of Neuroradiology.* 1998;19(4):796.

Beresford HR. Brain death. *Neurologic Clinics.* 1999;17(2):295.

De Tourtchaninoff M, Hantson P, Mahieu P, Geurit JM. Brain death in misleading conditions. *QJM.* 1999;92(7):407–14.

Flowers WM Jr, Patel BR. Accuracy of clinical evaluation in the determination of brain death. *Southern Med J.* 2000;93(2):203–6.

Flowers WM Jr, Patel BR. Persistence of cerebral blood flow after brain death. *Southern Med J.* 2000;93(4):364–70.

Grozovski E, Cohen J, Shapiro M, Kogan A, Michovitz R, Reches R, Singer P. Four year experience with brain-death determinations. *Transplantation Proc.* 2000;32(4):753–4.

Lovblad KO, Bassetti C. Diffusion-weighted magnetic resonance imaging in brain death. *Stroke*. 2000;31(2):539–42.

Powner DJ, Darby JM. Current considerations in the issue of brain death. *Neurosurgery*. 1999;45(5):1222–6;1226–7.

Rudolf J, Haupt WF, Neveling M, Grond M. Potential pitfalls in apnea testing. *Acta Neruochirurgica*. 1998;140(7):659–63.

Taylor RM. Reexamining the definition and criteria of death. *Seminars in Neurology*. 1997;17(3):265–70.

Truog RD. Is it time to abandon brain death? *Hastings Center Report*. 1997; 27(1):29–37.

Youngner SJ, Arnold RM, DeVita MA. When is "dead"? *Hastings Center Report*. 1999; 29(6):14–21.

Index

Note: entries printed in *italics* represent information contained in figures, illustrations, and tables.